Perioperative Management in Robotic Surgery

Perioperative Management in Robotic Surgery

Edited by

Alan David Kaye, MD, PhD, DABA, DABPM, DABIPP

Louisiana State University Medical Center, New Orleans, LA, USA

Richard D. Urman, MD, MBA, CPE

Harvard Medical School, Boston, MA, USA

CAMBRIDGE
UNIVERSITY PRESS

CAMBRIDGE
UNIVERSITY PRESS

University Printing House, Cambridge CB2 8BS, United Kingdom

One Liberty Plaza, 20th Floor, New York, NY 10006, USA

477 Williamstown Road, Port Melbourne, VIC 3207, Australia

4843/24, 2nd Floor, Ansari Road, Daryaganj, Delhi – 110002, India

79 Anson Road, #06-04/06, Singapore 079906

Cambridge University Press is part of the University of Cambridge.

It furthers the University's mission by disseminating knowledge in the pursuit of education, learning, and research at the highest international levels of excellence.

www.cambridge.org
Information on this title: www.cambridge.org/9781107143128
DOI: 10.1017/9781316534229

First published 2017

Printed in the United Kingdom by TJ International Ltd. Padstow Cornwall

A catalogue record for this publication is available from the British Library.

Library of Congress Cataloging-in-Publication Data
Names: Kaye, Alan David, editor. | Urman, Richard D., editor.
Title: Perioperative management in robotic surgery / edited by Alan David Kaye, Louisiana State University Medical Center, New Orleans, LA, USA, Richard D. Urman, Harvard Medical School, Boston, MA, USA.
Description: Cambridge, United Kingdom; New York, NY, USA: Cambridge University Press, 2017. |
Includes bibliographical references and index.
Identifiers: LCCN 2017007734 | ISBN 9781107143128 (hardback)
Subjects: LCSH: Surgical robots. | Robotics in medicine. | Therapeutics, Surgical. |
BISAC: MEDICAL / Anesthesiology.
Classification: LCC RD73.S785 P47 2017 | DDC 617.9/178–dc23
LC record available at https://lccn.loc.gov/2017007734

ISBN 978-1-107-14312-8 Hardback

Every effort has been made in preparing this book to provide accurate and up-to-date information that is in accord with accepted standards and practice at the time of publication. Although case histories are drawn from actual cases, every effort has been made to disguise the identities of the individuals involved. Nevertheless, the authors, editors, and publishers can make no warranties that the information contained herein is totally free from error, not least because clinical standards are constantly changing through research and regulation. The authors, editors, and publishers therefore disclaim all liability for direct or consequential damages resulting from the use of material contained in this book. Readers are strongly advised to pay careful attention to information provided by the manufacturer of any drugs or equipment that they plan to use.

To my mother Florence Susan Feldman, my brother Dr. Adam Kaye, and my sister Sheree Kaye Garcia, who have inspired me to be the man I have become, in the face of a childhood filled with adversity and challenge. Your kindness and love I can never adequately repay;

To my late stepfather Gideon Feldman whom I miss every day, thanks for all you did for us; we are sincerely grateful and will not forget;

To the members of the LSU Department of Anesthesiology, who are excellent at anesthesia and even greater people.

To my wife Kim Kaye, MD, and my children, Aaron and Rachel Kaye, who inspire me to work hard, who provide a morale compass for my soul, and who encourage me to try to be the best version of myself each day of my life.

To Sylvester Stallone for making *Rocky* and Dave Wottle for running his final gold medal miracle lap in the 1972 Olympics, sport and art that are very real to my heart.

Alan David Kaye, MD, PhD
New Orleans, Louisiana

To my patients who are the ultimate beneficiaries of this work;

To my colleagues from the Departments of Anesthesiology, Surgery and Nursing for their invaluable editorial input and collaboration;

To my parents Dennis and Tanya, my wife Zina Matlyuk-Urman, MD, for their encouragement and support, and to my daughters, Abigail and Isabelle.

Richard D. Urman, MD, MBA
Boston, Massachusetts

Contents

Contributors

Jan Akervall
William Beaumont Oakland University School of Medicine, Royal Oak, MI, USA

Jeffrey S. Barton
Louisiana State University School of Medicine, New Orleans, LA, USA

Enrico Benedetti
Professor and Chair, Department of Surgery, University of Illinois, Chicago

Elyse M. Cornett
Louisiana State University Health Sciences Center, Shreveport, LA, USA

Kurt G. Davis
University of the Health Sciences, Bethesda, MD, USA

Aladino De Ranieri
Advocate Illinois Masonic Medical Center, Chicago, IL, USA

Erin Dougher
LSU Department of OB/GYN, LSUHSC, New Orleans, LA

Fozia Ferozali
Cedars Sinai Medical Center, Los Angeles, CA, USA

Eric S. Fouliard
Advocate Illinois Masonic Medical Center, Chicago, IL, USA

Charles J. Fox
Louisiana State University Health Sciences Center, Shreveport, LA, USA

Michael Franklin
Louisiana State University Health Sciences Center, Shreveport, LA, USA

Elizabeth A.M. Frost
Professor of Anesthesiology Mount Sinai Medical Center, New York

Julie A. Gayle
Louisiana State University School of Medicine, New Orleans, LA, USA

Clifford M. Gevirtz
Medical Director Somnia, Inc., Adjunct Associate Professor, Department of Anesthesiology LSU Health Science Center

Farid Gharagozloo
Global Center for Advanced Thoracic Surgery, Orlando, FL, USA

Rainer W.G. Gruessner
Upstate Medical University, Syracuse, NY, USA

Barry Hallner
LSU Department of OB/GYN, LSUHSC, New Orleans, LA, USA

Daniel M. Herron
Icahn School of Medicine at Mount Sinai, New York, NY, USA

Phi T. Ho
University of Miami Miller School of Medicine, Miami, FL, USA

Paul Hoff
University of Michigan, Ann Arbor, MI, USA

Jim C. Hu
NewYork-Presbyterian Hospital, New York, NY, USA

Bassam Kadry
Stanford University School of Medicine, Stanford, CA, USA

Alan David Kaye
Louisiana State University School of Medicine, New Orleans, LA, USA

Pushpa Koyyalamudi
Louisiana State University Health Sciences Center, Shreveport, LA, USA

Ryan R. Krlin
Louisiana State University School of Medicine, New Orleans, LA, USA

Aaron A. Laviana
David Geffen School of Medicine at UCLA, Los Angeles, CA, USA

Alex Macario
Stanford University School of Medicine, Stanford, CA, USA

Tobias A. Mattei
Invision Health, Buffalo, NY, USA

Danica N. May
Louisiana State University School of Medicine, New Orleans, LA, USA

Russell Metcalfe-Smith
Cedars Sinai Medical Center, Los Angeles, CA, USA

Matthew Novitch
Medical College of Wisconsin, Milwaukee, WI, USA

Guy R. Orangio
Louisiana State University School of Medicine, New Orleans, LA, USA

John T. Paige
LSU Health New Orleans School of Medicine, New Orleans, LA, USA

Shilpadevi Patil
Louisiana State University Health Sciences Center, Shreveport, LA, USA

Lisa M. Peacock
LSU Department of Obstetrics and Gynecology, LSUHSC, New Orleans, LA

Robert Poston
St. Francis Medical Center, Trenton, NJ, USA

Amit Prabhakar
Louisiana State University Health Sciences Center, Shreveport, LA, USA

Maunak V. Rana
Advocate Illinois Masonic Medical Center, Chicago, IL, USA

Yury Rapoport
Louisiana State University Health Sciences Center, Shreveport, LA, USA

Cory Robertson
Louisiana State University Health Sciences Center, Shreveport, LA, USA

Ryan E. Rubin
Louisiana State University School of Medicine, New Orleans, LA, USA

Roya Saffary
Stanford University School of Medicine, Stanford, CA, USA

Amanda F. Saltzman
Louisiana State University School of Medicine, New Orleans, LA, USA

Laurence Schachter
St. Francis Medical Center, Trenton, NJ, USA

Sudipta Sen
Louisiana State University Health Sciences Center, Shreveport, LA, USA

Gurleen Sidhu
Louisiana State University Health Sciences Center, Shreveport, LA, USA

Jayne Smitten
University of Alberta, Canada

Katherine Stammen
Louisiana State University Health Sciences Center, Shreveport, LA, USA

Alisson R. Teles
Universidade de Caxias do Sul, Rio Grande do Sul, Brazil

Kiara Tulla
Department of Surgery, University of Illinois, Chicago, IL, USA

Ivo Tzvetanov
Associate Professor of Surgery, Chief Division of Transplantation, University of Illinois, Chicago

Richard D. Urman
Harvard Medical School, Boston, MA, USA

Preface

Few innovations in surgical technique have played as large a role in the growth of the field of laparoscopic surgery as has robotic-assisted surgery (RAS). Robotic systems offer many potential advantages to the surgeon, including providing a binocular, stereoscopic view of the surgical field, masking of surgical tremor by filtering hand movements, and allowing for 360 degree movement of the instruments, mimicking open surgery. There is ongoing research on patient outcomes and costs of care with RAS compared to laparoscopic and open surgery. Another promising application of robotic-assisted surgery is single port site surgery, and the number of surgical subspecialties using RAS is also increasing.

In this book we cover perioperative considerations for robot-assisted surgery (RAS), including preoperative, intraoperative, and postoperative management of the patient. We believe that ours is the first comprehensive, evidence-based clinical text that specifically focuses on the overall perioperative management of the patient, and not just technical surgical skills. Since minimally invasive surgery is now performed on many types of patients, including neonates, parturients, morbidly obese, trauma victims, and those with significant comorbidities, it is important to be adequately prepared in getting them through surgery.

Designed for practitioners, it is an easy to read, concise handbook rather than a large, complex textbook with an overwhelming amount of information. It covers physiologic effects and complications related to RAS, and has ample diagrams, tables, and figures to help organize the information for easy reference. Our book addresses preoperative evaluation, patient selection, common emergencies, complications, as well as pain management and recovery. We discuss patient management, describe the basics of various procedures and techniques, outline useful patient care protocols, and provide an overview of the perioperative issues that are unique to a given RAS procedure. We hope that a wide audience of healthcare practitioners will find it useful, including anesthesiologists, surgeons, allied health professionals, as well as medical proceduralists, biomedical engineers, nurses and physician assistants, and trainees from various disciplines. Each chapter contributor is an expert from a leading academic institution.

Introduction

The Surgeon's Perspective on Robotic Surgery

Rainer W. G. Gruessner

Since approval by the Food and Drug Administration was obtained in 2000, the robotic platform has revolutionized the advancement of minimally invasive surgery across all surgical specialties. Originally intended by NASA as a modality to replace the surgeon's physical presence and provide remote access care to astronauts or to soldiers in battlefields, the development of the first generation of robotic platforms started in the mid-1980s. Only after the evolution of the second and current generation of robotic systems, set up in a "master–slave" configuration, this new technique became clinical reality. The concept is as intriguing as it is radical: the "master" unit (the surgeon's console) controls a separate "slave" unit (several robotic arms with multiple degrees of freedom). The feasibility of the physical absence of the surgeon at the operating table was first proven in 2001 when a transcontinental robotic cholecystectomy was performed on a patient in Strasbourg, France, by surgeons located in New York City.

As of December 2015, the da Vinci surgical system (Intuitive Surgical, Inc., Sunnyvale, CA, USA) was the market leader in robotic platforms with 3,597 da Vinci surgical systems installed worldwide. According to a recent report (Wintergreen Research Company), robotic surgical systems collectively marketed $3.4 billion in 2014 and are anticipated to reach $20 billion by 2021.

After the first laparoscopic cholecystectomy was performed in 1985, laparoscopic techniques conquered the globe across all surgical fields because they resulted in shorter hospitalization, less postoperative pain, and quicker return to normal activity due to small incisions and limited tissue dissections. Over time, the limitations of laparoscopic surgery became apparent: decreased motion range of laparoscopic instruments (when compared to the human hand), impaired hand–eye coordination with the use of only two-dimensional screens, and an uncomfortable posture with increased ergonometric strain for the surgeon. In comparison to conventional laparoscopy, robotic surgery propelled minimally invasive surgery to a higher level of performance through the introduction of three-dimensional stereoscopic vision, elimination of hand tremor, better ergonomics for the surgeon, and increased dexterity, maneuverability, and precision via the Endo-Wrist technology. The wider application of robotic technologies is also the result of greater ease of use and comfort than with the laparoscopic setup once the operating staff is familiar and competent with the robotic platform. The da Vinci surgical system continues to be upgraded and now includes features such as near-infrared technology and a facilitated setup through single docking and single robotic port placement. The latest generation of less bulky robotic systems (Xi) even allows multiquadrant procedures. It is, therefore, not surprising that the robotic platform is replacing the laparoscopic approach in many surgical specialties.

As the number and variety of robotic surgeries continue to increase, interest of residents, fellows, and faculty in surgical training programs has also increased. Especially the current generation of residents, which I call respectfully the "Nintendo generation" (due to the exposure to computers and video games at a young age), appears to have a fast grasp on the technical intricacies that accompany robotic surgery. Training options for surgical residents and fellows have substantially improved over time, and many resident curricula now follow the robotic education curriculum, the Fundamentals of Robotic Surgery, which combines online didactics, dry lab simulation, and hands-on operating room experience. Studies have shown significant benefits of training on the da Vinci skills simulator, leading to an improvement in technical performance of robotic novices and shortening their learning curves. Surgical specialty organizations have published guidelines intended to lay a framework for hospitals that initiate new robotic credentialing and privileging programs. Hospitals will need to stay abreast with respect to technology updates and training guidelines.

Despite its apparent successes, robotic surgery is not free from controversy. In several meta-analyses comparisons, robotic surgery was shown to prolong operative times and costs. The former is associated with a steep learning curve. The latter includes primarily the high acquisition and maintenance costs and the repetitive costs of consumables. For that reason, and based on my own experience, robotic surgery is frequently not embraced by hospital administrations. During my tenure as Chairman of the Department of Surgery at the University of Arizona, a vision for widespread and innovative application of robotic surgery was developed in conjunction with all division chiefs but subsequently not supported by senior hospital administration. However, initial and temporary setbacks should not discourage surgeons interested in technical advances. Marketing has become a powerful tool and robotic surgery has strong allies not only in patients and payers but also in the media.

This textbook on perioperative management of the robotic surgery patient by Drs Alan Kaye and Richard Urman is an important tool to widen the application of robotic surgery by familiarizing anesthesiologists with this innovative technology. But this textbook is of importance to surgeons as well since they are frequently not fully aware of anesthesia-related concerns and the physiologic consequences of robotic surgery. The implications of pneumoperitoneum and Trendelenburg positioning can be complex and also dependent on factors such as intraabdominal pressure, degree and absorption of CO_2, and procedure duration. These factors impact cardiopulmonary and cardiovascular status, intracranial pressure, and the patient's neuroendocrine and immunologic status. Conversely, anesthesiologists may not be familiar with the surgeon's challenges, such as lack of tactile feedback and need of conversion to open procedure. These challenges in anesthesia and surgical management require close communication among the team before, during, and after the robotic surgery to decrease the potential morbidity associated with robotic surgery.

Robotic surgery is here to stay and will continue to expand across all surgical specialties. There will be further technological refinements in the future including less expensive, miniaturized, and lighter robotic devices, and anesthesiologists as well as surgeons need to be prepared for the next phase. This comprehensive textbook is of great value in improving provider proficiency as well as quality and outcome of robotic surgery now and in the future.

Chapter 1

Historical Overview of Robot-Assisted Surgery

Roya Saffary, Alex Macario, and Bassam Kadry

Development of Robots

In 1921, the Czech playwright Karel Capek introduced the term "robot" in his play *R.U.R.*, and while he has been credited for coining the term (1), he later acknowledged his brother, Josef Capek, as the real inventor (2). Originating from the Czech word *robota*, meaning "forced labor," this term referred to the type of labor that peasants had to perform in a feudalistic society. For his play, Capek used the term to describe manufactured humans or clones. In contrast, the current definition of the word describes "a machine capable of carrying out a complex series of actions automatically, especially one programmable by a computer" (3).

The word "robot" evokes different images for different people. Science fiction, both in print and in movies, has played a major role in shaping our understanding and familiarity with the idea of robots, which has ranged from helpful assistance completing small tasks to fully functioning, human-like machines. As their mechanical complexity and precision has improved, they have been deployed in a growing number of industries, with their usage likely to increase further. This chapter is intended to provide an overview of robotic development over time. In addition to providing a timeline (Box 1.1), this chapter also offers details about the specific models with a summary of the unique innovations in Table 1.1.

Box 1.1 Timeline

1921	Karel Capek introduces the term "robot"
1947	W. Grey Walter publishes his work on robots capable of phototaxis
1969	Victor Scheinman develops the "Stanford Arm"
1977	The Stanford Arm is sold to Unimate, leading to the development of the Programmable Universal Machine for Assembly (PUMA) system
1985	Kwoh et al. use the PUMA 200 to perform the first robot-assisted stereotactic brain biopsy; the subsequent model, PUMA 560, is used for prostate surgeries
1988	PROBOT is invented and used in prostate surgeries
1992	ROBODOC is invented and used for hip surgeries in Europe
1994	AESOP is invented and cleared by the Food and Drug Administration (FDA) for minimally invasive surgeries
1995	Zeus Robotic Surgical System (ZRSS) is developed and subsequently tested on animals
1998	Tubal reanastamosis and CABG are performed using the ZRSS system
2000	da Vinci model is approved by the FDA
2001	ZRSS is approved by the FDA
2001	Transcontinental robot-assisted cholecystectomy is performed
2008	ROBODOC receives FDA clearance
2014	Fourth-generation da Vinci system, the Xi model, receives FDA approval

Since the dawn of the field, robotic design has progressed from simple, repetitive functions to multistep complex tasks. One of the first roboticians, William Grey Walter, built two three-wheeled robots, Elmer and Elsie, which were capable of phototaxis (4). These machines, which consisted of a smooth shell and a sensor stalk, were equipped to mimic two senses, touch and sight. In the dark, Elmer and Elsie scanned their surroundings for light sources and slowly crawled forward with help from a battery-powered motor. Once they identified a light source, they were able to steer toward it. Similarly, when encountering a physical barrier, they were able to alter their trajectory to maneuver around it. Walter used these simple machines to illustrate how fairly complex behavior can be observed with such a simple system consisting of only two senses and two different motor activities.

While Walter tried to imitate life and characteristics such as spontaneity and purposefulness, George Devol focused on a specific task at hand and

Table 1.1 Timeline of new innovations in robotic systems

Year	Name	Use
1947	Elmer and Elsie	Capable of two senses, its goal was to emulate characteristics such as spontaneity, free will, purposefulness
1969	Stanford Arm	Use in assembly line and welding
1977	PUMA	Stanford Arm sold to Unimate and development of PUMA systems began
1985		PUMA 200 is used to perform brain biopsies
		PUMA 560 is used for prostatectomy
1988	PROBOT	Volume of resection preprogrammed by surgeon; no further input required from surgical team
1992	ROBODOC	Developed to improve precision of hip arthroplasty; robot capable of milling femur with superior precision
1994	AESOP	Allowed surgeon to operate camera with a hand or foot switch
1995	ZRSS	First master–slave system with surgical console and cart
2000	da Vinci	Most advanced master–slave system, with endowrist instruments

believed that the automated transfer of items would be useful in factories. In 1954, he invented Unimate, which became the first industrial robot when General Motors bought it in 1962 and installed it shortly thereafter to lift hot pieces of metal (5). This new development heralded a trend toward using robots to assist in industrial assembly lines.

The automobile industry was one of the first sectors to appreciate the vast opportunity that automation presented and began to rely on robotic arms to perform tasks that would be difficult and potentially dangerous for human workers. Over time, more industries discovered the utility of robots and have increasingly welcomed the integration of various types of robots. Here, we focus on the history of robots used in medicine.

First Robots Used in Medicine

The first laparoscopic cholecystectomy was performed in 1985 (6). This new technology provided a minimally invasive approach to surgery and resulted in shorter hospital stays and decreased postoperative pain due to smaller incisions and limited tissue dissection. With these obvious benefits, the list of surgeries performed laparoscopically quickly expanded and currently includes a variety of surgical specialties. However, despite its advantages, this surgical approach does carry limitations. During the surgery, the operator is confined to an uncomfortable posture and is required to view the surgical field on a screen, therefore making hand–eye coordination challenging. In addition, the images projected are two-dimensional, and the instrumentation does not allow for the same degree of tactile feedback as is possible with conventional surgeries. Perhaps most importantly, the range of motion of laparoscopic instruments is significantly limited when compared to that of the human hand, thereby restricting the surgical access and dexterity of the operator.

Some of these limitations have been addressed over time with the introduction of robots. Increasingly, more complex robotic systems have been introduced into the medical field and are able to perform more sophisticated surgical procedures. One interesting difference between robots used in medicine as compared to those used in other industries is the fact that robotic systems in the medical field continue to require human intervention. They are generally not expected to perform preprogrammed tasks independently. Instead, they are manipulated by the human operator either physically or through voice recognition and can be considered an extension of the operator's hand rather than as an autonomous actor in the classical sense.

The first medical robot was the PUMA 200. Initially developed in 1969 by Victor Scheinman, a mechanical engineering student at Stanford University, the robot was designed to assist with assembly and arc welding. In 1977, Scheinman sold his invention, known as the Stanford Arm, to Devol's company Unimation, which then used it to develop a series of PUMA robots. Although the 200 series was a desktop version, it was similar to the other versions as it consisted of a mechanical arm and a control system. In 1985, Kwoh et al. used the PUMA 200 to perform stereotactic brain biopsies (7). Using CT guidance, this system was able to determine its own depth through a negative feedback input. The same system and a more advanced model, the PUMA 560, were subsequently used for transurethral prostate resections by Davies et al. (8). However, both models still required guidance from the surgeon, and although they closely resembled the human arm, the greater flexibility came at a price of lower precision. These characteristics made the PUMA more suitable for assembly lines and welding where lack of precision cannot have detrimental effects as compared to patient care.

In 1988, researchers at the Imperial College London developed the PROBOT based on the PUMA system. The goal was to build a robot that would have a small enough working environment to allow safe operations within the human body (9). In contrast to previous robotic systems, this robot utilized a fixed path system that was programmed based on preoperative imaging. The robot was capable of moving in three different axes and contained a resectoscope that could move in a fourth axis. Prior to surgery, the length of the prostate was determined from the bladder neck to an anatomical landmark, the verumontanum. Surgery was limited to this area to prevent damage to the sphincter muscles. The robot was then positioned at the bladder neck and an ultrasound probe passed through the resectoscope acquired three-dimensional (3D) images in 5 mm intervals. Based on this 3D image, the surgeon then determined the exact region to be removed. Once programmed, the robot was then able to resect the predetermined tissue without any additional input from the surgeon, using small rough rotational movements. These movements resulted in resection of small, cone-shaped pieces of prostate tissue starting at the center and sequentially moving to the periphery by increasing the size of the cones. This process was repeated until the preprogrammed limits had been reached.

In the late 1980s, Howard A. Paul and William L. Barger collaborated to develop a robot that would increase the precision of hip arthroplasty. The resulting product consisted of a preoperative planning workstation (ORTHODOC) and a surgical assistant (ROBODOC) (10). Prior to surgery, a CT was obtained with fiducial markers. The images were then used to create 3D reconstructions of the bone that the surgeon could use to plan the operation. The initial exposure of the bone was similar to standard hip arthroplasty. However, once the bone had been exposed, the surgeon guided the surgical arm of ROBODOC toward the bone and the robot began milling the cavity for subsequent stem placement. Throughout the surgery, the surgeon had control over the robot and could both halt and redirect the surgical arm. Based on studies funded by the manufacturer, the precision of the cavity was significantly increased when compared to manual preparation (11). In 1992, the first total hip arthroplasty was performed in Europe; however, this system did not become commercially available in the United States until 2008 when it was finally approved by the FDA (11).

The next wave of new robots started with a growing interest in telesurgery. Researchers from NASA and the Stanford Research Institute collaborated to enable surgeries to be performed without the surgeon being physically present at the operating table (1). The goal was to enable remote access, without losing the physician–patient relationship. Once developed, the idea was to deploy this technology during wars and allow surgeons to remotely perform surgeries on wounded soldiers. This collaboration eventually led to the development of the automated endoscopic system for optimal positioning (AESOP). The device, which was cleared by the FDA in 1994, allowed the surgeon to operate the camera using a hand or foot switch instead of relying on an assistant, with later models being controlled by voice. A similar robot, the EndoAssist, was developed a few years later. The robot was able to adjust the camera based on the head movements of the surgeon, who wore an infrared headpiece. Compared to the AESOP, which was mounted on the operating room table and therefore moved with the table, the EndoAssist was free-standing and had to be adjusted when changes were made to the operating table (12). In both systems, the robot was limited to driving the camera, and the surgical instruments continued to be of laparoscopic type.

Advanced Robotic Systems

In 1995, the first master–slave robotic system was developed by Computer Motion. This robotic system consists of an input console (master) and a robotic surgical system (slave). The ZRSS consisted of three separate arms. The first arm was a voice-activated AESOP and provided the surgeon with a view of the surgical site. The other two arms were able to hold a variety of instruments and mimic the surgeon's hand movements. It was initially tested on animals, but by

1998, the first tubal reanastamosis and CABG had been performed using this system (13). In 2001, the ZRSS was cleared by the FDA, and at that time, the two robotic arms were able to hold twenty-eight different instruments. In 2003, a merger between Computer Motion and Intuitive Surgical, a rival company, led to the ZRSS being phased out with the aim to focus on the more advanced da Vinci Surgical System.

The first da Vinci model had been approved by the FDA and was introduced by Intuitive Surgical in 2000. Similar to the ZRSS, this system also consisted of a multi-arm patient-side cart and a surgeon console. As of 2015, the newest da Vinci system, the da Vinci Xi, has four arms that can hold the camera as well as a wide array of instruments. The surgical cart could be placed at any position around the patient; it comes with a laser targeting system that, when pointed at an area of interest, will optimally position the boom part of the system. The available endowrist instruments all have seven degrees of freedom (up/down, forward/back, right/left, wrist yaw, wrist pitch, wrist roll, grasp) and therefore provide the surgeon with significant surgical dexterity paralleling that of a human wrist. The surgeon is able to view 3D images of the surgical field within the surgeon console. Hand motions are scaled into micromovements to account for tremor and translated into movements of the surgical instruments. Although the system is referred to as a robot, it does not fulfill the abovementioned definition. Rather than performing a preprogrammed task, the da Vinci system is an example of a master–slave system and depends on the direct input from the operator without the ability to function independently.

Since its introduction, the da Vinci system has been used in an increasing number of procedures across multiple surgical specialties. In addition to urological and gynecological surgeries, more and more general surgical procedures, such as cholecystectomies and hernias, are being performed using the robotic system. In their 2014 annual report, the company noted that the yearly number of procedures had been steadily rising since 2009, and that the procedure growth for 2014 was 9 percent, with a 33 percent increase in general surgical procedures (14). These numbers indicate that robotic surgery not only has been widely accepted by the medical community but also is gaining popularity and is being used in an increasing number of surgical procedures. Figure 1.1 shows the steady increase in the number of surgeries performed using robotic systems over the last three years and, in particular, illustrates the increase in the number of departments that have started using the robotic system.

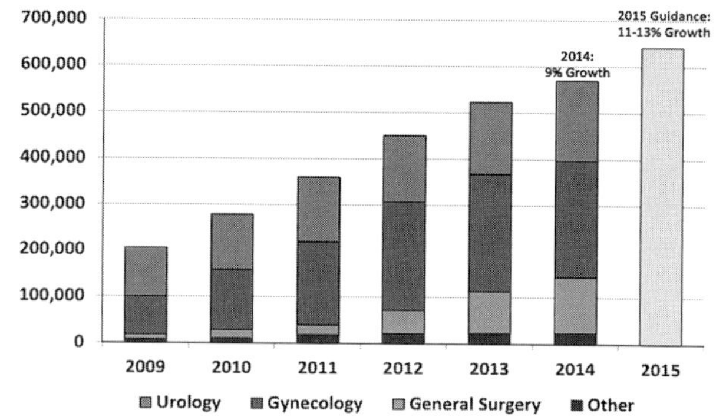

Figure 1.1 Annual utilization of robotic systems in different surgical departments (© 2017 Intuitive Surgical, Inc.; used with permission).

It is undeniable that robotic systems are no longer just used in the automotive industry and laboratories but are increasingly being used for a wide variety of medical procedures. Despite some technical limitations such as lack of tactile feedback posing a challenge (15), as advances are made in the technology and as our experience grows, gradually more complex cases will be performed using robotics. In 2001, a transcontinental robotic cholecystectomy was performed on a patient in Strasbourg (16). It is, therefore, not unreasonable to expect that, as the field of telesurgery improves, particularly with improved time lags for transmission, more complicated and uncommon surgeries might be performed in areas of the world where the surgical expertise is not accessible. In the most extreme case, technology might advance far enough that robots will be capable of performing surgeries autonomously.

References

1. Lanfranco AR, Castellanos AE, Desai JP, Meyers WC. Robotic surgery. *Ann Surg*. 2004; 239(1): 14–21
2. Satyam K, Chauhan S, Coelho RF, Orvieto MA, Camacho IR, Palmer KJ, Patel VR. History of robotic surgery. *J Robot Surg*. 2010; 4: 141–147
3. "Robot." *Oxford Dictionaries*. 2015. Available from www.oxforddictionaries.com/us/definition/american_english/robot [accessed July 31, 2015]
4. Walter WG. An imitation of life. *Sci Am*. 1947; 182(5): 42–45
5. Moran ME. Evolution of robotic arms. *J Robot Surg*. 2007; 1: 103–111

6. Blum CA, Adams DB. Who did the first laparoscopic cholecystectomy? *J Minim Access Surg*. 2011; 7(3): 165–168
7. Kwoh YS, Hou J, Jonckheere EA, Hayati S. A robot with improved absolute positioning accuracy for CT guided stereotactic brain surgery. *IEEE Trans Biomed Eng*. 1988; 35(2): 153–160
8. Davies B. A review of robotics in surgery. *Proc Inst Mech Eng*. 2000; 214: 129–140.
9. Imperial College London. 2015. Available from www3.imperial.ac.uk/mechatronicsinmedicine/research/theprobot [accessed October 23, 2015]
10. "Think surgical." 2015. California: Curexo Technology Cooperation. Available from www.robodoc.com/patient_about_history.html [accessed October 23, 2015]
11. Nakamura N, Sugano N, Nishii T, Kakimoto A, Miki H. A comparison between robotic-assisted and manual implantation of cementless total hip arthroplasty. *Clin Orthop Relat Res*. 2010; 468(4): 1072–1081
12. Gilbert JM. The EndoAssist robotic camera holder as an aid to the introduction of laparoscopic colorectal surgery. *Ann R Coll Surg Engl*. 2009; 91: 389–393
13. Reichenspurner H, Damiano RJ, Mack M, Boehm DH, Gulbins H, Detter C, Meiser B, Ellgass R, Reichart B. Use of the voice-controlled and computer-assisted surgical system Zeus for endoscopic coronary artery bypass grafting. *J Thorac Cardiovasc Surg*. 1999; 118(1): 11–16
14. *Annual Report 2014*. Sunnyvale, CA: Intuitive Surgical., 2014
15. Kroh M, Chalikonda S. *Essentials of Robotic Surgery*. Switzerland: Springer International Publishing, 2015
16. Marescaux J, Leroy J, Rubino F, Smith M, Vix M, Simone M, Mutter D. Transcontinental robot-assisted remote telesurgery: feasibility and potential applications. *Ann Surg*. 2002; 235(4): 487–492

Chapter 2

Credentialing for Robotic Surgery

Daniel M. Herron

Introduction: Why Is Robotic Privileging So Highly Charged?

The emergence of robotic surgery has perhaps had a more polarizing effect on surgeons and patients than any other new surgical technology in recent memory.[1] While some surgeons feel that robotic surgery is the new frontier of minimally invasive surgery, others feel its value is more as a marketing tool, with little or no concrete data to support its use. Proponents of robotic surgery claim that it is an enabling technology that improves surgical precision, speed, and outcomes while providing a more ergonomic operating environment for the surgeon. Critics emphasize the great financial cost associated with the use of robot and the dearth of controlled studies demonstrating any superiority of the technique over standard laparoscopic or thoracoscopic surgery.

This controversy is enhanced by the fact that, as of 2016, there is only one brand of surgical robot approved for clinical use, the Intuitive daVinci system. The lack of technological alternatives gives Intuitive a monopoly on surgical robotics, allowing the company to unilaterally set prices for the robot, its associated disposables, service contracts, and mandatory training programs. Intuitive has taken a very aggressive approach to marketing their devices, implying that hospitals and surgeons who do not adopt the robotic technology will become surgical dinosaurs, tantamount to the general surgeons of the 1990s who failed to adopt new laparoscopic procedures into their practice.

Many surgeons have used robotic surgery as a means of differentiating themselves from their competition, suggesting rightly or wrongly to patients that their practice is superior to others that do not offer robotic procedures. Vast amounts of such marketing materials become immediately evident upon performing an Internet search using the terms "robotic surgery" and the specialty or procedure of interest. This perceived value of robotic surgery as a marketing force, coupled with most surgeons' natural interest in trying out new technology, has the potential to encourage surgeons to initiate a robotic practice for reasons other than documented clinical benefit.

This eagerness for robotic surgery is often met with pushback from hospitals that may wish to limit the number of robotic procedures in order to limit costs. Additionally, there may be resistance to new robotic surgeons from existing robotic practices that have invested heavily in training and marketing to differentiate themselves. Finally, there may be concerns from all parties that surgeons are overly eager to start robotic surgery, eagerly seeking privileges to perform such surgery without first obtaining adequate training or supervised experience.

For these reasons, it is critical for hospitals to have appropriate and carefully vetted credentialing and privileging protocols in place to ensure that surgeons who will perform robotic procedures are appropriately trained

Background: Definition of Credentialing and Privileging

The terms "credentialing" and "privileging" are often used interchangeably by surgeons and are frequently confused. It is important to understand the differences between these terms. "Credentials" refers to the collection of documents and evidence that supports a surgeon's education, residency training, fellowship training, licensure, clinical experience, or other qualification that would impact his or her ability to perform a given procedure.[2–4] Credentialing is thus the process whereby a hospital, surgical center, or other health center confirms the veracity of a surgeon's training and experience.

"Privileges" is the term referring to the permission granted by a hospital to a surgeon to perform a particular group of services or procedures at a particular location or locations.[5] Thus, while it is common to hear a surgeon state "I am credentialed to perform this procedure," it would be more appropriate for the surgeon to state "the hospital completed my credentialing process by verifying my education, training and clinical experience, then granted me privileges to perform this procedure."

Why Are Attitudes about Robotic Privileging So Variable?

The process for credentialing and privileging is very dependent upon the scope of the privileges requested. Some categories of privileges are extremely broad, encompassing an entire medical or surgical specialty. As an example of a broadly specified category, my hospital grants "core general surgery privileges" to qualified general surgeons who have completed a general surgery residency program, are board-eligible or board-certified, and who meet the department's requisite criteria. Core general surgery privileges allow the surgeon to perform a broad range of abdominal and other procedures – as diverse as appendectomy, thyroidectomy, and esophagectomy – that would be considered to fall under the rubric of standard general surgery. This group of privileges gives the surgeon permission to perform a set of procedures appropriate to his or her specialty, but does not specify or limit how the procedures should be performed or what tools should be used to perform them. We can describe this broad-based category of privileges as a "specialty-based" one.

At the other end of the spectrum, the same hospital offers other categories of privileges that are extremely narrow in scope, focused more on a particular instrument than a medical specialty. One example is the use of various medical lasers. Surgeons or specialists in other departments may request privileges for one or more different types of laser, e.g., holmium laser, KTP laser, YAG laser. The applicant must demonstrate adequate training in the use of the specific laser and must confirm competence to a departmental preceptor at the hospital. The laser privilege confers permission to use a specific type of device but does not restrict the type of procedures for which the device is used. Thus, this category of privilege is device-limited, not specialty-limited. We can describe this type of privilege as a "tool-based" or "device-based" one.

These two different types of privileges – specialty-based vs. device-based – become critical to appreciate when we try to tackle the issue of robotic privileges. Asked plainly, is the robot a new tool or is it a new type of surgery? Are we considering "robotic surgery" to be its own subspecialty with a unique set of robotic operations? Or is it a new tool, albeit a complex and highly technology-intensive one, which, once mastered, can be used to perform any of the other procedures for which the surgeon is already privileged. Unfortunately, the only legitimate answer to this question is unsatisfyingly indeterminate: it depends!

More specifically, the answer depends upon what specialty we are addressing, as well as the background of the surgeons in question. Consider, for example, the typical young minimally invasive general surgeon at my hospital. Such a surgeon will have completed a residency in general surgery as well as a fellowship in minimally invasive or laparoscopic surgery. The surgeon will typically have privileges to perform both basic and advanced general surgical procedures via laparoscopic approach, i.e., using narrow instruments that are placed through a trocar into the peritoneal cavity. The surgeon will already be familiar with complex dissection techniques as well as with suturing, energy devices, and staplers that are deployed through a laparoscopic approach.

For this type of surgeon, the robot is not a new specialty but rather an advanced new tool. It brings incremental changes – some positive, some negative – to the procedures that the surgeon is already performing. The beneficial changes are debatable, but include features such as an improved hand-to-instrument interface and the ability to articulate at the wrist. However, the robot also eliminates certain advantages of traditional laparoscopy, such as the presence of haptic feedback, the ability to rapidly visualize and address all four quadrants of the abdomen, and the utility of changing the angle of view of the angled laparoscope. Nonetheless, it is a relatively straightforward process for the fellowship-trained laparoscopic surgeon to apply the robot – a novel tool – to the body of existing operations that he or she already performs. Once the details of the robotic tool are mastered, the tool can be applied to any appropriate procedure for which the laparoscopic surgeon is currently privileged.

In contrast, let us consider an older urologist who was trained in the era of open surgery and does not yet perform advanced laparoscopic procedures. This surgeon may have minimal or basic laparoscopic skills and be unfamiliar with complex laparoscopic dissection and suturing. If this surgeon adds robotic prostatectomy to his or her skill set, this represents an entirely new paradigm of operation – we are not introducing a new tool but rather an entirely new type of procedure. This surgeon is learning how to view tissues on a video monitor, operate through trocars, and utilize a completely new interface. In this situation, the surgeon is truly learning a new procedure, almost a new subspecialty. Clearly the privileging guidelines would need to reflect this difference.

Interestingly, the question of whether it matters if a surgeon has been trained in laparoscopic procedures before starting a robotic practice has been investigated. A 2013 study looked at the proficiency of laparoscopic-trained vs. robotic-trained surgeons who performed radical prostatectomy.[6] Interestingly, only minor differences in patient outcomes were seen between the two groups.

Guidelines from Specialty Organizations

A number of specialty organizations from diverse specialties – including general surgery, urology, and gynecology – have published guidelines intended to lay a framework for hospitals initiating a new robotic credentialing and privileging program.

The Society of American Gastrointestinal and Endoscopic Surgeons (SAGES) organized a consensus conference on robotic surgery in conjunction with the Minimally Invasive Robotic Association in 2006. One of the primary purposes of the meeting was to address the issues of training and credentialing/privileging in robotic surgery. A consensus document, including guidelines for surgeon training and credentialing, was included in the resultant publication.[7] One of the primary purposes of the document was to promote uniformity of standards. As stated in the consensus document:

> Uniform standards should be developed which apply to all medical staff requesting privileges to perform procedures utilizing these technologies. Criteria must be established which are medically sound, but not unreasonably stringent, and which are universally applicable to all those wishing to obtain privileges. The goal must be the delivery of high quality patient care. Surgical proficiency should be assessed for every surgeon, and privileges should not be granted or denied solely base on the number of procedures performed. Ongoing review of results and comparison to published data and/or recognized benchmarks is encouraged.[7]

The consensus document included an appendix entitled "Guidelines for Institutions Granting Privileges in Therapeutic Robotic Procedures," which was meant to serve as a basis for institutions seeking guidance in the development of their privileging processes. While the guideline requires that all applicants for robotic privileges must have completed an accredited surgical residency in the appropriate specialty, it accepts that adequate robotic training may be acquired during residency, fellowship, or by practical experience. The document also suggests that maintenance of privileges should require monitoring of performance and appropriate continuing medical education. Of note, there is no requirement that surgeons perform a specified minimum number of cases to maintain their privileges.

Similar guidelines have been put forth by other specialty organizations, including the American Urological Association (AUA), the Society of Urologic Robotic Surgeons, the American College of Obstetricians and Gynecologists (ACOG), and the American Association of Gynecologic Laparoscopists (AAGL).[2,8–11] While there are necessarily some minor differences among the different guidelines, the documents share many similarities. Each organization agrees that the privileging process remains the responsibility of the individual hospital, with the immediate oversight of the process being controlled by the chief of the appropriate service. Similarly, all agree that board certification or eligibility in the appropriate specialty, plus formal training in robotic procedures, whether through residency, fellowship, or practice experience, is mandatory.[12]

However, each organization's documents extend beyond these generally shared precepts. The AUA provides a very formalized protocol for currently practicing urologists who have had no formal training in robotic surgery, describing specific AUA curricula and intuitive surgical training modules that should be completed by the urologist applying for privileges.[11] The AAGL document describes separate privileging protocols for "basic" and "advanced" procedures and provides very specific recommendations for maintenance of robotic privileges, such as performance of at least "20 procedures each calendar year."[13]

A "Fundamentals of Robotic Surgery" course has been designed with the hope of standardizing the curriculum used in the training of robotic surgeons.[14] Similar in concept to the "Fundamentals of Laparoscopic Surgery" or FLS course initiated by

SAGES and now required as part of certification by the American Board of Surgery, the program could potentially provide a standardized, if basic, level of training.[15,16] Many other institutions have developed proprietary training programs to address robotic skill acquisition.[17–19]

A Typical Robotic Privileges Document

To better understand the details of the robotic privileging protocol, it may be helpful to review the process of robotic privileging as practiced in this particular author's hospital. While every hospital will have a slightly different process in place, in general there are more similarities than differences from one institution to another.[20]

Our institution has created a "Surgical Executive Committee" that manages all applications for robotic privileges. General surgeons applying for robotic privileges will apply for one of three privilege levels:

1. ***Provisional Privileges*** give the surgeon permission to perform cases under the direct supervision of a proctor.
2. ***Full Privileges*** are given to a surgeon who has performed three or more proctored cases without incident and obtained approval from the department chair or designated subordinate.
3. ***Proctor Privileges*** are given to a surgeon who holds full robotic privileges and has completed a minimum of fifteen robot-assisted privileges. The applicant must apply for the proctoring designation to the Surgical Executive Committee, which will consider the request.

All applicants must hold an MD or DO degree and be board-certified or board-eligible within their specialty. They must hold privileges to perform, using open or laparoscopic techniques, the same procedures for which they are requesting robotic privileges and must document that they have performed an adequate number of these open or laparoscopic procedures with acceptable outcomes.

All applicants must initially apply for provisional privileges. They must confirm that they have either successfully completed an ACGME/AOA-approved residency or fellowship with a structured experience in robotic surgery, or that they have undergone experiential, nonresidency-based training, including both formal didactic and practical lab experience.[14] Simulator experience is not required by the institution, but is part of the training protocol provided by Intuitive, and has been shown to have some predictive validity for skills.[21]

Once approved for provisional privileges, the applicant must perform a minimum of three proctored procedures, being supervised by a preceptor who holds proctor privileges and is privileged to perform the procedure being observed. The proctor then completes a proctor report form, which is submitted to the department chair for review. If approved by the chair, the file is forwarded to the Credentials Committee of the Medical Board.

At each reappointment cycle, the surgeon must document both volume and clinical outcomes for the robotic procedures. The decision to renew robotic privileges is then made in accordance with standard privileging processes as outlined in the medical staff bylaws. In order to facilitate the availability of proctors for future applicants for privileges, all surgeons who meet the numerical case requirements for preceptor privileges must agree to participate as proctors for future applicants.

Medicolegal Issues

Just as robotic surgery has attracted the attention of both surgeons and patients, it has also presented new opportunities to medical malpractice attorneys. A recent article in a journal for plaintiffs' attorneys noted that injuries from robotic surgery had more than doubled in the first eight months of 2013 compared to the same time period in 2012.[22] Potential targets include not only the robotic surgeons but the company manufacturing the robot and even proctoring surgeons.[23–25]

How Will Robotic Surgery Evolve? How Will This Affect Privileging?

At present, there is only a single surgical robotic system in clinical use, namely the Intuitive daVinci. Thus, our current conception of privileging guidelines must necessarily accommodate the existing technical paradigm that this single platform creates. This is to say that current privileging guidelines are set up to address a two-part surgical robot with a large, immersive console, in close proximity and connected by cables to a moveable, dockable, bedside console with independently actuated arms.[26]

It is highly likely that future robotic systems will be created using significantly different configurations. Some approaches that seem likely would include operating table rail-mounted arms, consoles that put the surgeon in closer proximity to the operative field, freestanding mechanical or electromechanical instruments with articulating wrists that are used in place of a standard laparoscopic instrument, etc. Just as was impossible to imagine thirty years ago that commonplace appliances like a washing machine or refrigerator would be equipped with high-powered microprocessors, one could easily imagine that the programmable microprocessors and high-powered electromechanical actuators that are now commonplace in cellphones, drones, and even electronic toys will make their way to the surgical instruments of the near future.

As these new tools evolve, it may become difficult to know exactly where the dividing line lies between robotic and traditional surgery. A standard surgical stapler is a highly complex mechanical device, yet is clearly considered to be a traditional surgical instrument. When this evolves into a powered device with a self-contained electrical supply, an internal microprocessor and electromechanical actuators that allow it to articulate, deploy its staples, and assess the adequacy of the firing, it is not so clear whether this is now a different type of surgical robot, albeit one with a highly focused purpose.[27] Does this advanced surgical stapler require a brief in-service with an explanation by the equipment representative? Or does it require additional formal training, with didactic and hands-on training components? Is it just a more advanced version of an existing surgical stapler, or does it require its own set of privileging guidelines? This is just one example of what will undoubtedly be many surgical tools that blur the boundaries between surgical instruments and robots.

The Future of Robotic Surgery and Mandates for Future Privileging

In the relatively near future, we will likely find ourselves in a surgical environment populated by many surgical "robots." These will likely not represent true robots that perform surgical tasks independently but rather advanced surgical tools that make use of advanced electronic and electromechanical components to improve or automate various surgical tasks such as tissue manipulation, dissection, suturing, and anastomosis. It will be necessary to make sure that privileging guidelines exist to promote the safe use of such instruments without creating an undue burden to hospitals and surgeons. Ultimately, the goal must be to use available surgical technology to optimize patient care in an appropriately monitored and controlled environment. Hospitals will need to stay abreast of updates in technology and guidelines from professional organizations so that privileging practices will evolve in a corresponding manner.

References

1. Griffen FD, Sugar JG. The future of robotics: a dilemma for general surgeons. *Bull Am Coll Surg.* 2013;98(7): 9–15. www.ncbi.nlm.nih.gov/pubmed/24010216.
2. Zorn KC, Gautam G, Shalhav AL, et al. Training, credentialing, proctoring and medicolegal risks of robotic urological surgery: recommendations of the society of urologic robotic surgeons. *J Urol.* 2009;182(3): 1126–1132. doi:10.1016/j.juro.2009.05.042.
3. Med Prot Co. Credentialing and privileging medical protective. 2014;March.
4. LaValley D (Ed.). Credentialing, privileging, & patient safety. *Crico/RMF Forum.* 2006;24(3):3–4.
5. NACHC. Human resources insights: tips for health center credentialing and privileging. *Natl Assoc Community Heal Centers.* 2013;May. www.nachc.com/hrclearinghouse/download-ch.cfm?df=Human Resources Insights May 201311.pdf&DID=195.
6. Kim B, Chang A, Kaswick J, et al. Achieving proficiency with robot-assisted radical prostatectomy: laparoscopic-trained versus robotics-trained surgeons. *Can Urol Assoc J.* 2013;7(11–12): E711–E715. doi:10.5489/cuaj.360.
7. Herron D, Marohn M. A consensus document on robotic surgery prepared by the SAGES-MIRA Robotic Surgery Consensus Group. *Surg Endosc.* 2007: 1–24. http://link.springer.com/article/10.1007/s00464-007-9727-5.
8. Lenihan JPJ. Flight plan for robotic surgery. *OBG Manag.* 2014;26(11): 44–48.
9. ACOG. Committee opinion: robotic surgery in gynecology. www.acog.org/Resources-And-Publications/Committee-Opinions/Committee-on-Gynecologic-Practice/Robotic-Surgery-in-Gynecology. Published 2015.
10. Decastro J, Trinh Q-D, Zorn K. Training and credentialing in robotic urologic surgery. In: Patel V, ed. *Robotic Urologic Surgery 2.* London: Springer Verlag; 2012: 19–33.
11. AUA. Standard operating practices for urologic robotic surgery. www.auanet.org/common/pdf/about/SOP-Urologic-Robotic-Surgery.pdf.

12. Intuitive. da Vinci training. 2016. www.intuitivesurgical.com/training.
13. AAGL. AAGL position statement: robotic-assisted laparoscopic surgery in benign gynecology. *J Minim Invasive Gynecol.* 2013;20(1): 2–9. doi:10.1016/j.jmig.2012.12.007.
14. Smith R, Patel V, Chauhan S, Satava R. Fundamentals of robotic surgery: outcomes measures and curriculum development. *NcsaglobalCom.* 2012;(Figure 1). https://ncsaglobal.com/sites/default/files/research/Fundamentals of Robotic Surgery Outcomes Measures and Curriculum Development.pdf.
15. Szold A, Bergamaschi R, Broeders I, et al. European Association of Endoscopic Surgeons (EAES) consensus statement on the use of robotics in general surgery. *Surg Endosc.* 2015;29(2): 253–288. doi:10.1007/s00464-014-3916-9.
16. Fundamentals of Laparoscopic Surgery Program. www.flsprogram.org/.
17. Dulan G, Rege R V, Hogg DC, et al. Developing a comprehensive, proficiency-based training program for robotic surgery. *Surgery.* 2012;152(3): 477–488. doi:10.1016/j.surg.2012.07.028.
18. Attalla K, Raza SJ, Rehman S, et al. Effectiveness of a dedicated robot-assiste surgery training program. *Can J Urol.* 2013;20(6): 7084–7090.
19. Sood A, Jeong W, Ahlawat R, et al. Robotic surgical skill acquisition: what one needs to know? *J Minim Access Surg.* 2015;11(1): 10–15.
20. Erickson BK, Gleason JL, Huh WK, Richter HE. Survey of robotic surgery credentialing requirements for physicians completing OB/GYN residency. *J Minim Invasive Gynecol.* 2012;19(5): 589–592. doi:10.1016/j.jmig.2012.05.003.
21. Culligan P, Gurshumov E, Lewis C, Priestley J, Komar J, Salamon C. Predicitive validity of a training protocol using a robotic surgery simulator. *Female Pelvic Med Reconstr.* 2014;20(1): 48–51.
22. Murphy DH. The current assessment. *Insid Med Liabil.* 2014;3: 2–4.
23. Price DJ. Robotic surgery : the human cost of the learning curve. *Prefer Prof Insur Co Case Rev.* 2015;4: 3–6. www.ppicins.com/wp-content/uploads/2015/04/Robotic-Surgery.pdf.
24. Weatherly LC. Medical malpractice law & strategy: is there a proctor in the house? *Law J Newsletters.* 2012; September.
25. Pradarelli JC, Campbell DA, Dimick JB. Hospital credentialing and privileging of surgeons: a potential safety blind spot. *JAMA.* 2015;313(13): 1313–1314. doi:10.1001/jama.2015.1943.
26. Lee JY, Mucksavage P, Sundaram CP, McDougall EM. Best practices for robotic surgery training and credentialing. *J Urol.* 2011;185(4): 1191–1197. doi:10.1016/j.juro.2010.11.067.
27. Echelon Flex Powered Surgical Stapler. www.ethicon.com/healthcare-professionals/products/staplers/endocutters/powered-echelon-flex.

Chapter 3

Robotic Technology

Phi T. Ho and Alex Macario

Introduction

In the late 1980s, surgical techniques focused on developing the field of minimally invasive surgery. With advances in video imaging, endoscopic technology, and instrumentation, many open procedures were converted into endoscopic ones.[1] Since the introduction of laparoscopy for general surgery in the 1990s, patients have benefited with fewer postoperative complications, shorter hospital stays, and higher patient satisfaction.[2–4] However, laparoscopic approaches pose challenges to surgeons due to decreased visualization of the surgical field and limited dexterity of the traditional instruments. These deficiencies led in part to the development of robot-assisted devices.[5]

In 2000, the Food and Drug Administration approved the use of the first surgical robot, the da Vinci Surgical System. The system was approved for pediatric and adult use in urological, general laparoscopic, and general noncardiovascular thoracscopic and thorascopically assisted cardiac procedures. Robotic-assisted surgery platforms offer several benefits over traditional laparoscopic equipment including:

- high definition (HD)
- three-dimensional (3D) visualization of the surgical field
- EndoWrist® instruments designed with seven degrees of freedom to allow for precision and ease of manipulation.[6]

Although a learning curve exists when using robotic-assisted surgery platforms,[7] surgeons equipped with a firm understanding of the robotic technology and proper training can perform robotic surgeries with acceptable procedure times and complication rates.[8]

The goal of this chapter is to provide a useful overview of the da Vinci platform and the application of robotic surgical technology.

Overview of the Robotic Surgical System

The da Vinci Surgical System, developed and commercialized by Intuitive Surgical, Inc., remains the most widely used robot-assisted surgery platform for minimally invasive procedures. The system was designed to mimic motion capabilities similar to its human operator. For example, when the operator's wrist is flexed or fingers move in a grasping motion, the surgical instrument simultaneously mimics these motions. The multiarticulated EndoWrist® instruments inserted into the patient pivot at a fixed point in the body wall designed thereby to minimize pressure and injuries to the body wall.

Additionally, the system is designed to have hand–eye alignment. Hand–eye alignment refers to the EndoWrist® instruments moving with respect to the camera in a similar manner as the hands of a surgeon would in relation to his or her eyes. This basic principle of surgery is disturbed when performing laparoscopic operations whereby the hand motions are not aligned with the orientation of the eyes looking at a monitor off-angle.

The da Vinci system has undergone several iterations over the past two decades. There are four different commercial models. The first-generation model is the da Vinci Standard System. However, it is no longer sold and is mainly used in laboratory and research centers.

The second model is the S Surgical System, which offers an integrated fourth arm for better access to larger surgical target areas and faster setup times, 3D HD visualization, and improved user interfaces.

The third-generation da Vinci system, the Si, entered the market in 2009 and introduced a dual-console feature that allows two consoles to be used simultaneously, allowing two surgeons to collaborate during surgery or enhance surgical education (student–driver model). It also improved the HD visualization with higher resolution and increased the range of motion of the instruments. The engineering of the product aims to continue to simplify and maximize ease-of-use. The objective is to optimize operating room turnaround times by having a motor-driven patient cart, streamlined draping, and easy setup.

Finally, the fourth-generation Xi Surgical System received FDA approval in 2014. The new overhead instrument arm architecture facilitates anatomical access from any position. The camera and endoscope are integrated and can be attached to any arm, adding flexibility for visualization. The arms are smaller and thinner, while the instrument shafts are longer, providing greater range of motion and operative reach. The Xi comprised 48% of units sold in 2014.[9,10]

The Firefly Technology was released in 2011 and is now a standard feature of the da Vinci Xi Surgical System. This imaging capability combines fluorescent dye (Indocyanine Green) with laser-based illuminators to allow surgeons to identify vasculature in 3D to better visualize important hepatobiliary anatomy, neurovascular bundles, tumor masses, and sentinel lymph nodes.[11–14]

The above-mentioned systems have the following three main components: the surgical console, the patient cart, and the vision cart. Each of the systems offers:

- wristed robotic instrumentation with seven degrees of freedom (move up and down, left and right, in and out, wrist yaw, wrist pitch, roll, and grasp)
- HD 3D imaging with up to ten times magnification
- intuitive operation with natural hand–eye alignment.

The following descriptions of the major components are based on the da Vinci® Si Surgical System as it is currently the most prevalent model in hospital operating rooms.

The da Vinci® Si Surgical Console

The console is the surgeon's workstation and includes the master controllers, stereo viewer, central touchpad, left and right pods, and footswitch panel. The operating surgeon sits at the surgical console, located outside of the sterile field within the operating room, and controls the movement of the robotic arms, the endoscope, and EndoWrist® instruments.

The instrument movement is streamed real-time to the stereo viewer and is aligned with the master controllers, where the surgeon's hands are located. The instrument movements mimic its human operator, thereby allowing for natural alignment of hand, eye, and surgical instrument. This provides surgical dexterity that is similar to open surgery but through a minimally invasive approach.

The *master controllers* are the control units of the robotic surgeon and work similarly to video gaming joysticks. The surgeon places their left and right hands in each controller to manipulate the movement of the robotic arm and the instrument within each arm. Each controller is built like a human arm, with finger grips and wrist and elbow/shoulder joints so that the movement of the patient cart instruments mimics the movement of the surgeon's hand, wrist, thumb, and middle or index finger. This concept is called the anthropomorphic principle. Clutch buttons on the master controllers can be accessed to disengage the controllers from the robotic instruments allowing for ergonomic repositioning of the master controllers without movement of the instruments inside the patient.

The *stereo viewer* provides the surgical video image to the surgeon and allows the surgeon to view the surgical site in 3D, as well as icon and text messages to provide additional information to the surgeon. Looking into the viewer, the system gives the surgeon the option to view in full-screen mode or to view in TilePro™ mode. This mode displays the 3D image along with up to two additional images. The image in the stereo viewer is duplicated on the monitor of the vision cart for the bedside personnel. The system also provides a two-way audio communication between the surgeon and the patient cart operator. A pair of speakers exists below the headrest and a microphone below the viewport.

The *central touchpad* is the main control interface for system functions. The home screen displays system status and control selections. Buttons on the touchpad control settings, such as zoom level, scope angle, and motion scaling. When using the dual-console mode, the touchpad is used to assign robotic arm control between the two surgical consoles.

The *left- and right-side pods* are located on either side of the master controllers. The *left-side pod* controls ergonomic positioning for the surgical console, which reduces unnecessary strain on the surgeon during long procedures. The *right-side pod* is equipped with emergency stop and power buttons.

The *footswitch panel* is located at the base of the surgical console and allows the surgeon to access system functions without having to move away from the stereo viewer. The three switches on the left control system function as robotic arm swaps, camera control, and the master clutch. Four colored pedals on the right are used to activate alternate energy sources for the use of cautery, ultrasonic shears, suction/irrigation, and other advanced instrumentation.

Two surgical consoles can be used simultaneously for one patient cart in the dual-console mode. Master controllers can be assigned control of different arms. This setup is particularly useful in a teaching situation. The da Vinci Skills Simulator can be attached to the surgical console. It provides exercises ranging from basic to advanced and which are applicable to any specialty to improve user proficiency. Exercises cover EndoWrist® manipulation, camera and clutching, fourth arm integration, needle control and driving, and others.

The da Vinci® Si Patient Cart

The patient cart is the operative component of the da Vinci Surgical System (Figure 3.1). The five main components are the setup joints, instrument arms, camera arm, EndoWrist® instruments, and an endoscope.

The *setup joints* of the da Vinci arms allow for flexible range of motion to position for sterile draping and docking of the instruments to the patient. Arm clutch buttons allow the user to rearrange the setup joints as needed during the surgery.

The *instrument arms* of the patient cart provide the interface for the EndoWrist® instruments, and the *camera arm* provides the same function for the endoscope. The surgical console operator controls the instruments and the camera remotely during the procedure. The bedside personnel will aid in installing, exchanging, and removing the camera and instruments.

EndoWrist® instruments are installed onto the instrument arms after docking the system to ports that are placed into the patient. Forceps, needle drivers, retractors, and other specialized instruments such as clip appliers and probe graspers aim to provide the surgeon with control inside the operative field (Figure 3.2). Although most instruments have an 8 mm diameter, 5 mm diameters are available for use in smaller access ports. The EndoWrist® Stapler is designed for resection, transection, and/or creation of anastomoses during surgery.

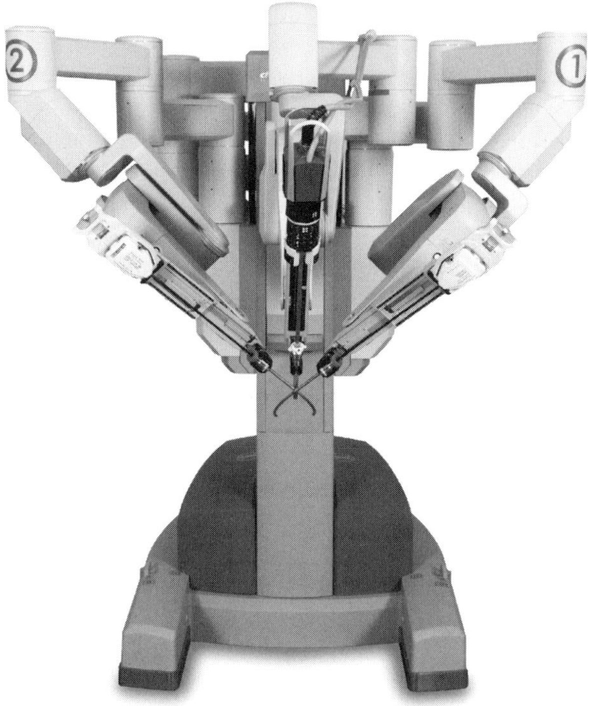

Figure 3.1 The da Vinci® Si Patient Cart provides a stable platform for the camera and instruments to be introduced into the patient. ©2017 Intuitive Surgical, Inc. Image available at www.intuitivesurgical.com/company/media/images/singlesite/SingleSite_PatientCart_4094.jpg. Used with permission.

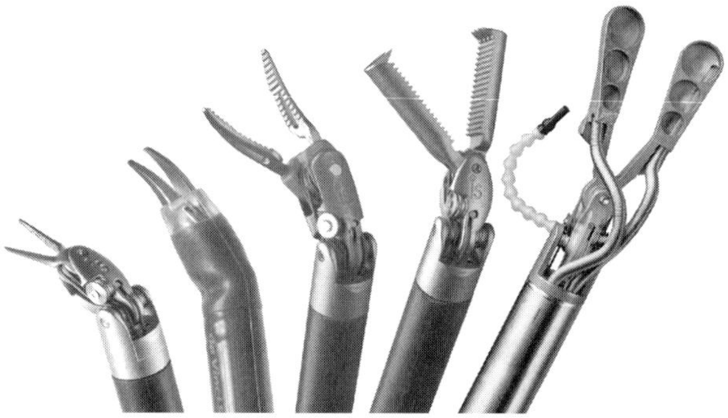

Figure 3.2 Instruments offer a range of motions similar to the human hand, with seven degrees of freedom and 90° of articulation. A wide variety of designs are available depending on the particular procedure. ©2017 Intuitive Surgical, Inc. Image available at www.intuitivesurgical.com/company/media/images/instruments/Instrument_array_fan_300.jpg. Used with permission.

The main characteristics of these instruments include the tip, the wrist, a long shaft, release levers for removal of the instrument, and instrument housing that engages in the sterile adapter of the patient cart instrument arm. The instruments are reposable, meaning that they can be reprocessed and used for a limited number of surgeries.

The da Vinci Si HD Vision System uses an 8.5 mm or 12 mm 3D rod lens endoscope with either a straight (0°) or angled (30°) tip. The illuminator emits light down the shaft of the endoscope projected onto the surgical field. Video image capture is through the left and right channels of the camera head. The camera head contains two separate cameras with independent focusing elements. This information is displayed on two monitors for the left and right eye on the surgical console, recreating a natural 3D image.

The da Vinci® Si Vision Cart

The vision cart houses the central processing and vision equipment for the system. A touchscreen monitor is available to activate telestration, calibrate the endoscope, and allow bedside personnel to view the surgical procedure. The cart has an integrated illuminator to provide lighting for the endoscope. It also houses visual equipment for central image processing from the camera through the camera control unit and audio equipment such as speakers and a microphone for verbal communication with the surgical console operator. There are adjustable shelves for ancillary surgical equipment such as insufflators and electrosurgical generators.[15–17]

The da Vinci® Xi System

The Xi System is the newest generation of the da Vinci Surgical System and has broader capabilities than prior generations, optimized for minimally invasive procedures and complex, multiquadrant surgeries. While the Xi surgeon console (Figure 3.3) and the Vision Cart (Figure 3.4) are similar to the Si, the main differences in the Xi are in the patient side system (Figure 3.5). The Xi expands upon core da Vinci system features, including EndoWrist® instruments, 3D HD visualization, and an ergonomic design.

The Xi System's key distinguishing features compared to prior generations include:

- A new overhead instrument arm architecture designed to provide better unobstructed access from virtually any position
- Four instrument arms and no designated camera arm. The endoscope and camera are integrated in one handheld design and can be placed in any instrument arm with no draping or focusing necessary
- A simpler, more compact endoscope design with improved visual definition and clarity
- An ability to attach the endoscope to any arm, providing flexibility in visualizing the surgical site
- Smaller, lighter arms with improved range of motion
- Longer instrument shafts designed to improve operative reach
- Compatible with Firefly Technology, a standard feature to visualize and assess vessels, bile ducts, and tissue perfusion in real-time.[18]

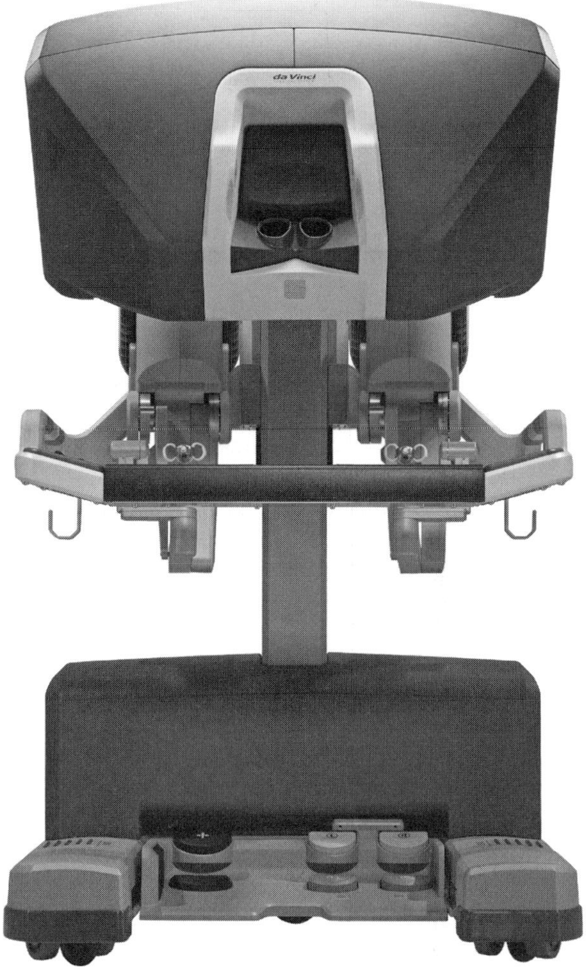

Figure 3.3 The da Vinci® Xi Surgical Console is the surgeon's workstation. ©2017 Intuitive Surgical, Inc. Image available at www.intuitivesurgical.com/company/media/images/xi/xi-surgeon-console-300dpi.png. Used with permission.

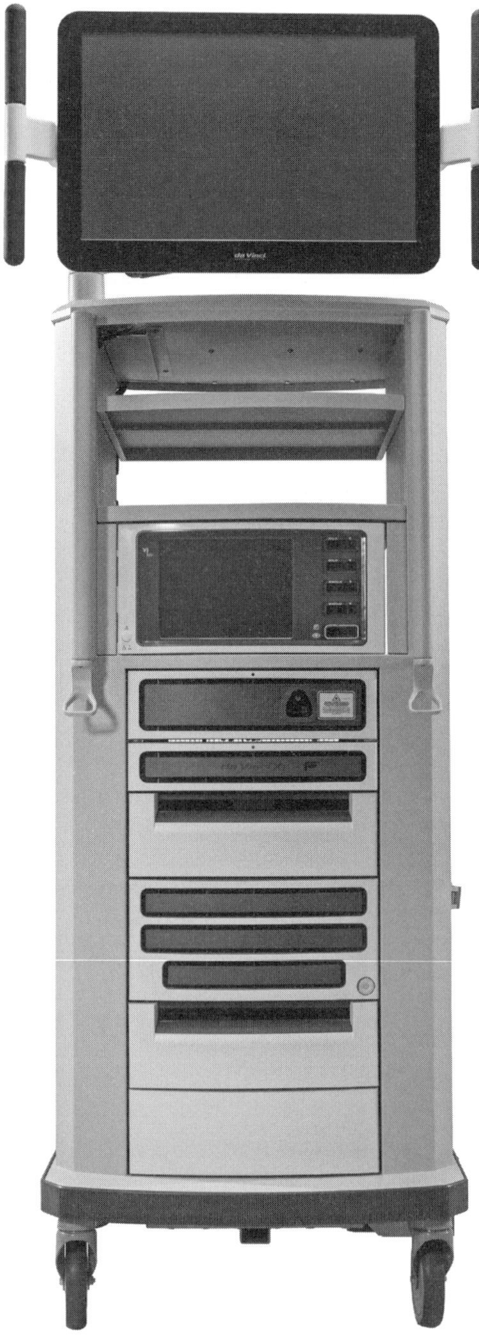

Figure 3.4 The Xi Vision Cart houses the central processing and vision equipment for the system. ©2017 Intuitive Surgical, Inc. Image available at www.intuitivesurgical.com/company/media/images/xi/crystal-clear-3D-HD-vision-300dpi.png. Used with permission.

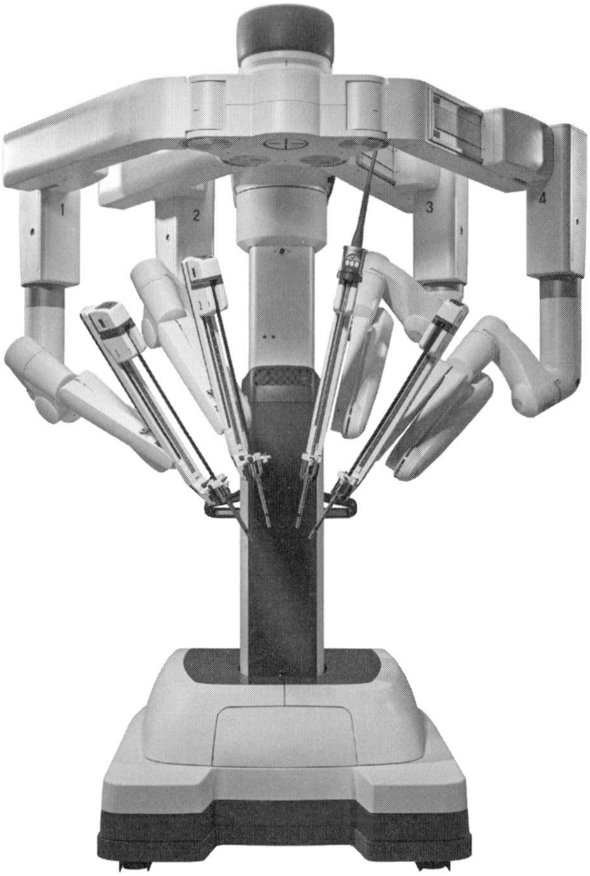

Figure 3.5 The Xi Patient Cart. ©2017 Intuitive Surgical, Inc. Image available at www.intuitivesurgical.com/company/media/images/xi/patient-cart-300dpi.png. Used with permission.

Other Systems

This chapter focused on technology behind the da Vinci Surgical Systems. Other robotic systems exist such as:

- The German Aerospace Center's Institute for Robotics and Mechatronics (DLR MIRO) is a second-generation versatile robot arm used for surgical applications. At 10 kg it has dimensions similar to that of a human arm, which allows it to be placed directly at the operating table and controlled remotely. While it has won numerous awards, there have been no reported cases on its application on humans.
- Titan Medical, Inc., a Canadian public company, is in the process of developing a system called SPORT™ (Single Port Orifice Robotic Technology). This is a surgeon-controlled robotic platform with a 3D HD vision system

and interactive multiarticulating instruments for performing minimally invasive procedures through a single port access. This system is expected to be commercially available at the end of 2016 in Europe and mid-2017 in the United States, pending government approval.

Summary

The da Vinci Surgical System has been at the forefront of technology innovation in robot-assisted surgery, including seven degrees of freedom, 3D HD visualization, and an impressive variety of instrument options. Robotic-assisted surgery will likely see further technological advances and new platforms.

References

1. Mack MJ. Minimally invasive and robotic surgery. *JAMA.* 2001;285(5), 568–572. doi:10.1001/jama.285.5.568
2. Cohn LH, Adams DH, Couper GS, et al. Minimally invasive cardiac valve surgery improves patient satisfaction while reducing costs of cardiac valve replacement and repair. *Ann Surg.* 1997;226(4):421–426.
3. Modi P, Hassan A, Chitwood WR. Minimally invasive mitral valve surgery: a systematic review and meta-analysis. *Eur J Cardiothorac Surg.* 2008;34(5):943–952.
4. Cox TC, Huntington CR, Blair LJ, et al. Laparoscopic appendectomy and cholecystectomy versus open: a study in 1999 pregnant patients. *Surg Endosc.*
5. Seco M, Cao C, Modi P, et al. Systematic review of robotic minimally invasive mitral valve surgery. *Ann Cardiothorac Surg.* 2013;2(6):704–716. doi:10.3978/j.issn.2225-319X.2013.10.18
6. Intuitive Surgical Products. www.intuitivesurgical.com/products/davinci_surgical_system/ Accessed November 29, 2015.
7. Shakir M, Boone BA, Polanco PM, et al. The learning curve for robotic distal pancreatectomy: an analysis of outcomes of the first 100 consecutive cases at a high-volume pancreatic centre. *HPB (Oxford).* 2015;17(7):580–586. doi:10.1111/hpb.12412
8. Angus AA, Sahi SL, McIntosh BB. Learning curve and early clinical outcomes for a robotic surgery novice performing robotic single site cholecystectomy. *Int J Med Robot.* 2014;10(2):203–207. doi:10.1002/rcs.1540
9. Intuitive Surgical Inc. Annual Report 2014. February 5, 2015. http://phx.corporate-ir.net/phoenix.zhtml?c=122359&p=irol-irhome. Accessed November 29, 2015.
10. Intuitive's (ISRG) CEO Gary Guthart on Q1 2015 Results – Earnings Call Transcript. April 21, 2015. http://seekingalpha.com/article/3088286-intuitives-isrg-ceo-gary-guthart-on-q1-2015-results-earnings-call-transcript. Accessed November 29, 2015.
11. Krane LS, Manny TB, Hemal AK. Is near infrared fluorescence imaging using indocyanine green dye useful in robotic partial nephrectomy: a prospective comparative study of 94 patients. *Urology.* 2012; 80(1):110–116.
12. Wagner OJ, Louie BE, Vallières E, Aye RW, Farivar AS. Near-infrared fluorescence imaging can help identify the contralateral phrenic nerve during robotic thymectomy. *Ann Thorac Surg.* 2012;94(2):622–625.
13. Marano A, Priora F, Lenti LM, Ravazzoni F, Quarati R, Spinoglio G. Application of fluorescence in robotic general surgery: review of the literature and state of the art. *World J Surg.* 2013; 37(12):2800–2811.
14. Holloway RW, Bravo RA, Rakowski JA, et al. Detection of sentinel lymph nodes in patients with endometrial cancer undergoing robotic-assisted staging: a comparison of colorimetric and fluorescence imaging. *Gynecol Oncol.* 2012;126(1):25–29.
15. Park CW, Portenier DD. Basic setup, principles, and troubleshooting in robotic surgery. In: Kroh M, Chalikonda S (eds.), *Essentials of Robotic Surgery.* Switzerland: Springer International Publishing, 2015:27–43.
16. Hagen ME, Curet MJ. The da Vinci Surgical Systems. In: Watanabe G (ed.), *Robotic Surgery.* Japan: Springer, 2014:9–19.
17. Hagen ME, Stein H, et al. Introduction to the robotic system. In: Kim KC (ed.), *Robotics in General Surgery.* New York: Springer Science+Business Media, 2014:9–15.
18. Intuitive Surgical Announces New da Vinci Xi Surgical System. April 1, 2014. http://investor.intuitivesurgical.com/phoenix.zhtml?c=122359&p=irol-newsArticle&ID=1914477. Accessed January 12, 2016.

Chapter 4

Physiologic Effects of Pneumoperitoneum and Positioning

Shilpadevi Patil, Pushpa Koyyalamudi, Cory Robertson, Elyse M. Cornett, Charles J. Fox, and Alan David Kaye

Introduction

Robotic-assisted surgery is also known as computer-assisted surgery or simply robotic surgery. This type of surgery allows a surgeon to utilize an instrument to perform a surgery (Vecchio, MacFayden, and Palazzo 2000) either from across the room for traditional robotic surgery or even from different places on Earth, referred to as "telepresence surgery."

The first documented robot-assisted surgery was in 1985 (Lanfranco et al. 2004) involving a non-laparoscopic robot called the Puma 560 (Kwoh et al. 1988). This robot was utilized to perform neurosurgical biopsies with greater precision. Soon after, this same robot was used for transurethral resection of the prostate, leading to the development of the PROBOT (Davies 2000). A major breakthrough in surgery began in 1987 with the first laparoscopic cholecystectomy. This procedure was minimally invasive and had numerous benefits, including smaller incisions, shorter hospital stays, lower risk of infection, shorter periods of convalescence, and decreased pain. One of the most popular robot surgical systems in the United States is the da Vinci system (Copeland et al. 2008). Approximately 1,000 robotic surgeries were performed across the world in 2000. By 2014, this number had climbed to 570,000. By the end of 2014, there were over 3,200 da Vinci systems being used internationally with over 2,200 located in the United States alone. In all, combining the techniques of robotic surgery and a laparoscopic approach has allowed for technical innovation while decreasing surgical invasiveness.

Nearly all laparoscopic procedures are performed with pneumoperitoneum (Perrin and Fletcher 2004). Pneumoperitoneum is the presence of gas in the peritoneal cavity of the abdomen, usually carbon dioxide. This is done to create a larger space inside the abdomen to make room for the tools to move around and function. However, the performance of pneumoperitoneum has multiple physiological sequelae that must be understood and controlled. Pneumoperitoneum is used for a wide range of surgeries. Laparoscopic procedures began as a diagnostic tool to obtain visual confirmation of pathology like liver disorders and abdominal trauma. Originally, gynecologic procedures were common endoscopic procedures. This practice continued until the first acknowledged laparoscopic cholecystectomy via four trochars in 1987 by Mouret. After the development of gas insufflation techniques, physicians could then work in the abdomen with sufficient operating space to not only have adequate visualization of structures but, additionally, to perform more technically difficult operations (Cheng et al. 2013).

Types of Surgeries Pneumoperitoneum Is Used For

General surgery cases were among the first to utilize pneumoperitoneum (Srivastava and Niranjan 2010). Types of surgeries include cholecystectomy, hernia repair, and removal of various organs, such as a colectomy. Obesity surgery has become more common with the advent of gastric banding, gastric bypass, and other forms of bariatric surgery. Certain repairs can also be achieved, such as fundoplication and bowel reanastamosis, as well as kidney transplants.

Gynecologic surgeries that can be performed include the basic procedures such as hysterectomy, oophorectomy, tubal ligation, and myomectomy. Different pathological conditions involve the removal of endometriosis, ectopic pregnancy, ovarian cysts, adhesions, and uterine fibroids. Other reparative conditions can involve uterine suspension for prolapse, bladder support for incontinence, and adnexal torsion correction (Miranda and Carvajal 2003).

Oncological procedures are performed under laparoscopy, which include removal of various tumors from virtually every abdominal and pelvic organ, including the stomach, small and large intestines, kidney, spleen, pancreas, uterus, ovary, cervix, bladder, and prostate (Clancy et al. 2015). Other procedures in this category can involve things like lymphadenectomy.

Urologic surgeons can perform many of the surgeries listed above, as well as correction of unique urinary tract pathology (Jackson 2001). Surgery to remove adrenal and renal tumors can easily be performed utilizing this technique. Additionally, other common uses include relieving urinary blockage along with removal of nephrolithiasis and kidney cysts.

Physiological Effects of Pneumoperitoneum

The physiologic consequences of pneumoperitoneum can be complex. They depend on the interaction between surgical factors such as magnitude of intraabdominal pressure, degree of CO_2 absorption, alteration in patient position, type and duration of surgical procedure. Also, the patient's preexisting cardiopulmonary status may play an integral role in their response to insufflation.

Cardiovascular Effects

The changes in cardiovascular function are attributed to the mechanical and neuroendocrine effects of pneumoperitoneum and the effects of absorbed CO_2. The degree to which increased intraabdominal pressure affects hemodynamics is in turn dependent on several factors, including intravascular volume status, level of intraabdominal pressure, and patient position. Most studies investigating the cardiovascular changes associated with laparoscopic surgery report an increase in systemic vascular resistance (SVR), mean arterial pressure (MAP), and myocardial filling pressures, accompanied by a fall in cardiac index (CI), with little change in heart rate (Table 4.1; O'Malley and Cunningham 2001). Increased intraabdominal pressure causes compression of abdominal venous and arterial vasculature. The compressive effects on the arterial vasculature and capillaries contribute to an increase in SVR and afterload. Studies have shown that at low right atrial pressures the inferior vena cava is compressed, causing a decrease in venous return. Conversely, at high right atrial pressures the vena cava resists compression and increased intraabdominal pressures serve to augment venous return. Overall, the increased cardiac filling pressures, CVP and PCWP, may reflect increased intrathoracic pressures caused by pneumoperitoneum. Dexter et al. (1999) randomized patients to insuffulation pressures of 7 or 15 mmHg during laparoscopic cholecystectomy. Both groups showed an increase in heart rate and MAP, but the cardiac output and stroke volume were significantly more depressed in the 15 mmHg group. Kraut et al. (1999) found similar decrease in cardiac output and stroke volume, but the addition of 10 cm of PEEP exaggerated these reductions to a statistically significant level.

The hemodynamic changes that occur during abdominal robotic surgery appear to be similar to those observed during laparoscopic surgery. Most of the studies evaluating such changes are performed in patients undergoing prostatectomy in steep head down position. Peritoneal insuffulation combined with 40-degree trendelenburg position caused an increase in CVP, SVR, and MAP, while other hemodynamic variables remain within acceptable limits (Kalmar et al. 2010). A recent study by Lester et al. found that although cardiac filling pressures were increased two- to three-fold, the cardiac performance indices (stroke volume, cardiac output, mixed venous oxygenation) as well as echocardiographic cardiac dimensions were maintained in relatively healthy patients undergoing robotic-assisted prostatectomy with patients in 45° head down tilt and pneumoperitoneum with IAP 12 mmHg (figures 1–3; Lestar et al. 2011). However, in patients with severe cardiac dysfunction, there may be significant reduction in CI and hemodynamic deterioration. Safran et al. noted increases in MAP and SVR with significant reduction of CO subsequent to intraperitoneal insuffulation pressure of 15 mmHg in patients with severe heart disease (ASA III or IV) undergoing laparoscopy (Safran, Sgambati, and Orlando 1993).

Hypercarbia by itself causes hemodynamic changes due to the direct action of CO_2 on the cardiovascular system and its indirect effect on the autonomic nervous system. At a PCO_2 of 55–70 mmHg, hypercarbia and acidosis cause vasodilatation, myocardial depression, pulmonary vasoconstriction, and lower arrhythmia threshold. These effects are counteracted by a centrally mediated sympathetic stimulation that causes tachycardia and systemic vasoconstriction. Wittgen et al. compared the effects of CO_2 pneumoperitoneum during laparoscopic cholecystectomy in patients with normal preoperative cardiopulmonary status and previously diagnosed cardiac or pulmonary disease (Wittgen et al. 1991; ASA classes II, III). No differences in ET-CO_2 were found but significant increases in $PaCO_2$ and decreases in pH were

Table 4.1 Cardiovascular Responses to Pneumoperitoneum

Measurement method	MAP	SVR	HR	PCWP	CVP	CI/CO	Patient population	Reference No.
TEE	↑	↑	↔		↑	↓	18 ASA I/II	80
ED	↑	↑	↔			↓	8 ASA I/II, 2 ASA III	45
TEE	↑		↑			↓	14 ASA I/II	27
TBC	↑	↑	↔			↔	16 ASA I/II	16
PAC	↑	↑			↑	↑	15 ASA III >75 years	24
PAC	↑	↑	↔	↑	↑	↓	12 ASAI I/II, 10 elderly with cardiac risk	125
PAC	↑		↔	↑	↑	↓	15 ASA I/II	63
PAC	↑		↔	↑	↑	↓	20 ASA I/II	48
TBC	↔	↑	↔	↓		↓	22 ASA I/II	71
PAC	↑	↑	↔	↑		↓	15 ASA III/IV, preexisting heart and/or lung disease	37
ED	↑		↔			↓	Patients with/without cardiac disease	31
TBC	↑					↓	10 ASA I/II	115
PAC	↑	↑		↑		↓	17 ASA III/IV	46
PAC	↑	↑				↓	15 ASA III/IV	100
TBC	↔	↑	↔			↓	16 ASA I/II	57
PAC	↑	↑	↔			↓	20 ASA I/II	61

MAP, mean arterial blood pressure; SVR, systemic vascular resistance; HR, heart rate; CVP, central venous pressure; PCWP, pulmonary capillary wedge pressure; CI/CO, cardiac index/cardiac output; PAC, pulmonary artery catheter; ED, esophageal Dopper probe; TEE, transesophageal echocardiography; TBC, transthoracic bioimpedence cardiography; ASA, American Society of Anesthesiologists.
↑, increase, ↓, decrease, ↔, no change.

demonstrated in patients with preexisting cardiopulmonary disease.

Stretching of peritoneal lining and local irritation by CO_2 can sometimes produce reflex vagal stimulation causing bradycardia. Other rare complications, including CO_2 gas embolism, hypoxemia, arrhythmias, hypotension, and cardiac arrest, have been reported with these procedures. Overall, while the CO_2 pneumoperitoneum–induced physiologic changes are well tolerated by most healthy patients, they could have adverse consequences in patients with limited cardiopulmonary reserve.

Respiratory Effects

Changes in pulmonary function are largely attributed to the effects of pneumoperitoneum on lung mechanics and gas exchange. Both FRC and lung compliance decrease with supine positioning and general anesthesia. Abdominal insuffulation coupled with trendelenburg position causes cephalad shift of diaphragm, further decreasing FRC and vital capacity, resulting in atelectasis, ventilation-perfusion (V/Q) mismatch, and potential hypoxemia. Controlled ventilation with application of PEEP decreases the risk of hypoxemia by recruitment of alveoli at the lung bases and minimizing alveolar atelectasis. Also, an increase in minute ventilation is needed in most cases to maintain ET-CO_2 within normal limits. However, in the patient undergoing abdominal insufflation, this may lead to an increase in peak airway pressure. Changes in pulmonary mechanics induced by pneumoperitoneum are summarized in Table 4.2 (Grabowski and Talamini 2009) and in figure 4 of Kalmar et al. (2010).

Although strategies such as helium insufflation or abdominal wall lift have been proposed, most of the laparoscopic surgical procedures are routinely performed by insufflating CO_2 into the abdomen. Following insuffulation, CO_2 is absorbed transperitoneally and the rate at which this occurs depends on gas solubility, perfusion of the peritoneal cavity, and duration of pneumoperitoneum. Mullet and colleagues found that CO_2 absorption reaches a plateau

Table 4.2 Alterations of Hepatic Blood Flow during CO_2 Laparoscopy

Study	Model	Method	IAP (mmHg)	Total hepatic flow	Portal venous flow	Hepatic arterial flow	Reversibility
Gutt et al.	Rats	Transit-time US	2	ND	−22.3%	ND	Yes
			4		−35.3%		
			6		−48.4%		
			12		−84.4%		
Jakimowicz et al.	Humans	Dopper US	7	ND	−37%	ND	Yes
			14		−53%		
Junghans et al.	Pigs	Transit-time US	8	↓	↓	=	Yes
			16	↓↓	↓↓		
Klopfenstein et al.	Pigs	Transit-time US	15	=↑	=	+49%	Yes
Odeberg et al.	Humans	Intravascular	11–13	=	ND	ND	ND
Rasmussen et al.	Pigs	?	25	ND	−34%	ND	ND
Sala et al.	Pigs	IGC	15	ND	−76%	ND	ND
Schäfer et al.	Rats	Microspheres	4/10	−37.2%	−46.2%	=	Yes
Schilling et al.	Humans	Dopper US	10	=	ND	ND	Yes
			15	−39%			
Takagi et al.	Humans	Dopper US	> 10	ND	↓	ND	ND
Tunon et al.	Pigs	IGC	14	↓↓	ND	ND	ND
Windberger et al.	Pigs	?	7	=	=	=	Yes
			14	↓	−17.7%	=	

IAP, intraabdominal pressure; US, ultrasonography; IGC, indocyanine green clearance; ND, not defined.

Table 4.3 Changes in Pulmonary Mechanics Because of Insufflation

Respiratory factor	Change
Functional residual capacity	Decrease
Alveolar dead space	Increase
Peak airway pressures	Increase
Pulmonary compliance	Decrease
Forced expiratory volume in 1 second (FEV_1)	Decrease
Forced vital capacity	Decrease
Peak expiratory flow	Decrease

within 10 to 15 minutes after initiation of intraperitoneal insuffulation and thus is not influenced by the duration of surgery. However, it continues to increase progressively throughout extraperitoneal CO_2 insuffulation (Mullett et al. 1993).

Although laparoscopic surgery is associated with increased CO_2 absorption, the changes in arterial CO_2 ($PaCO_2$) concentrations remain clinically insignificant in healthy patients. However, in patients with severe cardiopulmonary disease, the resultant rise in $PaCO_2$ may be significant despite adjusting minute ventilation and refractory hypercapnia, and acidosis can supervene (Wittgen et al. 1991). Kalmar et al. found that in patients undergoing robot-assisted prostatectomy in steep Trendelenburg position, ET-CO_2 values may underestimate arterial CO_2 levels, and maintaining ET-CO_2 between 25 and 35 mmHg will result in $PaCO_2$ levels of 35–45 mmHg (Kalmar et al. 2010). Interestingly, the absorption and excretion pattern of CO_2 in morbidly obese patients appear to be similar to nonobese population (Nguyen and Wolfe 2005). However, in obese patients placed in head down position, arterial oxygenation and alveolar-arterial oxygen gradient are impaired (Meininger et al. 2006). Despite the seemingly deleterious respiratory effects of pneumoperitoneum, patients undergoing open procedures had significantly more impairment in pulmonary function tests (including FVC, FEV1, and oxygen saturation) than patients undergoing laparoscopic abdominal procedures (Hasukić et al. 2002).

Subcutaneous emphysema, pneumomediastinum, and pneumothorax may occur due to incorrect positioning of gas insuffulation needles and trocar, anatomical anamolies, or by gas diffusion across weak tissue planes. Care must be taken to prevent endobronchial movement of the endotracheal tube. This may occur with insufflation by cephalad movement of lungs and carina in relation to the fixed endotracheal tube.

Renal Effects

The mechanical compressive and neuroendocrine effects of pneumoperitoneum may account for reduction in renal blood flow (RBF), glomerular filtration (GFR), and urine output commonly observed in patients undergoing laparoscopic surgery. The effect of increased intraabdominal pressure on cardiac output and renal function was investigated by Harman et al. by inflating intraperitoneal bags in anesthetized dogs (Harman et al. 1982). When the intraabdominal pressures were elevated to 20 mmHg, RBF and GFR decreased to less than 25 percent of normal. There was an increase in systemic and renal vascular resistance, while the cardiac output was reduced to 37 percent of normal. When the cardiac output was returned to baseline with a volume expander, the renal effects persisted, suggesting that the renal effects were independent of the hemodynamic changes. Shuto et al. showed that compression of renal vessels and parenchyma occurred with an insufflation pressure of 20 mmHg. This resulted in a significant decrease in RBF (Shuto et al. 1995). London et al. (2000) measured the RBF in pigs using a renal artery flow probe during IAP of 15 mmHg. Pigs were given maintenance fluids, bolus fluids, or hypertonic saline (Ortega et al. 1996). A drop in RBF and oliguria was found in those receiving only maintenance fluids. Such change was not noticed in well-hydrated animals with adequate volume loading, but impairment of creatinine clearance persisted (figures 5 and 6).

Neurohormonal factors also influence renal perfusion and function as they affect flow through other intraabdominal organs. Studies show that pneumoperitoneum is associated with oliguria and increased levels of plasma arginine vasopressin (AVP), ADH, renin, and aldosterone (Dolgor et al. 1998). Vasopressin exerts its antidiuretic effect by activating renal V2 receptors, thereby promoting reabsorption of water in the distal tubule and collecting ducts and leading to the formation of more concentrated urine. The study by Dolgar et al. investigated the role of AVP in the pathogenesis of oliguria due to pneumoperitoneum (Dolgor et al. 1998). They found that blocking the effects of vasopressin using a V2 receptor antagonist (OPC-31260) partially reversed the oliguria seen in rats during insuffulation, despite unaltered GFR.

The majority of data from animal studies show only a transient decline in renal function during insuffulation. Krisch et al. used insuffulation pressures of either 5 or 10 mmHg in a rat pneumoperitoneum model (Kirsch et al. 1994). They reported a significant increase of serum creatinine in rats within the 10 mmHg group. Creatinine level, however, returned to baseline after 2 hours following desuffulation (Hazebroek et al. 2003). Examination of kidneys procured after exposure to pneumoperitoneum has by and large failed to show any significant histologic damage (Hashikura et al. 1994). The measurable decrease in RBF and renal function caused by pneumoperitoneum does not appear to be deleterious and has little or no postoperative significance.

Splanchnic Effects

Splanchnic circulation is shown to be affected during raised IAP. It is presumed that both increased intraabdominal pressure and hypercapnia are the main factors underlying these disturbances. Increased IAP impairs hepatic perfusion and decreases blood flow to the mesenteric artery, the intestinal mucosa, and the kidney (Bongard et al. 1995). Bongard et al. found a positive correlation between duration and extent of increased IAP and a decrease in bowel mucosal oxygen tension (Knolmayer et al. 1998). Gastric intramucosal pH is used as a monitor of splanchnic perfusion, and intramucosal acidosis signifies inadequate perfusion. Knolmayer et al. studied the effects of pneumoperitoneum on gastric blood flow and traditional hemodynamic measurements in anesthetized swine models (Knolmayer et al. 1998).

This study showed that with increasing insufflation pressures, arterial pH decreased, arterial CO_2 increased, mixed venous CO_2 increased, and gastric intramucosal pH decreased significantly, suggesting that gastric blood flow is adversely affected. These effects were more pronounced at IAP >15 mmHg (Schäfer and Krähenbühl 2001). The decrease in splanchnic perfusion is mediated partly by mechanical compression of the mesenteric vasculature in addition to humorally mediated vasoconstriction.

However, some of these effects may be counterbalanced by the direct splanchnic vasodilatation caused by hypercapnia. Schäfer et al. (2001) studied the alterations in hepatic and splanchnic circulation during laparoscopy in rats. Reduction in organ blood flow was found to be different for hollow viscus versus solid organs. Although small and large bowel blood flow was reduced significantly (26.6 and 23.9 percent, respectively), gastric blood flow remained unchanged. The decreases in liver, spleen, pancreas, and kidney circulation were 29–37.2, 37.6–64.6, 51.2–57.5, and 34.8–40.6 percent, respectively, with a significant decrease in portal blood flow by about 53.8 percent. Only partial restoration of organ blood flow following desuffulation was noted (Schäfer and Krähenbühl 2001). The clinical importance of reduction in hepatic blood flow is still under debate. Elderly patients with generalized atherosclerosis and preexisting liver disease may be at increased risk of hepatic ischemia and its consequences. But, the majority of patients undergoing various laparoscopic procedures do not exhibit any increased intraoperative or postoperative morbidity. Further studies are needed to reveal whether reduced microcirculation in diseased organs (i.e., liver cirrhosis, small bowel ileus, kidney transplantation) and prolonged operating times may have potential adverse effects for the laparoscopic approach.

Central Nervous System

Pneumoperitoneum has a well-documented impact on intracranial pressure (ICP). Both experimental and clinical studies have demonstrated an increase in ICP associated with pneumoperitoneum. Several theories have been proposed to account for the rise in ICP observed during pneumoperitoneum.

One hypothesis incorporates the modified Monroe–Kellie doctrine, by which a change in one intracranial compartment (among three compartments, namely vascular, cerebrospinal fluid, and parenchymal) results in a compensatory change in the other compartment. Rapid changes in one compartment, however, may preclude compensation, resulting in a rising ICP (Josephs et al. 1994). Este-Mcdonald et al. postulated that abdominal insufflation can increase intrathoracic pressure, leading to the obstruction of venous outflow from the spinal cord via lumbar and pelvic plexuses (Este-McDonald et al. 1995). The increased volume of the vascular intracranial compartment induces a rise in ICP. Others have theorized that impaired absorption of CSF accounts for an increase in ICP.

Conversely, Rosenthal et al. have postulated that a rise in ICP is mediated by a two-phase mechanism (Rosenthal et al. 1997):

1. early, passive, venous effect
2. late, active, arterial effect

In the early mechanical stage, increased intraabdominal pressure results in the compression of IVC with a resultant increase in CVP. This in turn impairs venous drainage from the lumbar plexus, thereby raising ICP. In the late stage, hypercarbia, due to ventilation–perfusion mismatch and peritoneal absorption of CO_2, causes vasodilation of intracranial vessels and a rise in ICP. Furthermore, acute elevation in ICP elicits a central nervous system response (Cushing reflex) mediated by the release of catecholamines and vasopressin. The Cushing's reflex yields an increased MAP and SVR while reducing splanchic and visceral blood flow to ameloriate central venous return. Collectively, this array of hemodynamic changes may be accounted for by rise in ICP.

The clinical significance of these observations in patients without preexisting intracranial disease is unknown, although, to date, no cases of significant neurological impairment directly attributable to pneumoperitoneum have been reported. However, for patients with a head injury or an intracranial lesion, the potential for increased ICP during CO_2 pneumoperitoneum could be dangerous. As such, laparoscopy may be contraindicated in these patients or should be undertaken only under conditions of low intraabdominal pressure or gasless laparoscopy to avoid potentially dangerous elevations in ICP. Additionally, the use of intraoperative ICP monitoring in this situation is prudent (Halverson et al. 1998).

Immune System

The effect of pneumoperitoneum on immune and metabolic responses has been extensively studied, primarily based on alterations in cytokines and other immune response mediators. Although correlation of these findings with actual immune function and clinical complication has not been forthcoming, alterations in stress and immune response to laparascopic surgery may provide insight into the observed clinical outcomes. Alterations in stress and immune response correlate with the severity or extent of injury; as such, the physiological response to laparoscopic surgery may differ from that of open surgery. The primary mediators of the acute phase response are the inflammatory cytokines interleukin (IL-1), interleukin-6 (IL-6), and tumor necrosis factor, which is released from the peritoneal macrophages (Cruickshank et al. 1990).

The hepatic component of the acute phase response is regulated by IL-6, which stimulates the production of acute phase proteins, including C-reactive protein, which is the primary marker. TNF and IL-1 mediate the nonhepatic manifestations of the acute phase response, such as fever and tachycardia (Pullicino et al. 1990). A number of investigators have compared IL-6 levels after laparoscopic and corresponding open operations. Numerous studies have demonstrated significantly higher levels of IL-6 with open as compared with laparoscopic cholecystectomy.

The influence of specific gas used for insufflation on immune function has been addressed experimentally. Chekan and colleagues (1999) compared the immune competence of mice, as determined by their ability to clear an intraperitoneally administered intracellular pathogen, Listeria monocytogenes, after undergoing abdominal laparotomy or laparoscopy using either CO_2 or helium as an insufflant. Although all interventions were associated with impaired cell-mediated immunity (decreased clearance of interperitoneal bacteria), CO_2 pneumoperitoneum resulted in a lower bacterial clearance rate than either laparotomy or helium pneumoperitoneum, with helium pneumoperitoneum demonstrating the best clearance rates. West and colleagues demonstrated significantly lower levels of TNF and IL-1 in response to bacterial lipopolysaccharides when macrophages were incubated in CO_2 compared with air or helium (West, Baker, and Bellingham 1996).

Effects of CO_2

The most commonly used gas for insufflation is CO_2. It is noncombustible, rapidly soluble in the blood, and relatively inexpensive. Because CO_2 is the main byproduct of cellular metabolism, humans have an efficient mechanism for its elimination. A small portion of CO_2 is dissolved in blood and is delivered directly to the lungs. The majority of CO_2 combines with water in red blood cells to form carbonic acid, which then dissociates into hydrogen and bicarbonate.

$$CO_2 + H_2O = H_2CO_3 = H^+ + HCO_3$$

The produced hydrogen ions complex with hemoglobin, and the bicarbonate diffuses into the plasma.

CO_2 absorbed through the peritoneum is handled in the same manner and, ultimately, is eliminated by respiratory exchange in the lungs. Insufflation increases the delivery of CO_2 to the lungs by as much as 50 percent, which necessitates a compensatory increase in minute ventilation to maintain eucapnia. While under general anesthesia, minute ventilation volumes must be increased by up to 16 percent to maintain normocarbia. Even if the increase in $PaCO_2$ is not fully compensated by hyperventilation, most healthy patients are easily able to adapt to the transient increase in end-tidal CO_2 and slight decrease in pH by maximizing the use of their intracellular and plasma buffering systems and increasing the rate of CO_2 transport. Some patients, however, have less homeostatic reserve and are unable to tolerate the increased CO_2 load during insufflation. Patients particularly at risk are those with decreased pulmonary function (i.e., severe chronic obstructive pulmonary disease), reduced cardiac output, or a high metabolic and cellular respiratory rate (i.e., septic patients). These patients require strict monitoring of end-tidal CO_2 and arterial blood pH to avoid significant hypercarbia and acidemia and subsequent complications.

References

Bongard, F, N Pianim, S Dubecz, and S R Klein. 1995. "Adverse Consequences of Increased Intra-Abdominal Pressure on Bowel Tissue Oxygen." *The Journal of Trauma* 39 (3): 519–24; discussion 524–5. www.ncbi.nlm.nih.gov/pubmed/7473918.

Chekan, E G, C Nataraj, E M Clary, T Z Hayward, F J Brody, J C Stamat, M C Fina, W S Eubanks, and C J Westcott. 1999. "Intraperitoneal Immunity and Pneumoperitoneum." *Surgical Endoscopy* 13 (11): 1135–8. www.ncbi.nlm.nih.gov/pubmed/10556454.

Cheng, Y, J Lu, X Xiong, S Wu, Y Lin, T Wu, and N Cheng. 2013. "Gases for Establishing Pneumoperitoneum during Laparoscopic Abdominal Surgery." *The Cochrane Database of Systematic Reviews* 1(January): CD009569. doi:10.1002/14651858.CD009569.pub2.

Clancy, C, D P O'Leary, J P Burke, H P Redmond, J C Coffey, M J Kerin, and E Myers. 2015. "A Meta-Analysis to Determine the Oncological Implications of Conversion in Laparoscopic Colorectal Cancer Surgery." *Colorectal Disease : The Official Journal of the Association of Coloproctology of Great Britain and Ireland* 17(6): 482–90. doi:10.1111/codi.12875.

Copeland, D R, C Boneti, E R Kokoska, R J Jackson, and S D Smith. 2008. "Evaluation of Initial Experience and Comparison of the Da Vinci Surgical System with Established Laparoscopic and Open Pediatric Nissen Fundoplication Surgery." *Journal of the Society of Laparoendoscopic Surgeons/Society of Laparoendoscopic Surgeons* 12(3): 238–40. www.pubmedcentral.nih.gov/articlerender.fcgi?artid=3015888&tool=pmcentrez&rendertype=abstract.

Cruickshank, A M, W D Fraser, H J Burns, J Van Damme, and A Shenkin. 1990. "Response of Serum Interleukin-6 in Patients Undergoing Elective Surgery of Varying Severity." *Clinical Science (London, England 1979)* 79 (2): 161–5. www.ncbi.nlm.nih.gov/pubmed/2167805.

Davies, B. 2000. "A Review of Robotics in Surgery." *Proceedings of the Institution of Mechanical Engineers. Part H, Journal of Engineering in Medicine* 214 (1): 129–40. www.ncbi.nlm.nih.gov/pubmed/10718057.

Dexter, S P, M Vucevic, J Gibson, and M J McMahon. 1999. "Hemodynamic Consequences of High- and Low-Pressure Capnoperitoneum during Laparoscopic Cholecystectomy." *Surgical Endoscopy* 13 (4): 376–81. www.ncbi.nlm.nih.gov/pubmed/10094751.

Dolgor, B, S Kitano, T Yoshida, T Bandoh, K Ninomiya, and T Matsumoto. 1998. "Vasopressin Antagonist Improves Renal Function in a Rat Model of Pneumoperitoneum." *The Journal of Surgical Research* 79(2): 109–14. doi:10.1006/jsre.1998.5409.

Este-McDonald, J R, L G Josephs, D H Birkett, and E F Hirsch. 1995. "Changes in Intracranial Pressure Associated with Apneumic Retractors." *Archives of Surgery (Chicago, IL 1960)* 130 (4): 362–5; discussion 365–6. www.ncbi.nlm.nih.gov/pubmed/7710333.

Grabowski, J E, and M A Talamini. 2009. "Physiological Effects of Pneumoperitoneum." *Journal of Gastrointestinal Surgery : Official Journal of the Society for Surgery of the Alimentary Tract* 13 (5): 1009–16. doi:10.1007/s11605-008-0662-0.

Halverson, A, R Buchanan, L Jacobs, V Shayani, T Hunt, C Riedel, and J Sackier. 1998. "Evaluation of Mechanism of Increased Intracranial Pressure with Insufflation." *Surgical Endoscopy* 12 (3): 266–9. www.ncbi.nlm.nih.gov/pubmed/9502709.

Harman, P K, I L Kron, H D McLachlan, A E Freedlender, and S P Nolan. 1982. "Elevated Intra-Abdominal Pressure and Renal Function." *Annals of Surgery* 196 (5): 594–97. www.pubmedcentral.nih.gov/articlerender.fcgi?artid=1352794&tool=pmcentrez&rendertype=abstract.

Hashikura, Y, S Kawasaki, Y Munakata, S Hashimoto, K Hayashi, and M Makuuchi. 1994. "Effects of Peritoneal Insufflation on Hepatic and Renal Blood Flow." *Surgical Endoscopy* 8 (7): 759–61. www.ncbi.nlm.nih.gov/pubmed/7974101.

Hasukić, S, D Mesić, E Dizdarević, D Keser, S Hadziselimović, and M Bazardzanović. 2002. "Pulmonary Function after Laparoscopic and Open Cholecystectomy." *Surgical Endoscopy* 16 (1): 163–5. doi:10.1007/s00464-001-0060-0.

Hazebroek, E J, R W F de Bruin, N D Bouvy, R L Marquet, F Bonthuis, I M Bajema, D P Hayes, J N M Ijzermans, and H J Bonjer. 2003. "Long-Term Impact of Pneumoperitoneum Used for Laparoscopic Donor Nephrectomy on Renal Function and Histomorphology in Donor and Recipient Rats." *Annals of Surgery* 237 (3): 351–7. doi:10.1097/01.SLA.0000055272.96210.A0.

Jackson, C L. 2001. "Urologic Laparoscopy." *Surgical Oncology Clinics of North America* 10 (3): 571–8. www.ncbi.nlm.nih.gov/pubmed/11685928.

Josephs, L G, J R Este-McDonald, D H Birkett, and E F Hirsch. 1994. "Diagnostic Laparoscopy Increases Intracranial Pressure." *The Journal of Trauma* 36 (6): 815–18; discussion 818–19. www.ncbi.nlm.nih.gov/pubmed/8015003.

Kalmar, A F, L Foubert, J F A Hendrickx, A Mottrie, A Absalom, E P Mortier, and M M R F Struys. 2010. "Influence of Steep Trendelenburg Position and CO(2) Pneumoperitoneum on Cardiovascular, Cerebrovascular, and Respiratory Homeostasis during Robotic Prostatectomy." *British Journal of Anaesthesia* 104 (4): 433–9. doi:10.1093/bja/aeq018.

Kirsch, A J, T W Hensle, D T Chang, M L Kayton, C A Olsson, and I S Sawczuk. 1994. "Renal Effects of CO_2 Insufflation: Oliguria and Acute Renal Dysfunction in a Rat Pneumoperitoneum Model." *Urology* 43 (4): 453–9. www.ncbi.nlm.nih.gov/pubmed/8154067.

Knolmayer, T J, M W Bowyer, J C Egan, and H J Asbun. 1998. "The Effects of Pneumoperitoneum on Gastric Blood Flow and Traditional Hemodynamic Measurements." *Surgical Endoscopy* 12 (2): 115–18. www.ncbi.nlm.nih.gov/pubmed/9479723.

Kraut, E J, J T Anderson, A Safwat, R Barbosa, and B M Wolfe. 1999. "Impairment of Cardiac Performance by Laparoscopy in Patients Receiving Positive End-Expiratory Pressure." *Archives of Surgery (Chicago, IL 1960)* 134 (1): 76–80. www.ncbi.nlm.nih.gov/pubmed/9927136.

Kwoh, Y S, J Hou, E A Jonckheere, and S Hayati. 1988. "A Robot with Improved Absolute Positioning Accuracy for CT Guided Stereotactic Brain Surgery." *IEEE Transactions on Bio-Medical Engineering* 35 (2): 153–60. doi:10.1109/10.1354.

Lanfranco, A R, A E Castellanos, J P Desai, and W C Meyers. 2004. "Robotic Surgery: A Current Perspective." *Annals of Surgery* 239 (1): 14–21. doi:10.1097/01.sla.0000103020.19595.7d.

Lestar, M, L Gunnarsson, L Lagerstrand, P Wiklund, and S Odeberg-Wernerman. 2011. "Hemodynamic Perturbations during Robot-Assisted Laparoscopic Radical Prostatectomy in 45° Trendelenburg Position." *Anesthesia and Analgesia* 113 (5): 1069–75. doi:10.1213/ANE.0b013e3182075d1f.

London, Eric et al. 2000. "Effect of Intravascular Volume Expansion on Renal Function during Prolonged CO2 Pneumoperitoneum." *Annals of Surgery* 231(2):195–201. Retrieved (https://www.ncbi.nlm.nih.gov/pmc/articles/PMC1420986/#).

Meininger, D, B Zwissler, C Byhahn, M Probst, K Westphal, and D H Bremerich. 2006. "Impact of Overweight and Pneumoperitoneum on Hemodynamics and Oxygenation during Prolonged Laparoscopic Surgery." *World Journal of Surgery* 30 (4): 520–6. doi:10.1007/s00268-005-0133-7.

Miranda, C S, and A R Carvajal. 2003. "Complications of Operative Gynecological Laparoscopy." *Journal of the Society of Laparoendoscopic Surgeons/Society of Laparoendoscopic Surgeons* 7 (1): 53–8. www.pubmedcentral.nih.gov/articlerender.fcgi?artid=3015471&tool=pmcentrez&rendertype=abstract.

Mullett, C E, J P Viale, P E Sagnard, C C Miellet, L G Ruynat, H C Counioux, J P Motin, J P Boulez, D M Dargent, and G J Annat. 1993. "Pulmonary CO_2 Elimination during Surgical Procedures Using Intra- or Extraperitoneal CO_2 Insufflation." *Anesthesia and Analgesia* 76 (3): 622–6. www.ncbi.nlm.nih.gov/pubmed/8452278.

Nguyen, N T, and B M Wolfe. 2005. "The Physiologic Effects of Pneumoperitoneum in the Morbidly Obese." *Annals of Surgery* 241 (2): 219–26. www.pubmedcentral.nih.gov/articlerender.fcgi?artid=1356906&tool=pmcentrez&rendertype=abstract.

O'Malley, C, and A J Cunningham. 2001. "Physiologic Changes during Laparoscopy." *Anesthesiology Clinics of North America* 19 (1): 1–19. doi:10.1016/S0889-8537(05)70208-X.

Ortega, A E, J H Peters, R Incarbone, L Estrada, A Ehsan, Y Kwan, C J Spencer, E Moore-Jeffries, K Kuchta, and J T Nicoloff. 1996. "A Prospective Randomized Comparison of the Metabolic and Stress Hormonal Responses of Laparoscopic and Open Cholecystectomy." *Journal of the American College of Surgeons* 183 (3): 249–56. www.ncbi.nlm.nih.gov/pubmed/8784319.

Perrin, M, and A Fletcher. 2004. "Laparoscopic Abdominal Surgery." *Continuing Education in Anaesthesia, Critical Care & Pain* 4 (4): 107–10. doi:10.1093/bjaceaccp/mkh032.

Pullicino, E A, F Carli, S Poole, B Rafferty, S T Malik, and M Elia. 1990. "The Relationship between the Circulating Concentrations of Interleukin 6 (IL-6), Tumor Necrosis Factor (TNF) and the Acute Phase Response to Elective Surgery and Accidental Injury." *Lymphokine Research* 9 (2): 231–8. www.ncbi.nlm.nih.gov/pubmed/1692598.

Rosenthal, R J, J R Hiatt, E H Phillips, W Hewitt, A A Demetriou, and M Grode. 1997. "Intracranial Pressure. Effects of Pneumoperitoneum in a Large-Animal Model." *Surgical Endoscopy* 11 (4): 376–80. www.ncbi.nlm.nih.gov/pubmed/9094281.

Safran, D, S Sgambati, and R Orlando. 1993. "Laparoscopy in High-Risk Cardiac Patients." *Surgery, Gynecology & Obstetrics* 176 (6): 548–54. www.ncbi.nlm.nih.gov/pubmed/8322127.

Schäfer, M, and L Krähenbühl. 2001. "Effect of Laparoscopy on Intra-Abdominal Blood Flow." *Surgery* 129 (4): 385–9. doi:10.1067/msy.2001.110224.

Shuto, K, S Kitano, T Yoshida, T Bandoh, Y Mitarai, and M Kobayashi. 1995. "Hemodynamic and Arterial Blood Gas Changes during Carbon Dioxide and Helium Pneumoperitoneum in Pigs." *Surgical Endoscopy* 9 (11). doi:10.1007/BF00210922.

Srivastava, A, and A Niranjan. 2010. "Secrets of Safe Laparoscopic Surgery: Anaesthetic and Surgical Considerations." *Journal of Minimal Access Surgery* 6 (4): 91–4. doi:10.4103/0972-9941.72593.

Vecchio, R, B V MacFayden, and F Palazzo. 2000. "History of Laparoscopic Surgery." *Panminerva Medica* 42 (1): 87–90. www.ncbi.nlm.nih.gov/pubmed/11019611.

West, M A, J Baker, and J Bellingham. 1996. "Kinetics of Decreased LPS-Stimulated Cytokine Release by Macrophages Exposed to CO_2." *The Journal of Surgical Research* 63 (1): 269–74. doi:10.1006/jsre.1996.0259.

Wittgen, C M, C H Andrus, S D Fitzgerald, L J Baudendistel, T E Dahms, and D L Kaminski. 1991. "Analysis of the Hemodynamic and Ventilatory Effects of Laparoscopic Cholecystectomy." *Archives of Surgery (Chicago, IL 1960)* 126 (8): 997–1000; discussion 1000–1001. www.ncbi.nlm.nih.gov/pubmed/1830738.

Chapter 5

Considerations in Patients with Comorbidities, Pregnant and Pediatric Patients

Shilpadevi Patil, Michael Franklin, Yury Rapoport, Elyse M. Cornett, Charles J. Fox, and Alan David Kaye

Introduction

Endoscopic procedures have been described in the literature for over 200 years [1]. The first known case was performed in veterinary medicine in 1805 [2]. These procedures were performed infrequently until the early 1980s when the first laparoscopic appendectomy was performed in 1982. In the 1990s, laparoscopic procedures such as appendectomy, cholecystectomy, and hysterectomy became routine, and more difficult procedures were attempted occasionally [2]. Since then, the demand for minimally invasive techniques has grown, citing possible benefits such as smaller incisions, fewer wound complications, reduced postoperative pain, faster recovery, and shorter hospital stays [3,4].

The latest addition to laparoscopic surgery has been robot-assisted surgery, which has become increasingly more common since the da Vinci Surgical System received FDA approval in 2000 [3–5]. In 2012, there were more than 400,000 da Vinci robotic-assisted surgical procedures performed in the United States, covering a variety of surgical subspecialties, such as urology, otolaryngology, gynecology, cardiothoracic, and others, in addition to general surgery [3,6]. Like other laparoscopic surgical techniques, robot-assisted laparoscopic surgery requires insufflation of the abdomen, which provides room for the surgeon to work and have a better view of anatomic structures [2,7]. Insufflation is achieved by pumping carbon dioxide (CO_2) into the abdomen through a port, inflating the abdomen to a desired pressure. While it is effective, rare complications can arise as the increased intra-abdominal pressure and CO_2 may alter the patient's physiology [8]. The anesthesia provider and surgeon should be cognizant of these possibilities.

Metabolic complications related to insufflation include acidosis secondary to absorption of CO_2, which can theoretically affect the fetus in pregnant patients [7–9]. Increased intraabdominal pressure is a consequence of insufflation; however, this is more problematic in obese patients, who have increased intraabdominal pressure at baseline. Furthermore, this procedure can have adverse effects on airway pressure during positive pressure ventilation, as well as the cardiovascular circulation [10,11]. The effects of insufflation on pediatric patients are similar, but are generally well tolerated [12]. Patients with known medical comorbidities (especially ASA classes III and IV) are at additional risks of developing intraoperative complication during robotic cases, due to distorted physiology. Preoperative counseling along with thorough evaluation is prudent in this group. In addition, pediatric and pregnant patients exhibit unique features that may make robotic surgery challenging. These features are discussed later in the chapter.

General Concerns and Regulations in Robotic-Assisted Surgery

Each patient must have a thorough history and physical examination before robotic surgery. Many medical conditions require unique implications for preoperative screening, optimization, and intraoperative anesthetic management. Cardiac conditions (systolic and diastolic failure, valve regurgitation, dilated cardiomyopathy, coronary artery disease), pulmonary pathology, renal insufficiency, mesenteric ischemia, intracranial pathology, ocular pathology, and glaucoma can be impacted by robotic procedures.

Step Trendelenburg positioning can cause significant dependent edema, so the preanesthetic evaluation should primarily address potential problems that may occur with intraocular pressure, intracranial pressure, hemodynamics, ventilation, or volume loading as a result of positioning. Since postoperative edema of the face, eyes, and larynx might delay extubation or necessitate reintubation, any known or suspected preoperative airway challenges will be magnified in the postoperative period. Hence, a good preoperative airway exam is of paramount importance. A thorough preoperative neurological evaluation is paramount because preexisting undiagnosed peripheral nerve injuries are not unusual. The patient should be thoroughly examined and all preexisting deficits should be documented. Electrophysiological and imaging studies may be indicated for further evaluation prior to surgery.

Age

Age has not affected the adult population outcomes for robotic surgery. Robotic surgery can be performed in the elderly population with low mortality, acceptable morbidity, and short hospital stay. Age should not be a contraindication to robotic surgery [13].

Lung Pathology

The synergistic effect of CO_2 pneumoperitoneum and steep Trendelenburg position, especially during pelvic procedures, can affect patients with virtually any thoracic cavity pathology. The diaphragm is pushed cephalad, which decreases lung compliance, thoracic volume, and functional residual capacity (FRC), while increasing work of breathing and peak inspiratory pressure. Normal lungs have a remarkable capacity to withstand the aforementioned changes and maintain adequate oxygenation, but any underlying lung pathology can distort adaptation mechanisms and lead to atelectasis and pulmonary interstitial edema. This may result in respiratory failure and hypoxia. A routine preoperative pulmonary function testing is advised if a patient shows signs of chronic lung pathology. The risks of developing hypercarbia and acidosis are significantly higher while undergoing robot-assisted procedures if compromised pulmonary function exists. For these cases, an arterial line should be placed prior to the start of the surgical procedure for frequent blood gas monitoring. Patients with COPD, reactive airway disease, and OSA must be counseled for postoperative recovery, CPAP, or ICU ventilation.

Musculoskeletal

Cervical spine disease and limited range of motion may be a factor if the patient is in the lateral position with flexion. This position may cause lateral displacement of the cervical spine with potential stretch of the brachial plexus or exacerbation of spinal stenosis. Lateral flexion of the lumbar spine might exacerbate forminal stenosis, back pain, or radiculopathy. Any calf pain, myopathies, or use of statin drugs should be considered whenever the legs are elevated and compressed in leg holders.

Morbid Obesity

Patients who are morbidly obese are at increased risk of sleep apnea, restrictive lung disease, difficult intubation, delayed gastric emptying, difficult vascular access, cardiovascular disease, diabetes mellitus, degenerative joint disease, thromboembolic events, and reduced wound healing. Lastly, they are at increased risk for conversion to open or aborted procedures.

The multiple airway changes due to obesity are the first and foremost concern of the anesthesiologist. They may be difficult to ventilate and intubate. Morbidly obese patients have reduced vital capacity, functional residual capacity, and forced expiratory volume at 1 second, together with increased closing capacity leading to increased shunting. The introduction of anesthesia and steep Trendelenburg positioning negatively impacts the respiratory physiology and, when combined with obesity, profoundly affects their pulmonary physiology. Because of these respiratory issues, they desaturate quickly and are more prone to atelectasis. Pressure control mode of ventilation might be helpful to prevent barotrauma from high peak pressures [14].

Peripheral Neuropathy

All patients undergoing robotic surgery should be evaluated for preexisting neurological abnormalities. Acquired peripheral nerve damage is a well-documented complication after robotic surgery, particularly in patients with increased BMI or severe comorbidities (ASA class IV, including diabetes, vascular diseases, or anatomic anomalies). Of note, positioning and increased operative duration are the major contributing factors for developing postoperative neurologic injuries. A recent study assessing the rate of neurologic complications following robotic-assisted urological surgeries found that 6.6 percent of patients experienced a nerve injury due to improper positioning, and 23 percent of these nerve injuries persisted for longer than 6 months [15].

Anesthesiologists may lessen the incidence of brachial plexus injury, a debilitating neurological complication of robotic procedures, by proper positioning. Lateral flexion and dorsal extension of the head, along with abduction, external rotation, or extension of the arms, should be avoided during robotic cases. Straps placed across the chest secure the patient's position and prevents sliding. This method is preferred. The use of shoulder braces may increase the rate of brachial plexus injury.

Cardiovascular Pathology

Preexisting cardiovascular abnormalities may be exaggerated during robotic surgery. Steep Trendelenburg position increases preload due to facilitated venous return from gravity effects. This position along with pneumoperitoneum can cause concomitant aortic compression and increase in SVR (afterload). Therefore, the overall effects on circulation are reduced cardiac output and increases in myocardial oxygen demand and mean arterial pressure.

Patients with CAD, heart failure, and/or valve dysfunction may have difficulties after positioning. Because of this, preoperative cardiovascular risk should be meticulously assessed. The patient's cardiac symptoms, medications, studies, and exercise tolerance must be identified before surgery. Current American Heart Association/American College of Cardiology (AHA/ACC) guidelines should be followed when determining whether a patient has been optimized for surgery [16]. Beta-blocker medication should be continued perioperatively. Echo or stress testing in high-risk patients helps the anesthesiologist to select optimal drug combinations in the light of SVR and PVR effects of pneumoperitoneum and Trendelenburg position. It is also helpful in evaluating cardiac valvular dysfunction since it may profoundly alter hemodynamics. Furthermore, attention should be paid to patients presenting with anticoagulation therapy. The risks and benefits must be weighed against the possibility of intraoperative stent thrombosis and the challenge of management during robotic surgery [17].

Diabetes

Diabetic patients must get a preoperative blood glucose level before robotic surgery. Intraoperative glucose monitoring might be necessary in insulin-dependent diabetics especially in robotic cases of lengthy duration. These patients are at increased risk for nerve injury, so a preoperative neurological exam documenting preexisting abnormalities is critical.

Cancer

Cancer patients may experience certain unique issues while undergoing robotic surgery. Patients with renal cell carcinoma have a 10–40 percent chance of paraneoplastic syndromes. If a patient has a paraneoplastic syndrome, the tumor may secrete ectopic hormones such as erythropoietin, renin, insulin, or glucose during surgery. Cancer patients previously treated with radiation therapy may experience more difficulties during surgical resection. Fibrosis of tissue from radiation therapy may prolong surgical dissection and ultimately increase surgical bleeding and incidence of other complications.

Chemotherapy can result in a number of systemic complications that affect intraoperative planning. Patients may have significant weight loss, anemia, and a predisposition to clot formation resulting in electrolyte abnormalities, hypothermia risk, decreased protein, malnutrition, and embolism. Anesthetic planning should account for decreased protein binding and volume of distribution for medications; these changes may significantly alter pharmacokinetics. Additionally, a history of exposure to agents such as doxorubicin (cardiomyopathy) and bleomycin (pulmonary fibrosis) necessitates further preoperative testing. At a minimum, preoperative studies for robotic cancer surgery should include electrocardiogram, chest radiograph, and blood work, notably blood counts, coagulation studies, renal function and basic electrolytes, and blood type and screen. Reflux, infection, and deep vein thrombosis prophylaxis should be considered with nonparticulate antacid, antibiotics (within 1 hour of surgical incision), subcutaneous heparin, and sequential compression devices, respectively.

Pregnant Patients

A slightly less steep Trendelenburg position, as opposed to 30° lithotomy position required during urologic procedures, is acceptable for gynecological robotic surgeries [18]. While most concerns are somewhat similar to other robotic procedures, operating on pregnant patients poses additional risks for mother and fetus and deserves further attention. While there are some surgical procedures that must be performed urgently or emergently, regardless of whether or not the patient is pregnant, it is recommended that all elective surgeries should be postponed until after delivery, and all other procedures should be postponed until the second trimester, if possible, as the risk of teratogenicity and miscarriage is lower at this point [19].

The risk of developmental abnormalities is highest in the first trimester, and the risk of spontaneous abortion is highest in the third trimester [20]. It is also advisable to consult the OB/GYN service prior to proceeding to the operating room to discuss the possibility of fetal monitoring, which should be at least considered [19,21]. Laparoscopic surgery, both conventional and robotic-assisted, has been performed safely in pregnant patients. Some advantages to performing procedures laparoscopically, as opposed to open (i.e., laparotomy), include less need for narcotic analgesics, which can affect the fetus as well as the mother, shorter hospital stay, lower risk of thromboembolism, less manipulation of gravid uterus, and fewer wound infections. However, it should also be noted that uterine perforation is a significant risk, particularly while placing the trocar for the surgical port. Labor and preterm birth can also be induced if the uterus is accidentally insufflated, rather than the abdomen. The risk of miscarriage may also be higher than with open procedures.

In addition to anesthetic and surgical management of the mother, there is a second patient to keep in mind as well, and potential effects on the fetus must be considered. To ensure a favorable outcome, one must be diligent to maintain adequate oxygenation and uteroplacental perfusion, as well as avoiding teratogenic medications or medications that may otherwise negatively affect the fetus in the anesthetic plan. Maternal hyperventilation should be avoided as it can decrease venous return, which can lead to decreased uterine blood flow. When treating hypotension, short-acting ephedrine and phenylephrine are agents of choice, whereas other agents such as epinephrine may reduce uterine blood flow [22]. It has been suggested that, with CO_2 insufflation that is used for laparoscopic procedures, fetal acidosis secondary to CO_2 absorption and hypoxia may occur [7,9]. However, while this has been described in sheep models, the same results have not been found in humans [9,23].

The robotic-assisted surgical system provides several advantages over conventional laparoscopic surgery. The operator will be able to utilize superior camera magnification and visualization, as well as more precise movements with the camera and instruments. This could potentially lead to less inadvertent manipulation of gravid uterus, which could potentially decrease risk to the fetus. While there are also disadvantages, such as higher cost and a greater time commitment for training physicians to safely and effectively operate the equipment, robotic surgery does appear to be as safe as conventional laparoscopy, both for the mother and the fetus. However, the number of cases described in the literature is small [24].

Pediatric Patients

With the number of robotic-assisted surgeries growing exponentially, they are gaining more popularity among pediatric surgeons as well, and there has been a recent trend to that effect [25]. Robotic approach has been utilized extensively by pediatric surgeons in a variety of specialties, including general surgery, urology, and thoracic surgery, safely and successfully, and surgeons are performing procedures with a progressively increasing complicity as time passes [26]. However, it still remains somewhat less common as in adult patients, and choosing the best modality is sometimes a subject for debate [27]. As with adult patients, the robot offers potentially greater dexterity, visualization, and ability to operate in difficult spaces, and this may be of even greater benefit in pediatric patients, given their relatively small abdominal cavity [26,28,29]. However, the major challenge lies in the light of inability to change patient's position or even get any access to the patient until the robot is fully detached. As with any laparoscopic surgical technique, there are metabolic, respiratory, and hemodynamic concerns in children with the only difference that children have limited physiologic reserve and timing is usually crucial as delay may result in critical complications. Hemodynamic changes that have been reported secondary to pneumoperitoneum include intraoperative tachycardia and hypertension, with a decrease in cardiac index and aortic blood flow. It has also been demonstrated that, by maintaining intraabdominal pressures at 5 mmHg or below, these effects may be less significant [30].

The alterations to respiratory mechanics with abdominal insufflation may be considerable. Increased intraabdominal pressure, in the similar fashion as in adult patients, may restrict the movement of diaphragm, causing increased airway resistance and a reduction in tidal volume and overall minute ventilation. This can ultimately lead to decreased oxygenation and even hypoxemia. Additionally, pediatric patients may have an increased rate of bronchospasm during pneumoperitoneum secondary to insufflation [31]. Early recognition of the problems intraoperatively by an anesthesiologist along with adequate surgical team training for fast de-docking of the robotic system is required, should the necessity for emergent intervention ensue.

Conclusion

Clearly, the application of robot-assisted technics will continue its integration into the majority of surgical subspecialties, increasing the number of patients requiring this approach, including vulnerable and high-risk patient populations. Anesthesiologists should be alongside with this tendency and be ready to provide better care for patients undergoing robot-assisted surgery. As this modality poses unique risks intraoperatively, a careful patient selection and thorough preoperative assessment should be employed in identifying patients in whom risks of robot-assisted surgical approach may outweigh the benefits of the procedure, or who may require optimization of the medical status prior to the procedure. Common considerations include the following complications: positioning nerve injuries, especially in obese and patients with diabetes or vascular diseases, cardiopulmonary compromise in patients with preexisting heart failure, coronary artery disease, or lung pathology. Patients with decreased functional reserve including pediatric population should be monitored closely as robot needs to be fully detached before any action or repositioning could be implemented. Pregnant patients may safely undergo robot-assisted procedures; however, elective procedure should be postponed at least until second trimester. Finally, good communication and teamwork among the medical staff are essential in providing patient safety and preventing intraoperative complications.

References

1. S. J. Spaner and G. L. Warnock, "A brief history of endoscopy, laparoscopy, and laparoscopic surgery," *J. Laparoendosc. Adv. Surg. Tech. A*, vol. 7, no. 6, pp. 369–73, 1997.
2. W. E. Kelley, "The evolution of laparoscopy and the revolution in surgery in the decade of the 1990s," *JSLS*, vol. 12, no. 4, pp. 351–7, 2008.
3. FDA, "MedSun survey report: da Vinci surgical system," pp. 1–16, 2013.
4. J. R. Lee, "Anesthetic considerations for robotic surgery," *Korean J. Anesthesiol.*, vol. 66, no. 1, pp. 3–11, 2014.
5. E. Singer, "The slow rise of the robot surgeon," *Technol. Rev.*, 2010.
6. L. Tanner, "FDA takes fresh look at robotic surgery," *USA Today*, April 2013.
7. M. J. Curet, D. A. Vogt, O. Schob, C. Qualls, L. A. Izquierdo, and K. A. Zucker, "Effects of CO2 pneumoperitoneum in pregnant ewes," *J. Surg. Res.*, vol. 63, no. 1, pp. 339–44, 1996.
8. S. J. Neuhaus and D. I. Watson, "Pneumoperitoneum and peritoneal surface changes: a review," *Surg. Endosc.*, vol. 18, no. 9, pp. 1316–22, 2004.
9. K. Uemura, R. J. McClaine, S. G. de la Fuente, R. J. Manson, K. A. Campbell, D. J. McClaine, W. D. White, J. S. Stamler, W. S. Eubanks, and J. D. Reynolds, "Maternal insufflation during the second trimester equivalent produces hypercapnia, acidosis, and prolonged hypoxia in fetal sheep," *Anesthesiology*, vol. 101, no. 6, pp. 1332–8, 2004.
10. S. H. Loring, N. Behazin, A. Novero, V. Novack, S. B. Jones, C. R. O'Donnell, and D. S. Talmor, "Respiratory mechanical effects of surgical pneumoperitoneum in humans," *J. Appl. Physiol.*, vol. 117, no. 9, pp. 1074–9, 2014.
11. N. T. Nguyen and B. M. Wolfe, "The physiologic effects of pneumoperitoneum in the morbidly obese," *Ann. Surg.*, vol. 241, no. 2, pp. 219–26, 2005.
12. D. Meininger, C. Byhahn, S. Mierdl, M. Lehnert, K. Heller, B. Zwissler, and D. H. Bremerich, "Hemodynamic and respiratory effects of robot-assisted laparoscopic fundoplication in children," *World J. Surg.*, vol. 29, no. 5, pp. 615–9; discussion 620, 2005.
13. N. C. Buchs, P. Addeo, F. M. Bianco, S. Ayloo, E. F. Elli, and P. C. Giulianotti, "Safety of robotic general surgery in elderly patients," *J. Robot. Surg.*, vol. 4, no. 2, pp. 91–8, 2010.
14. P. Greenland, J. S. Alpert, G. A. Beller, E. J. Benjamin, M. J. Budoff, Z. A. Fayad, E. Foster, M. A. Hlatky, J. M. Hodgson, F. G. Kushner, M. S. Lauer, L. J. Shaw, S. C. Smith, A. J. Taylor, W. S. Weintraub, N. K. Wenger, and A. K. Jacobs, "2010 ACCF/AHA guideline for assessment of cardiovascular risk in asymptomatic adults: executive summary: a report of the American College of Cardiology Foundation/American Heart Association Task Force on Practice Guidelines," *Circulation*, vol. 122, no. 25, pp. 2748–64, 2010.
15. J. T. Mills, M. B. Burris, D. J. Warburton, M. R. Conaway, N. S. Schenkman, and T. L. Krupski, "Positioning injuries associated with robotic assisted urological surgery," *J. Urol.*, vol. 190, no. 2, pp. 580–4, 2013.
16. A. Sharma and A. Berkeley, "Intraoperative drug-eluting stent thrombosis in a patient undergoing robotic prostatectomy," *J. Clin. Anesth.*, vol. 21, no. 7, pp. 517–20, 2009.

17. S. Shenoy, P. Ward, and T. Wigmore, "Surgical management of urological malignancy: anaesthetic and critical care considerations," *Curr. Anaesth. Crit. Care*, vol. 20, no. 1, pp. 22–7, 2009.
18. K. Gupta, Y. Mehta, A. Sarin Jolly, and S. Khanna, "Anaesthesia for robotic gynaecological surgery," *Anaesth. Intensive Care*, vol. 40, no. 4, pp. 614–21, 2012.
19. T. G. Cheek and E. Baird, "Anesthesia for nonobstetric surgery: maternal and fetal considerations," *Clin. Obstet. Gynecol.*, vol. 52, no. 4, pp. 535–45, 2009.
20. S. Y. Park, W. S. Ham, H. J. Jung, W. Jeong, W. T. Kim, and K. H. Rha, "Robot-assisted laparoscopic partial nephrectomy during pregnancy," *J. Robot. Surg.*, vol. 2, no. 3, pp. 193–5, 2008.
21. M. K. Stewart and K. P. Terhune, "Management of pregnant patients undergoing general surgical procedures," *Surg. Clin. North Am.*, vol. 95, no. 2, pp. 429–42, 2015.
22. M. A. Rosen, "Management of anesthesia for the pregnant surgical patient," *J. Am. Soc. Anesthesiol.*, vol. 91, no. 4, p. 1159, 1999.
23. D. C. Shay, K. Bhavani-Shankar, and S. Datta, "Laparoscopic surgery during pregnancy," *Anesthesiol. Clin. North America*, vol. 19, no. 1, pp. 57–67, 2001.
24. S. Carter, S. Depasquale, and S. Stallings, "Robotic-assisted laparoscopic ovarian cystectomy during pregnancy," *AJP Rep.*, vol. 1, no. 1, pp. 21–4, 2011.
25. T. P. Cundy, H. J. Marcus, A. Hughes-Hallett, S. Khurana, and A. Darzi, "Robotic surgery in children: adopt now, await, or dismiss?," *Pediatr. Surg. Int.*, 2015.
26. T. P. Cundy, K. Shetty, J. Clark, T. P. Chang, K. Sriskandarajah, N. E. Gattas, A. Najmaldin, G.-Z. Yang, and A. Darzi, "The first decade of robotic surgery in children," *J. Pediatr. Surg.*, vol. 48, no. 4, pp. 858–65, 2013.
27. N. E. Bruns, O. S. Soldes, and T. A. Ponsky, "Robotic surgery may not make the cut in pediatrics," *Front. Pediatr.*, vol. 3, no. 10, pp. 1–3, 2015.
28. S. H. Song and K. S. Kim, "Current status of robot-assisted laparoscopic surgery in pediatric urology," *Korean J. Urol.*, vol. 55, no. 8, pp. 499–504, 2014.
29. D. B. Camarillo, T. M. Krummel, and J. K. Salisbury, "Robotic technology in surgery: past, present, and future," *Am. J. Surg.*, vol. 188, no. 4, pp. 2–15, 2004.
30. E. E. C. De Waal and C. J. Kalkman, "Haemodynamic changes during low-pressure carbon dioxide pneumoperitoneum in young children," *Paediatr. Anaesth.*, vol. 13, pp. 18–25, 2003.
31. C. F. Bannister, K. K. Brosius, and M. Wulkan, "The effect of insufflation pressure on pulmonary mechanics in infants during laparoscopic surgical procedures," *Paediatr. Anaesth.*, vol. 13, no. 9, pp. 785–9, 2003.

Chapter 6

Anesthetic Considerations for Robotic-Assisted Surgery

Julie A. Gayle, Ryan E. Rubin, Richard D. Urman, and Alan David Kaye

Introduction

Robotic-assisted surgery has gained popularity as demand for minimally invasive surgeries continues to grow. Robotic-assisted surgery offers the patient smaller surgical incisions and minimally invasive instrumentation, as well as less surgical blood loss and presumably less postoperative pain. Shorter recovery room times and hospital stays are also beneficial for most patients.[1,2] Robotic-assisted surgeries offer the surgeon a unique, magnified, three-dimensional view of the operative field with degrees of motion and maneuverability not offered with conventional laparoscopy.[3] Areas of concern for the anesthesiologist specific to robotic-assisted surgery are many and are equally applicable to most types of operations utilizing robotic assistance. These include all phases of the perioperative period from patient selection and screening to intraoperative considerations and postoperative care. Prolonged surgical time with restricted access to the patient, extremes of patient positioning combined with insufflation and the resultant physiologic and hemodynamic disturbances during robotic-assisted surgery present unique anesthetic management challenges for the anesthesiologist. Anticipation, recognition, and prompt management of the more common complications associated with robotic-assisted surgery is a must. Subcutaneous emphysema, venous gas embolism, airway edema, nerve injury, and hypothermia are a few of the complications related to robotic-assisted surgery.

Anesthetic Management

Preoperative Considerations

Careful patient selection and preoperative assessment is crucial to minimizing perioperative complications in patients scheduled to undergo robotic-assisted surgery.[4] A systematic and thorough review of the patient's history and physical, medications, allergies, surgical, and anesthetic history is required prior to robotic-assisted surgery. Risk factors to be considered are patient co-morbidities and the complexity of the surgical case.[5,6] Specific factors that may increase patient's risk associated with prolonged pneumoperitoneum and/or extremes of position need to be elicited. Patients with significant cardiovascular and/or respiratory disease should be considered for alternative surgical methods to robotic-assisted surgery.[2]

Patients with obesity (body mass index [BMI] over 30) may have conditions that warrant serious deliberations prior to undergoing robotic- assisted surgery. Obese patients may come with conditions such as obstructive sleep apnea and restrictive airway disease in addition to difficulties with intubation and vascular access. Decreased gastric emptying and higher risk for aspiration are real areas of concern in the obese patient. Co-morbidities such as cardiac disease and diabetes further complicate matters for the obese patient. Also, risk of conversion to an open procedure is increased for the obese patient. As the BMI approaches or surpasses 40, the above risks become even more of a concern for the anesthesiologist.[1]

Patients with cardiovascular disease require further investigation prior to robotic-assisted surgery. Areas to consider in addition to history and physical examination include exercise tolerance, symptoms, medications and laboratory results, and cardiac studies. Patients with heart failure are likely to experience an exacerbation of their condition during the extremes of position that are required during robotic-assisted surgery.[1] Patients with preexisting cardiac disease should be optimized prior to surgery. In patients with cardiac stents, a careful weighing of the risks and benefits of surgical bleeding with anticoagulation versus discontinuation of the anticoagulation and the associated risk of stent thrombosis should be considered.[1] Patients with moderate to severe mitral insufficiency are subject to worsening of the regurgitant lesions with extreme positioning and insufflation.[7]

Patients with pulmonary disease may not tolerate the physiologic changes associated with the extremes of position during robotic-assisted surgery.[1] History of chronic obstructive pulmonary disease, bullous emphysema, and spontaneous pneumothorax may contraindicate robotic-assisted surgery and warrant further investigation.

Patients with known intracranial lesions, increased intracranial pressure, and intraocular pressure (IOP) are at risk for exacerbation of their underlying condition with positioning during robotic-assisted surgery.[1] History of cerebrovascular accident, presence of cerebral aneurysm, elevated intracranial pressure, or glaucoma require further investigation prior to robotic-assisted surgery. Patients with preexisting ocular problems are at risk for retinal detachment and periorbital edema and development of dangerous ocular pressures due to the prolonged extremes of position associated with robotic-assisted surgery.[1]

Patients with a history of cancer and radiation therapy are at higher risk for difficult surgical resection due to fibrosis and increased bleeding. History of chemotherapy may present with weight loss and anemia and a predisposition to hypothermia and clot formation. Other considerations in patients with cancer history and chemotherapy include electrolyte abnormalities, malnutrition, and risk of embolism. Certain chemotherapy agents such as doxorubicin and bleomycin put the patient at risk for cardiomyopathy and pulmonary fibrosis, respectively. History of exposure to chemotherapy agents warrants further investigation prior to robotic-assisted surgery.[1]

Patients with renal insufficiency require optimization prior to robotic-assisted surgery. Positioning, fluid restriction, and mechanical obstruction put patients with renal dysfunction at high risk for exacerbation of their underlying condition. Risks and benefits of robotic-assisted surgery in patients with renal insufficiency deserve careful consideration prior to proceeding to the operating room.[1] Renal protective strategies, such as avoidance of nephrotoxic drugs and renal hypoperfusion, should be employed.

Intraoperative Considerations

Spatial limitations, intraoperative monitoring, and intravenous access as well as prolonged length of surgery require special consideration in preparation for robotic-assisted surgery. The physical space required for the robotic equipment and the orientation of this bulky equipment in the operating room may compromise movement of personnel and visualization of placement sites of intravenous lines, monitors, and the endotracheal tube.[1] Standard ASA monitors are indicated as well as additional monitoring and intravenous lines depending on the patient's comorbidities, complexity of surgery, risks of bleeding, and the surgeon's level of experience with robotic-assisted surgery. It is important to reliably secure the endotracheal tube and all monitors and intravenous lines as visual inspection may be unavailable once the robot is locked into place. Furthermore, intravenous lines should have sufficient length to provide access far from the insertion site.

Standard intravenous induction of anesthesia and intubation is acceptable with adjustments as needed for a patient's medical condition. As indicated above, the endotracheal tube should be secured properly keeping in mind limitations of access once surgery is underway and the risk of tube migration with extremes of patient positioning. In addition, robotic equipment presents a risk of accidental dislodgement of the endotracheal tube, making meticulous attention to securing the tube even more important. Mechanical ventilation to manage hypercarbia and muscle relaxation to prevent patient movement is utilized throughout robotic-assisted surgery. It is imperative the patient remain immobile throughout the procedure until the robot is undocked.[1] Securing the eyelids closed with a film dressing and ointment helps protect the patient from corneal injury and desiccation. Gastric decompression helps to reduce the risk of facial and ocular burns from passive regurgitation of stomach contents. Since the surgery is typically prolonged, use of a volatile agent such as Desflurane with a shorter half-life should be considered. An adjunct opioid, such as a remifentanil infusion, provides a balanced anesthetic technique and is well tolerated during robotic-assisted surgery.

Patients are at risk for nerve injury from stretching and compression. Meticulous attention to patient positioning, padding, and protection from movement is required due to positioning needs to optimize surgical views. Ventilation is complicated by decreased compliance and changes in lung volumes due to extremes of patient position used in robotic-assisted surgery. Further discussion of physiologic and hemodynamic perturbations encountered during robotic-assisted surgery is covered later in this chapter. Fluid management is important to minimize facial and airway edema. Temperature monitoring and management are required to avoid hypothermia.

Emergence from anesthesia should be timed correctly. It is recommended to maintain anesthetic levels and muscle relaxation until the robot is undocked. Reversal of neuromuscular blockade, emergence from anesthesia, and extubation can then proceed as appropriate. Special attention should be paid to the possibility of residual hypercarbia and delayed emergence, atelectasis, and airway edema.

Surgical injury and occult blood loss are a concern and should be anticipated. In addition, robotic malfunction and/or failure have occurred. Use of checklists is recommended to prevent equipment malfunction.[1]

Box 6.1 Major Concerns for the Anesthesiologist during Robotic-Assisted Surgery

Limitation of access
Length of surgical case
Inexperience of surgeon, surgical assistants, and/or team
Extremes of patient positioning
Cardiopulmonary effects of extremes of position and pneumoperitoneum
Fluid management
Temperature control
Occult surgical injury
Occult blood loss

Postoperative Considerations

Being cognizant of the possible need for postoperative reintubation and providing adequate pain control are priorities in the postoperative period.[1] Standard monitoring techniques following general anesthesia apply. Following robotic-assisted surgery, specific considerations include management of pain, evaluation and management of cardiopulmonary complications, and treatment of hypothermia and oliguria. Mental status should return to baseline prior to discharging to the next phase of care. Furthermore, a preliminary evaluation for nerve injury should be performed. Occult injury and/or blood loss should be suspected if patients complain of significant postsurgical pain unrelieved with typical pain medications or if vital signs suggest hemodynamic decompensation.

Specific Anesthetic Considerations Associated with Robotic-Assisted Surgery

Robotic-assisted surgery offers a means to provide minimally invasive surgical intervention by way of robotic technology. Robotic-assisted surgery allows the surgeon to maneuver in small, enclosed spaces with precision accuracy. The surgeon operates from a distance with three extra degrees of motion that are lost during conventional laparoscopy. The surgeon has a three-dimensional stereoscopic view of the operative field with adjustable magnification and a controlled camera platform.[3] Surgical specialties such as urology, gynecology, cardiac and thoracic, abdominal, and head and neck surgery all have procedures that utilize robotic-assisted surgery. Reduced pain, shorter hospital stay, and smaller surgical incision sites are potential advantages associated with robotic-assisted surgery.[2] Potential disadvantages include extremes of patient positioning, perturbations in normal physiology, limitation of access, longer surgical times, and inexperience of the surgical team.

Restricted Access to the Patient

During robotic-assisted surgery, access to the patient is limited. Once the robot has been docked, the patients' position cannot be easily or quickly modified. The robotic arms and platform are locked in a fixed position.[8] Overall arrangement of the operative equipment and personnel during robotic-assisted surgery conflicts with the conservative basis of anesthesia care. Spatial restrictions due to bulky equipment requiring excessive space are another key consideration. Once the robot is docked, the anesthesiologist cannot readily access the patient. All lines, monitors, and patient positioning and protective devices must be functional and secured. If changes to the above are necessary, the robot must be detached first, which may result in related delays and complications. Early detection of any problems and/or complications is imperative since robotic detachment takes time. Emergency situations require advanced training of the entire surgical and anesthesia team to ensure quick detachment of the robotic system.[8] Certain robotic-assisted surgeries require the patient head, and airway, be situated away from the anesthesiologist. Upper abdominal, thoracic, and head and neck robotic-assisted surgeries require the patients' head be situated away from the anesthesia workstation.[8,9] Mediastinal procedures require the operating table to be rotated 90 degrees away from the anesthesiologist. During these types of surgeries, access to the airway is almost impossible and field avoidance methods must be implemented.[9]

Patient Positioning

Patient positioning is of critical importance in robotic-assisted surgery. Patient outcomes and surgical conditions rely on proper patient positioning and port placement. The crucial nature of proper positioning stems from the reality that once surgery begins, the patient cannot be moved to any other position throughout the robot portion of the procedure. Once the robotic trocars and instruments are fixed, movement of the patient in any way could be catastrophic. To avoid having to repeat the positioning process multiple times, it is recommended to standardize the positioning process. Intraoperative patient movement not related to positioning must be prevented by the use of muscle relaxants.[10]

Steep Trendelenburg

Robotic-assisted surgeries of the lower abdomen and pelvis require extremes of position for optimal surgical exposure. Proper patient positioning on the surgery table is necessary to allow for optimal surgical exposure and to prevent neuromuscular injury.[11] In the extreme head down position, cardiac, pulmonary, and nervous systems are affected. Steep Trendelenburg between 30 and 45 degrees for prolonged periods of time can lead to significant physiologic perturbations. Consequences of steep Trendelenburg include cephalad displacement of the diaphragm, decreased pulmonary compliance, decreased functional residual capacity (FRC), worsening of ventilation/perfusion mismatch, and pulmonary edema.[10] Trendelenburg position is associated with a 30–40 percent reduction of cardiac output and elevation of pulmonary capillary wedge pressure. Patients with compromised systolic function are at risk for development of heart failure with steep Trendelenburg. Patients with coronary artery disease may develop demand ischemia due to the hemodynamic changes associated with positioning for robotic-assisted surgery. Creation of pneumoperitoneum – air within the peritoneal cavity – exacerbates the conditions described above. Furthermore, steep Trendelenburg leads to increases in cerebral blood flow and intracranial pressure as well as decreased venous outflow.[1] Steep Trendelenburg for prolonged periods of time can result in laryngeal edema, cerebral edema, and facial swelling.[11,12] Trendelenburg position can also lead to endobronchial intubation due to the cephalad displacement of the trachea and resultant atelectasis if uncorrected.[12]

Protecting the patient from injury requires meticulous attention to positioning. Stretching and compression along with improper padding and positioning can result in nerve injury. Common nerve injuries encountered after robotic-assisted surgery include injuries to the brachial plexus, ulnar, and lateral femoral cutaneous nerves. For robotic-assisted surgery in which the patient is in steep Trendelenburg with lithotomy, arms and hands should be padded well and tucked in the neutral position at the patient's side.[1] Degree of limb extension, stirrup location, and duration of immobility and padding of bony prominences require particular consideration. Careful attention to the function of monitors and intravenous lines is important during positioning because once the robotic part of surgery is underway, manipulation is impossible. Methods to prevent patient shifting include braces, leg suspension, iliac supports, and antiskid material. Unfortunately, any of these methods can result in nerve injury.[10] To prevent upward sliding, padding with egg crate or a beanbag in the form of an "X" binds the patient's chest. Shoulder braces should be used with caution to prevent brachial plexus nerve injury during prolonged head down positioning.[1] Patient sliding risks stretching and tearing of incisions as well as risk of incisional hernia. Movement or shifting of the trunk may lead to improper positioning of the extremities, which increases the risk of nerve injury from stretching and compression. Other complications include acute compartment syndrome and rhabdomyolysis from prolonged lithotomy positioning, hypothermia, unrecognized surgical injury, and occult blood loss.[10] The lower extremities are at risk for hypoperfusion in steep Trendelenburg and may result in postoperative rhabdomyolysis. Overlying tight table straps and improperly positioned leg holder straps add to the risk of rhabdomyolysis. Risk factors for developing compression injury and subsequent rhabdomyolysis include extreme patient positions, morbid obesity, hypertension, diabetes, and peripheral vascular disease.[11]

Steep Trendelenburg causes IOP to rise to levels similar to that of untreated glaucoma.[13] Rising IOP in addition to increased end-tidal CO_2 levels may make robotic-assisted surgery unsuitable for patients with glaucoma. Prolonged steep Trendelenburg, as used with robotic-assisted surgery, can result in posterior ischemic optic neuropathy. Increases in central venous pressure, intracranial pressure, and IOP associated with steep Trendelenburg over prolonged periods put the patient at risk for permanent blindness.[14]

Laryngeal edema as a result of steep Trendelenburg for prolonged periods is a major concern. Edema of the supraglottic airway structures, including the vocal cords, arytenoids, and epiglottis, may result in stridorous or no respirations after the endotracheal tube is removed. The need for emergent reintubation and swollen airway structures makes for a dangerous combination. Therefore, it is recommended to ensure the patient can breathe around the endotracheal tube with the cuff deflated prior to extubation.[9,13]

Pneumoperitoneum

The presence of air or gas within the peritoneal cavity is known as pneumoperitoneum. CO_2 is the gas most commonly used to create pneumoperitoneum. Other gases such as oxygen, helium, argon, and nitrous oxide are problematic due to their combustible nature and/or the possibility of intravascular embolism on insufflation.[10] For pelvic and lower abdominal robotic-assisted surgery, intraperitoneal insufflation with CO_2 is performed with the patient in the Trendelenburg position. After the trocars are inserted, intraabdominal pressures are increased to 20 mmHg with CO_2 insufflation, then reduced to 12–15 mmHg after the ports are positioned.[1] Changes in respiratory mechanics and hemodynamics resulting from pneumoperitoneum present a special challenge for the anesthesia provider.

One of the main concerns during pneumoperitoneum is proper ventilation. Effects on respiratory mechanics are significant and include decreases in lung compliance, mean pulmonary arterial pressure, and pulmonary capillary wedge pressure. Increases in end-tidal CO_2 tension, peak inspiratory, and plateau pressures occur with pneumoperitoneum. Decreases in total lung capacity (TLC) and FRC create various ventilation problems. Areas of the lung in which there is perfusion but no ventilation result in decreases in both oxygenation and CO_2 exchange. Increased closing capacity and decreased FRC lead to atelectasis.[13] To compensate for high pressures and hypercapnia, titration of respiratory rate to alter minute ventilation is preferred. It is desirable to maintain lower tidal volumes to improve surgical view.[1] Because shunting and hypoxia often occurs, it is important to attempt to improve gas exchange. Careful implementation of peak end-expiratory pressures (PEEP) should be considered as long as peak pressures remain below safe limits.[1] PEEP helps to decrease atelectasis and improve lung mechanics and oxygenation. PEEP also hinders venous blood return from the lower extremities and decreases cardiac output. However, extreme Trendelenburg mitigates these effects. PEEP also contributes to the risk of development of facial, laryngeal, and oropharyngeal edema.[8] Risk of barotrauma and pneumothorax makes adequate ventilation of the patient a challenge. It may be difficult to control the level of CO_2 in the blood ($PaCO_2$) due to increases in ventilation to perfusion mismatch, decreased lung volumes, and restrictions on tidal volumes in the presence of high peak airway pressures. Respiratory acidosis results in a host of hemodynamic changes. These include sympathetic nervous system stimulation, myocardial depression, increases in cerebral blood flow, and intracranial pressure.[13] Exogenous CO_2 in addition to the patients' own CO_2 production may pose a problem in the postoperative period for patient with certain co-morbidities. Patients with chronic obstructive pulmonary disease (COPD) are unable to eliminate excessive CO_2 and may require prolonged postoperative mechanical ventilation due to respiratory hypercarbia and acidosis.[10]

Pneumoperitoneum results in hemodynamic changes as a result of increased intraabdominal pressure. These changes include increased systemic vascular resistance (SVR), increased mean arterial pressures (MAP), increased filling pressures, and a 50 percent decrease in cardiac index (CI). Increase in heart rate can also occur. After about 10 minutes, SVR and CI normalize. Pneumoperitoneum in addition to steep Trendelenburg can decrease cardiac output by 10–30 percent.[1] Increases in intraabdominal pressure activates the renin-angiotensin system, which results in increased SVR and increased blood pressure. Decreased urine output aids in increasing intravascular volume. Pneumoperitoneum causes decreased splanchnic blood flow, which also augments increases in intravascular volume and blood pressure. However, intraabdominal pressures over 15 mmHg results in the compression of inferior vena cava and decreases in MAP by way of decreased venous return, preload, and cardiac output.[13] Blood flow to intraabdominal organs such as liver, kidneys, and intestines is decreased due to decrease in flow to portal and systemic circulation as a result of pneumoperitoneum.[1]

Risk of venous gas embolism is present immediately upon insufflation. Gas emboli risk is minimized by the use of CO_2, which has a high diffusion coefficient. While rare, the consequences of venous gas embolism are catastrophic and include severe cardiovascular failure, reduction in pulmonary blood flow, and death. The mechanism of venous gas embolism upon insufflation is thought to be infiltration of insufflated CO_2 into the venous/lymphatic channels. Clinical manifestations are a sudden increase, then a rapid fall in end-tidal CO_2 level, hypotension, tachycardia, localized diminished breath sounds, cyanosis, and a "mill-wheel" murmur associated with gas embolization. Should venous gas embolism occur, treatment involves rapid deflation of pneumoperitoneum, hyperventilation with 100 percent oxygen, left lateral decubitus and Trendelenburg, cardiopulmonary resuscitation followed by attempted aspiration of the embolism through a multiport central venous catheter in the right atrium.[1,10] Other potential complications include cardiac arrhythmias and vagal reactions as a result of insufflation and peritoneal distension or viscus manipulation. Asystole cardiac arrest can result from vena cava compression and subsequent diminished cardiac preload. Cardiac arrhythmias may result from hypercapnia or hypoxia.

Pneumoperitoneum, in addition to steep Trendelenburg, presents even more of a challenge to the anesthesiologist, more so than each individual maneuver. The risks to the patient undergoing robotic-assisted surgery involved with positioning and hemodynamic perturbations as discussed above are magnified when insufflation and steep Trendelenburg (25–40 degrees) are combined. Significant hypercapnia (ET-CO_2 >45 mmHg) and significant intraoperative hypoxemia (SpO_2 <90 percent) can occur.[13] Atelectasis and ventilation/perfusion mismatch is exacerbated by steep Trendelenburg with pneumoperitoneum. Decreased pulmonary compliance, decreased FRC, and increases in peak airway pressures are more pronounced with insufflation in the steep Trendelenburg position. Subcutaneous emphysema occurs frequently in the steep Trendelenburg position, resulting in significant amounts of CO_2 absorption.[8,10] An increase in end-tidal CO_2 levels larger than 25 percent or if occurring 30 minutes after insufflation suggests the development subcutaneous emphysema.[15] Hyperventilation to decrease the levels of CO_2 in blood and resultant respiratory acidosis is limited due to the steep Trendelenburg position and higher ventilator inspiratory pressures during robotic-assisted surgery. In addition, diaphragmatic excursion is limited by abdominal CO_2 insufflation. Therefore, increased airway pressures are primarily a result of decreased thoracic compliance due to the pressure of the abdominal contents on diaphragm and the pressure exerted with abdominal insufflation. Elevated peak and plateau inspiratory pressures are measured at the mouthpiece and do not reflect the pressure in the alveoli nor the transmural pressure across the alveoli.[15] Although there is no proven superior form of ventilation in the setting of increased airway pressures, recommendations involve the use of pressure-controlled ventilation. Lower peak airway and plateau pressures with higher lung compliance and larger tidal volumes for a given inspired pressure have been reported using pressure-controlled ventilation in patients undergoing robotic-assisted surgery and in whom adequate oxygenation if difficult to achieve.[10,16] In patients with high end-tidal CO_2 even with optimization of ventilator settings, permissive hypercapnia can be safely tolerated.[8]

Pneumoperitoneum combined with steep Trendelenburg (45 degrees) result in marked increases in MAP, right and left ventricular filling pressures, and pulmonary capillary wedge pressure (PCWP) in both healthy patients and patients with cardiac disease. Although pneumoperitoneum combined with steep Trendelenburg results in two- to three-fold increases in filling pressures, cardiac performance seems to be unaffected in ASA I and II patients.[17] Further studies are needed to establish perioperative risk for patients with existing cardiac disease.[17]

Increased intracranial pressure is made worse by steep Trendelenburg during insufflation. The proposed mechanism is increased intraabdominal and intrathoracic pressure of the Trendelenburg position, in addition to impaired cerebral fluid absorption from insufflation inhibits lumbar venous plexus drainage. Impaired venous plexus drainage induces an increase in intracranial pressure.[15] Furthermore; hypercarbia causes dilation of cerebral vessels, which also increases intracranial pressure. Despite increases of hydrostatic pressure in the cerebral vessels, an intact blood–brain barrier helps prevent interstitial edema in the central nervous system. Therefore, patients with conditions that might disrupt the blood–brain barrier (e.g., brain tumor) placed in steep Trendelenburg with insufflation carry unknown risk.[18]

Box 6.2 Physiologic Effects of Steep Trendelenburg Combined with Pneumoperitoneum[2,17]

Cardiovascular
- Increased systemic vascular resistance, mean arterial pressure, central venous pressure, pulmonary capillary wedge pressure, myocardial O_2 consumption
- Decreased renal perfusion, splanchnic perfusion, portal blood flow

Respiratory
- Increased ventilation/perfusion mismatch, peak airway pressure
- Decreased functional residual capacity, vital capacity, pulmonary compliance
- Hypercarbia
- Pulmonary edema
- Respiratory acidosis

Central nervous system
- Increased intracranial pressure, intraocular pressure, cerebral blood flow

Gastrointestinal
- Increased intragastric pressure

Endocrine
- Increased catecholamine release, renin–angiotensin activity

Steep Trendelenburg with increases in intraabdominal pressure from insufflation causes increased intragastric pressure. Risk of pulmonary aspiration is increased. Risk of passive regurgitation of gastric fluids may result in injury to the eyes. The risk of passive aspiration and eye injury is lessened with gastric decompression by an orogastric tube.[13] Conjunctival edema and corneal abrasions are other potential complications. Conjunctival edema causes the upper and lower eyelids to separate and can result in corneal desiccation and abrasion even when the eyes are taped closed.[19] The use of ophthalmic ointment acts as a shield protecting the cornea and should be considered for use during robotic-assisted surgery in addition to securing the lids.[13] In addition, a preoperative dose of ranitidine may reduce the risk of gastric reflux and should be considered for all patients.

Fluid Management

Excessive fluid administration during robotic-assisted surgery is known to be associated with facial edema and swelling of the airway and conjunctiva. Whether or not colloids carry an advantage over crystalloids remains speculative.[15] Due to the fact that edema of the face and airway is known to develop over time in the steep Trendelenburg position, it is recommended to avoid overzealous administration of fluids. It has also been suggested that a standardized, more restrictive fluid management is beneficial for patients undergoing certain types of robotic-assisted surgery.[9,20] Because increased intraabdominal pressure such as that which occurs with insufflation leads to oliguria, urinary output is a poor indication of volume status during robotic-assisted surgery.

Hypothermia

Development of hypothermia during robotic-assisted surgery is multifactorial. Typical operating room conditions coupled with altered thermoregulatory mechanisms while under anesthesia promote heat loss. Long surgical time, CO_2 insufflation, and exposure exacerbate heat loss. Therefore, active warming techniques are of great importance. These include temperature monitoring, warm intravenous fluids, warm humidified gases, air warming device, and operating room temperature control.[21]

Pain Management

Multimodal approaches to pain management have been shown to decrease length of hospital stay and improve patient satisfaction.[22] Use of acetaminophen and nonsteroidal anti-inflammatory drugs, if no contraindication exists, are recommended. As needed, opioids are acceptable if indicated. Epidural analgesia is not typically needed for robotic-assisted surgical pain.[1] Epidural analgesia is said to have no advantage for postoperative pain control following robot-assisted surgery. Epidural anesthesia should not be used intraoperatively since the steep Trendelenburg position can cause a high block and cardiovascular instability.[2]

The Learning Curve

While robotic-assisted surgeries have a number of technical advantages, such as favorable field of view and minimally invasive instrumentation, variable learning curves and associated risks are discussed in the literature. As surgeons pursue lengthier and more complex robotic-assisted cases, the morbidity risk to the patient becomes greater.[5,23] In the initial phase of practice, extended surgical time required for the surgical team to use the robot is known as the "learning curve."[1] Ongoing training in robotic-assisted surgery for surgical support staff should mirror the complexity of the surgery being performed.[24] The number of cases required for surgical proficiency remains unclear. Most agree that the number of cases to become proficient depends on surgical skill and type of procedure performed.[25]

Communication among Team Members

Communication among all team members, including the surgeon, anesthesiologist, nurses, and operative assistants, is imperative to establish and maintain safe and effective environment. Ensuring quality of communication is an active process in robotic-assisted surgery. Because the surgeon sits behind a console away from the operative field, communication with the operative assistant and the anesthesia provider presents a challenge. In order to facilitate transmission of the surgeons' voice, audio speakers are added to the video tower.[2] Simulation environments, continuous training, and emergency drills offer opportunities to improve communication among team members and outcomes and prevent complications.[26]

Box 6.3 Complications Associated with Robotic-Assisted Surgery

Pneumoperitoneum: subcutaneous emphysema, venous gas embolism, pneumothorax, capnothorax, pneumomediastinum, endotracheal tube displacement, intraabdominal fire

Steep Trendelenburg: patient slippage, facial trauma, corneal abrasion, facial edema, laryngeal edema, rhabdomyolysis

Neurologic: cerebral hemorrhage, posterior ischemic optic neuropathy, paradoxical cerebral air embolism

Neuromuscular: peripheral nerve injury (i.e., median, radial, ulnar, brachial plexus, sciatic, obturator, peroneal, lateral femoral cutaneous), compartment syndrome

Cardiovascular: arrhythmias, congestive heart failure, myocardial infarction, refractory hypertension

Pulmonary: barotrauma, pulmonary edema, atelectasis, pneumothorax, elevated central venous pressure, respiratory acidosis

Gastrointestinal: passive regurgitation/aspiration, burns to face/eyes

Renal: rhabdomyolysis, renal dysfunction/failure

Development of a perioperative protocol for all phases of anesthetic management is recommended for patients undergoing robotic-assisted surgery to help ensure patient safety and satisfaction as well as optimal clinical care and provider satisfaction.[27]

Conclusion

Robotic-assisted surgery presents unique anesthetic challenges for the anesthesiologist. Despite the risks inherent to prolonged extremes of position coupled with insufflation and associated perturbations of normal physiology, robotic-assisted surgery has been successfully performed in a large number of patients. Anticipation and recognition of risks and complications unique to robotic-assisted surgery by the anesthesiologist is essential to successful perioperative management. Common complications include subcutaneous emphysema, venous gas embolism, hypothermia, facial and airway edema, cardiopulmonary compromise, and nerve injury, to name a few. Vigilance on the part of the anesthesiologist lessens the potential for these complications. Furthermore, efficient communication and teamwork between the anesthesiologist and the surgical team also minimizes development of complications, preserves patient safety, and improves surgical conditions and patient outcomes.

References

1. Berger JS, Alshaer T, Lukula D, Dangerfield R. Anesthetic Considerations for Robot-Assisted Gynecologic and Urology Surgery. *J Anesth Clinic Res.* 2013;4(8): 1–7.
2. Irvine M, Patil V. Anaesthesia for Robot-Assisted Laparoscopic Surgery. *Cont Edu Anaesth Crit Care and Pain.* 2009;9(4): 125–129.
3. Lee JR. Anesthetic Considerations for Robotic Surgery. *Korean J Anesthesiol.* 2014;66(1): 3–11.
4. Massachusetts Board of Registration in Medicine, Quality and Patient Safety Division. Preoperative Assessment and Coordination of Care, 2013. Available at www.mass.gov/eohhs/docs/borim/physicians/pca-notifications/coordination-care.pdf.
5. Buchs NC, Addeo P, Bianco FM, Gorodner V, Ayloo SM, Elli EF, Oberholzer J, Benedetti E, Giulianotti PC. Perioperative Risk Assessment in Robotic General Surgery: Lessons Learned from 884 Cases at a Single Institution. *Arch Surg.* 2012;147(8): 701–708.
6. SAGES-MIRA Robotic Surgery Consensus Group. A Consensus Document on Robotic Surgery, Position

Papers/Statements, 2007. Available at www.sages.org/publication/id/ROBOT/.

7. Haas S, Haese A, Goetz AE, Kubitz JC. Haemodynamics and Cardiac Function during Robot-Assisted Laparoscopic Prostatectomy in Steep Trendelenburg Position. *Int J Med Robot.* 2011;7(4): 408–413.

8. Badawy M, Beique F, Al-Halal H, Azar T, Akkour K, Lau SK, Gotlieb WH. Anesthesia Considerations for Robotic Surgery in Gynecologic Oncology. *J Robotic Surg.* 2011;5(4): 265–269.

9. Sullivan MJ, Frost EAM, Lew MW. Anesthetic Care of the Patient for Robotic Surgery. *ME J Anesth.* 2008;19(5): 967–982.

10. Kaye AD, Vadivelu N, Ahuja N, Mitra S, Silasi D, Urman RD. Anesthetic Considerations in Robotic-Assisted Gynecologic Surgery. *Ochsner J.* 2013;13(4): 517–524.

11. Ghomi A. Robotics in Practice: New Angles on Safer Positioning. *Contemporary OB/GYN.* 2012;57(10): 26.

12. Chang CH, Lee HK, Nam SH. The Displacement of the Tracheal Tube during Robot-Assisted Radical Prostatectomy. *Eur J Anaesthesiol.* 2010;27(5): 478–480.

13. McLarney JT, Rose GL. Anesthetic Implications of Robotic Gynecologic Surgery. *J Gynec Endosc Surg.* 2011;2: 75–78.

14. Weber ED, Colyer MH, Lesser RL, Subramanian PS. Posterior Ischemic Optic Neuropathy after Minimally Invasive Prostatectomy. *J Neuroophthalmol.* 2007;27: 285–287.

15. Kalmar AF, DeWolf AM. Hendrickx JFA. Anesthetic Considerations for Robotic Surgery in the Steep Trendelenburg Position. *Advances in Anesthesia.* 2012;30: 75–96.

16. Oksar M, Akbulut Z, Ocal H, Balbay MD, Kanbak O. Anesthetic Considerations for Robotic Cystectomy: A Prospective Study. *Rev Bras Anestesiol.* 2014;64(2): 109–115.

17. Lestar M, Gunnarsson L, Lagerstrand L, Wiklund P, Odeberg-Wernerman S. Hemodynamic Perturbations during Robot-Assisted Laparoscopic Radical Prostatectomy in 45 Degrees Trendelenburg Position. *Anesth Analg.* 2011;113(5): 1069–1075.

18. Pandey R, Garg R, Darlong V, Punj J, Chandralekha, KA. Unpredicted Neurological Complications after Robotic Laparoscopic Radical Cystectomy and Ileal Conduit Formation in Steep Trendelenburg Position: Two Case Reports. *Acta Anaesthesiol Belg.* 2010;61(3): 163–166.

19. Kim K, Kim HJ, No JH, Kim TW, Kim YB, Suh CS. Increased Risk for Post-Operative Corneal Injuries in Patients Who Undergo Laparoscopic Gynecologic Surgery. *Acta Anaesthesiol Scand.* 2012;56: 504–506.

20. Piegeler T, Dreessen P, Graber SM, Haile SR, Schmid DM, Beck-Schimmer B. Impact of Intraoperative Fluid Administration on Outcome in Patients Undergoing Robotic-Assisted Laparoscopic Prostatectomy—A Retrospective Analysis. *BMC Anesthesiology.* 2014;14: 61.

21. Diaz M, Becker D. Theromoregulation: Physiological and Clinical Considerations during Sedation and General Anesthesia. *Anesth Prog.* 2010;57: 25–33.

22. Elvir-Lazo OL, White PF. The Role of Multimodal Analgesia in Pain Management after Ambulatory Surgery. *Curr Opin Anaestheiol.* 2010;23(6): 697–703.

23. Zorn KC, Gautam G, Shalhav AL, et al. Training, Credentialing, Proctoring and Medicolegal Risks of Robotic Urologic Surgery: Recommendations of the Society of Urologic Robotic Surgeons. *J Urol.* 2009;182(3): 1126–1132.

24. Advisory on Robot-Assisted Surgery. Commonwealth of Massachusetts Board of Registration in Medicine. Quality and Patient Safety Division. March 2013. Available at www.mass.gov/eohhs/docs/borim/physicians/pca-notifications/robot-assisted-surgery.pdf

25. AAGL Position Statement: Robotic-Assisted Laparoscopic Surgery in Benign Gynecology. *J Minimally Invasive Gynecol.* 2012. Available at www.jmig.org.

26. Sharmim KM, Ahmed K, Gavazzi A, Gohil R, Thomas L, Poulsen J, Ahmed M, Jaye P, Dasgupta P. Development and Implementation of Centralized Simulation Training: Evaluation of Feasibility, Acceptability and Construct Validity. *BJU International.* 2013;111(3): 518–523.

27. Prabhakar A, Donnenfeld BL, Kaye AD, Felmate CM, Urman RD. Concepts in Creating Evidence-Based Anesthetic Protocol for Robotic-Assisted Laparoscopic Pelvic Surgery. *J Med Pract Manage.* 2015;30(6): 18–23.

Chapter 7

General and Colorectal Robotic Surgery of the Abdomen and Pelvis

Guy R. Orangio, Jeffrey S. Barton, and Kurt G. Davis

Introduction

This chapter will discuss the application of the robotic surgical platforms (RSPs) utilized today by general surgery (GS) and colon and rectal surgery (CRS) on abdominal and pelvic procedures. The chapter is divided into preoperative, intraoperative, and postoperative management of patients undergoing RSP procedures. The preoperative section will discuss preoperative considerations of patients with comorbidities that could be exacerbated by the positioning and the effect of pneumoperitoneum on cardiovascular, pulmonary, and cerebral systems

The intraoperative section will focus on the RSP application in hepatobiliary, pancreatic, esophageal, gastric, splenic, and colorectal diseases. The chapter will discuss RSP application in benign and malignant disease from the historical perspective to current-day procedures. It will discuss safety and feasibility and economic considerations of the application of the RSP to complex abdominal procedures.

The postoperative section will discuss the advantages of the RSP and the utilization of enhanced recovery after surgery (ERAS) protocols, including early ambulation, postoperative pain management, onset of dietary intake, and the goal of decreasing length of stay (LOS) and decreasing hospital readmission rates.

Historical Perspectives

The first application of the robot in surgery was in 1988, for CT-guided brain biopsy [1]. Since then, the field of robotic engineering for medical use has been evolving at a rapid pace. This development was in part due to the rapid utilization of minimally invasive procedures in GS and CRS. The developers of robotic engineering were aware of the limitations of minimally invasive surgical instrumentation, loss of tactile sensation, only four degrees of freedom movement, amplification of physiologic tremors of the surgeon, difficulty with suturing, and camera fatigue. Although the application of minimally invasive surgery is accepted and tremendous technological advances have been made, there are still technical and ergonomic limitations of the standard minimally invasive equipment.

As far back as the early 1980s and 1990s, there was a belief in the potential of the clinical application of robotic surgery in abdominal and pelvic surgery.

There were significant developments for the robotically assisted laparoscopic surgery era; for example, the Automated Endoscopic System for Optimal Positioning (AESOP) and the ZEUS Robotic Systems (telemanipulator system) from the American Company Computer Motion (Goleta, CA) both began to utilize robotic arms for stability and integration into imaging technology [2,3].

During this era, the da Vinci Robotic Surgical System from Intuitive Surgical (Sunnyvale, CA) was forging ahead with engineering milestones, offering surgeons seven degrees of freedom with a robotic arm that replicated the human wrist. The concept of "telerobotic" surgery was first developed with grants from the US Department of Defense. The Department of Defense hoped to develop a robotic surgical system to permit combat surgeons to operate from a remote location on wounded soldiers on the battlefield. This system represented the transition from "laparoscopic instrumentations," with lack of articulation, inadequate precision, and nonintuitive motion, to a robotic platform that electronically controls an articulating tip of an instrument, which improved range of motion and dexterity. For the Intuitive Surgical Company, a series of licensing agreements gave them rights to patents that allowed them to develop a robotic system that is software-driven, which provides intuitive control of seven-degrees-of freedom laparoscopic instruments, stereoscopic vision system, and an architecture composed of redundant sensors to provide maximum safety during operation [4]. The Intuitive Surgical Company has continued to redesign and engineer the most sophisticated user-friendly and patient-safe robotic platform systems, which has revolutionized its application in the clinical setting to date.

Robotic Abdominal Surgery Platforms

The evolution from standard laparoscopic abdominal surgery to Laparoendoscopic Single-Site Surgery (LESS)/ Single-Incision Laparoscopic Surgery (SILS), and the affect that this technology has had on the robotic platforms and the development of the Robotic Laparoendoscopic Single-Site Surgery (R-LESS)/ Robotic Single-Site (RSS) platforms (RSSPs), has advanced minimally invasive surgery over a very short time. The development of LESS has reduced the number and size of incisions, which decreases postoperative pain, shortens convalescence, and improves the cosmetic outcome.

The technique of LESS is much more challenging than standard laparoscopic surgery (SLS), especially for suturing. For example, LESS requires crossing instrumentation at the abdominal wall in order to facilitate dissection, which has resulted in reverse handedness for the surgeon. Combine this with the already counterintuitive approach intrinsic to laparoscopic procedures and the LESS technique can be quite a mental strain. This problem has limited further proliferation of LESS into laparoscopic armamentarium of the laparoscopic surgeon.

Standard Robotic-Assisted Surgery (SRAS) has several advantages over SLS: improved optics, ergonomics, dexterity, and precision, which has enhanced its use in a wider patient population and more difficult procedures [5]. The early R-LESS platform did have the problem of instrument clashing due to the coaxial alignment of instruments and the current bulky robotic arms. To minimize this, Joseph et al. crossed the robotic instruments at the abdominal wall and, at the console, switched the controls so that the left actuator was directing the right robotic arm [6]. Intuitive Surgical Inc. developed a set of R-LESS-specific instruments: a multichannel access platform with four port channels and insufflation valve. Two of the ports have curved cannulas for the robotic instruments (which are also curved) and two straight ports for the endoscope and assistant instruments. These innovations have effectively minimized instrument collisions during multiple procedures. In GS, the most clinical experience with R-LESS has been with cholecystectomy.

General Comments on Abdominal and Pelvic Robotic Surgery

Preoperative Management

Multiple unique considerations come into play for the anesthesiologist prior to initiation of robotic abdominopelvic and retroperitoneal surgery. Indeed, presurgical time comprises a significant portion of total operating room time in robotic surgery [7–9]. Adequate preparation can reduce the time to initiation of surgery and in turn reduce the total anesthetic time for the patient [7].

In order to create a working space for the surgeon, current platforms in robot-assisted abdominopelvic and retroperitoneal surgery require the initiation of a pneumoperitoneum. While the choice of induction agent of general anesthetic is unimportant, adequate muscle relaxation is necessary to facilitate both pneumoperitoneum and ease of mechanical ventilation during the procedure [10,11]. In a prospective, randomized trial, Yoo et al. compared deep versus moderate neuromuscular blockade (NMB) in 67 patients undergoing robot-assisted laparoscopic prostatectomy [12]. Deep NMB was associated with successful completion of the operation under intraabdominal pressure (IAP) of 8 mmHg more often than moderate NMB (88 percent vs. 25 percent, p <0.001). Madsen et al. found that the use of deep NMB and low IAP significantly decreased the incidence of postoperative shoulder pain in laparoscopic hysterectomy when compared with moderate NMB (28.6 percent vs. 60 percent, p = 0.002) [13]. Deep NMB has also been shown to provide superior working space for the operating surgeon in both RS and LS [12–15].

Currently available robotic platforms allow for limited access to the patient following docking. Adequate intravenous access, as well as plethysmography and blood pressure monitoring devices, should be placed prior to positioning and rechecked following positioning to ensure function before docking [8,10,16]. Additional noninvasive or invasive monitoring is left to the discretion of the anesthesiologist. However, access for intraoperative placement of invasive monitoring devices will be limited, and so consideration should take place prior to docking.

Of even greater concern, access to the airway may be limited, particularly in cases where docking positions of the robot or its arms are above the patient's head, or where the table must be repositioned with the head away from the anesthesiologist [16,17].

Positioning of the endotracheal tube should be ensured after patient positioning and following docking by auscultation. Procedures requiring the use of steep Trendelenburg position shorten the trachea, increasing the risk of endotracheal tube displacement [16]. In an emergency setting, the presence of the robot can preclude rapid evaluation of the patient and initiation of CPR. However, an experienced team can accomplish undocking quickly in order to facilitate patient access and appropriate resuscitation [16].

Following bag-mask ventilation, the patient stomach may demonstrate significant distension. A gastric tube may be placed for intraoperative decompression with particular attention toward manipulation of the tube in cases of upper GI surgery [8,18]. Patient warming devices and corneal protection (plastic goggles with a form frame) should be placed in the standard fashion to prevent intraoperative hypothermia and corneal abrasions, respectively.

Patient Positioning

Positioning the patient is critical for the completion of abdominopelvic surgery. Because the current robotic platforms do not allow the patient's position to change without undocking, this often leads to prolonged periods of pressure under moderate to deep NMB. The range of positions for robotic abdominal surgery varies considerably, from steep Trendelenburg to reverse Trendelenburg, lateral decubitus, lithotomy, supine or split-leg depending on the region of interest [18–21]. In fact, some cases require multiple dockings with a change in position mid-way to facilitate exposure of additional quadrants of the abdomen, although newer robotic platforms are beginning to allow for up to 180-degree access within the abdomen [19,21]. With each position comes more potential for neuropathic injury. A bevy of upper and lower extremity neuropathies has been described following robotic surgery [20–23].

Safe patient positioning for robotic surgery requires a team approach to prevent position-related injuries and includes the primary surgeon, operative nursing staff, and the anesthesiologist. Positioning the patient can take a considerable amount of time, therefore, most high-volume robotic surgical centers train the nursing and anesthesiology staff in patient positioning to decrease time wasted in the OR. All patients must be well padded on major pressure points, no matter which position is required for the operation, in order to prevent position-related injury. In the past, the primary responsibility of the anesthesiologist was to secure the patient's endotracheal tube and protect the patient's eyes. They are now confronted with making sure they have "unrestricted access" to the endotracheal tube, intravenous lines, and blood pressure monitoring while being confronted with maximally protected arms and radically "fixed" patient positions. Especially during procedures that involve laparoscopic and robotic approaches requiring radical Trendelenburg positioning and the different docking positions of the robotic arms. It has become a challenge for anesthesiologists to adapt to the various "fixed" positions of patients with operations that have prolonged procedural times. They must also be ready for any adverse event that would require emergency undocking and emergency conversion to laparotomy.

The vast majority of position-related injury studies have come from the urology and gynecology literature, because these specialties have the most experience with robotic surgical procedures [7,8]. The position-related injuries are classified as cutaneous, musculoskeletal, neurologic, and vascular. The goal is to eradicate or minimize all of these position-related injuries. The incidence of position-related injuries varies in the literature, but in 2014, DiPierro looked at position-related injuries in patients undergoing Robotic-assisted Radial Prostatectomy (RARP) with Extended Pelvic Lymph Node Dissection (EPLND) classifying complications using a modified Clavian–Dindo surgical grading system. The patients were placed into four groups, and the overall minor complication rate was 75 percent (86 of 115 patients). The position-related injuries in groups 1–4 were 31, 29, 29, and 7 percent, respectively. The differences were statistically significant in groups 1–3 and group 4 (p = .023). Overall, 24 percent of the patients showed position-related injuries: 21 percent with Clavien grade 1, 2 percent with Clavien grade 2, and 1 percent with Clavien grade 3. After 60 patients, the grade 3 position-related injuries disappeared. The only variable that was associated with positioning injuries was time (p= .039) and CCI (p= .007). The injuries were pressure skin redness and neuropathies that were all Clavien grades 1 and 2 [24].

Just as the robotic platforms have advanced, surgical industry has advanced in minimizing position-related injuries with different types of padding materials to protect the patients, for example, gel foam and eggcrate foam. There are vacuum mattresses that conform to patient position; there are many nonslip materials that prevent patient migration during procedures. Combinations of these materials are utilized by experienced robotic teams in order to prevent position-related injuries.

The Perineolithotomy Position

Placing a patient in the perineolithotomy position is the most challenging of all positions, so it deserves a separate discussion because it defines the difficulty in preventing position-related injuries and exemplifies the importance of team approach. It begins when the patient self-transfers from the stretcher to the operating room table on one of the "nonslip" devices, which are secured to the operating room bed. The arms are placed on arm boards at 60 degrees to the bed and secured with Velcro soft restraints. The patient then moves down on the bed until the sacrum is in the middle of the bed and the lower edge of the buttocks is just below the lower break in the bed. The legs are carefully transferred simultaneously and placed in the stirrup boots (Yellow Fin by Allen Medical Systems is the most commonly utilized), making sure the heel is in the base of the boot and minimal pressure is on calf muscles and lateral tibia. The ankle and knee are placed in alignment with the contralateral shoulder in order to minimize external rotation. The knee is then flexed to approximately 90 degrees. The patient is then examined to ensure symmetry and that the pelvis is level. The patient's arms are then safely placed on the operating table with the thumbs up on a gel foam pad, then either eggcrate foam or another gel foam pad is placed on lateral and medial sides of the arm, especially protecting the elbow and medial epicondyle. Prior to wrapping the arm with the top sheet, anesthesiologist will check the IV lines, blood pressure cuff, and oxygen saturation monitor. The hands are usually formed into a fist around a piece of foam, then wrapped in foam to protect them from injury. If the patient is morbidly obese and it is not possible to place the arms on the table, there are surgical arm shields that can hold the arms or they can be placed on arm boards that are angled less than 90 degrees at the patient's side.

Attention is then turned to securing the patient at the level of the thorax, in order to minimize the patient slipping toward the head of the table during the procedure while in the very radical Trendelenburg position. A soft surgical restraint is placed firmly over the nipple line with eggcrate foam to protect the patient's skin. Usually silk tape or a strap is then placed firmly across the surgical restraints from opposite sides of the bed. Anesthesiologist then covers the eyes with protective plastic glasses. At this point, the surgeon should reexamine the patient, ask anesthesiologist to put the patient into Trendelenburg position, and reexamine all extremities and chest restraints. Then the patient is returned to the supine position and the prep started.

Physiologic Changes in Robotic Surgery

The combined effects of positioning, increased IAP from pneumoperitoneum, and use of CO_2 can be significant in robotic surgery. Separating out these effects is challenging because they can act synergistically or antagonistically depending on the position and procedure, and individual measurements in vivo would prove challenging. Nevertheless, measurable physiologic effects are present during robotic surgery in numerous organ systems and should be considered by the anesthesiologist during the operation.

Pulmonary System

The initiation of CO_2 pneumoperitoneum has numerous effects on the pulmonary system. Most abdominal operations are performed with an IAP goal between 8 and 15 mmHg. The increased IAP decreases functional residual capacity (FRC) [10,11]. When combined with Trendelenburg position, the cephalad migration of intraabdominal contents combines with IAP to decrease pulmonary compliance by as much as 68 percent [10]. The associated increase in atelectasis and pulmonary dead-space can lead to associated hypoxemia [25]. Increased peak and plateau pressures are observed in the setting of pneumoperitoneum, with increases as high as 50 percent [25]. Balick-Weber et al. compared volume-controlled and pressure-controlled ventilation systems in LS and found a small but significant decrease in peak airway pressures associated with pressure-control ventilation [25]. In a similar study, Choi et al. found that pressure control ventilation was associated with lower peak airway pressures and greater dynamic compliance than volume control ventilation [26]. Despite these significant differences, both studies failed to demonstrate clinical differences or changes in patient outcome with different ventilator settings [25,26]. CO_2 remains the most commonly used gas to generate pneumoperitoneum. It is noncombustible and is rapidly absorbed by the peritoneum, leading to shortened duration of pain associated with pneumoperitoneum [13,17]. Excess CO_2 leads to a mild respiratory acidosis, which is countered by multiple buffering systems in the body, the largest of which is in bone. These systems have the capacity to absorb upwards of 120 L of excess CO_2 in order to maintain normal pH [27]. After the body's buffering system is saturated, hypercarbia and metabolic acidosis can worsen. Increasing minute ventilation by 10–15 percent through increases in tidal volume and respiratory rate can correct hypercarbia, and close intraoperative monitoring of end-tidal CO_2 can guide these adjustments [28].

The principle contributor to hypercarbia during CO_2 pneumoperitoneum is decreased pulmonary compliance [29]. As such, patients with comorbidities such as asthma, chronic obstructive pulmonary disease, or obesity are at greater risk of developing metabolic acidosis during robotic intraabdominal surgery. Surgical risk factors include positioning in steep Trendelenburg and prolonged operative times [10,17]. Knowledge of both patient and operative risk factors can help guide the anesthesiologist in assessing the patient pre- and intraoperatively. Retroperitoneal and extraperitoneal dissection may contribute to the absorption of CO_2. Meininger et al. observed a significantly faster rise in $PaCO_2$ during extraperitoneal insufflation as compared with intraperitoneal insufflation [30]. Additionally, patients in this study had a higher plateau of $PaCO_2$ which suggests that the larger absorptive surface area of extraperitoneal space more readily absorbed CO_2[30]. A subsequent comparison of transabdominal preperitoneal (TAPP) and total extraperitoneal (TEP) herniorrhaphy by Sumpf et al. demonstrated increase rate of CO_2 uptake in extraperitoneal surgery. In this study, the degree of subcutaneous emphysema correlated with CO_2 uptake, again suggesting a contribution from the increased surface area. In addition, the authors suggest that a disruption of extraperitoneal microvasculature may contribute to more rapid CO_2 uptake and greater hypercarbia [31].

While these effects are relatively small in healthy patients, patients with underlying pulmonary disease may see greater consequences of the physiologic changes of pneumoperitoneum [17]. Decreasing the IAP associated with pneumoperitoneum can reduce the absorption of CO_2 and allow anesthesiologists time to treat and adjust for hypercarbia or reduce peak airway pressures required for ventilation to reduce these risks.

Cardiovascular System

Initiation of pneumoperitoneum for robotic surgery can have profound and immediate effects on the cardiovascular system. Hemodynamic changes can be related to increased IAP or secondary to hypercarbia of CO_2 pneumoperitoneum. Insufflation of abdomen leads to a stretch of the peritoneum, which is innervated by the vagus nerve [27]. Rapid peritoneal stretch can cause a vasovagal response, leading to bradycardia and occasionally hypotension [28]. This effect is most commonly seen with pressures above 12 mmHg and usually resolves quickly with cessation of pneumoperitoneum, with judicious application of intravenous fluids or a vagolytic agent (i.e., atropine) when necessary. The rise in IAP associated with pneumoperitoneum leads to a direct compression of intraabdominal inferior vena cava (IVC) [27]. Compression of the vena cava at IAP above 15 mmHg can lead to decreased venous return and increase the risk of cardiovascular collapse due to decreased venous return, particularly in patients who are hypovolemic preoperatively. Central venous pressure (CVP) measurement may rise due to the transmission of increased IAP to the thoracic cavity or remain unchanged [27,32]. Lestar et al. found that while pneumoperitoneum alone did not change CVP, the combination of pneumoperitoneum and Trendelenburg position led to a greater than two-fold increase in CVP, mean pulmonary artery pressure, and pulmonary capillary wedge pressure (p <0.001). These changes resolved rapidly following desufflation of the abdomen [30,32].

A secondary effect of the compression of IVC is engorgement of lower extremity and pelvic blood vessels and associated venous stasis [27]. The physiologic effect of stasis is an increased risk of venous thromboembolic disease. The use of compression stockings or sequential compression devices or administration of pharmacologic VTE prophylaxis preoperatively counteracts this effect. In fact, in a large retrospective analysis, the National Surgical Quality Improvement Program (NSQIP) has suggested that minimally invasive techniques convey lower risk of VTE than open procedures (AOR 1.33, p<0.01) [33,34].

Increased IAP associated with pneumoperitoneum leads to an increase in systemic vascular resistance (SVR) due to the compression of aorta [35]. Lestar et al. observed a 20 percent rise in SVR following initiation of pneumoperitoneum in their case series ($p < 0.05$). In their case series, the initiation of steep Trendelenburg position returned SVR to basal values [32]. Hypercarbia associated with the use of CO_2 pneumoperitoneum also has an effect of increasing SVR. The increased SVR and associated rise in afterload can lead to an overall decrease in stroke volume (SV) [10,11,17].

Changes in venous return and SVR associated with pneumoperitoneum can lead to alterations in cardiac output (CO) [10,27]. Indeed, Chow et al. observed a reduction of CO by 37 percent with the combination of steep Trendelenburg and pneumoperitoneum [10]. Contrary to this, Lestar and Flabella both observed no significant change in CO on initiation of pneumoperitoneum or changes in positioning, while Haas et al. found an increase in CO of 22.5 percent ($p < 0.05$) [32,35,36]. Reverse Trendelenburg position may worsen the changes in CO and cardiac index (CI), due to worsened venous return combined with increased cardiac afterload [21,37].

The physiologic effect of pneumoperitoneum on heart rate (HR) is multifactorial, and so like CO, the resulting effect can be mixed. In addition to vagal-mediated bradycardia, the use of CO_2 can affect HR. Physiologically, hypercarbia can produce tachycardia and an associated increase in myocardial oxygen demand [27]. While this response was observed by Meininger et al., multiple studies both prior and subsequent to this failed to note a statistically significant change in HR due to either pneumoperitoneum or altered positioning [29,32,35,37].

The cardiovascular perturbations associated with robotic abdominopelvic surgery are generally well tolerated by healthy patients and by those with cardiac comorbidities. Speicher et al. examined NSQIP between 2005 and 2011, specifically evaluating patients with congestive heart failure undergoing abdominal procedures. After adjustment for other comorbidities, logistic regression analysis found that 30-day mortality was lowered in laparoscopic versus open procedures (OR 0.45, $p = 0.038$) [38]. Extrapolating data from laparoscopy to robotics, this suggests that robotic abdominopelvic and retroperitoneal surgery is safe in patients with preexisting cardiac disease.

Cerebrovascular System

The effects of positioning and CO_2 pneumoperitoneum on the cerebrovascular system are intimately linked. When inspected individually, each of increased IAP, hypercarbia, and extreme positioning has an effect on cerebral perfusion and oxygenation. The combination of these effects may be enough to overcome cerebrovascular autoregulation and alter cerebral perfusion.

CO_2 pneumoperitoneum can lead to hypercarbia, as previously described. Elevated serum CO_2 leads to cerebrovascular dilation, increasing cerebral perfusion [39,40]. The rise in IAP associated with pneumoperitoneum is transmitted across the diaphragm, increasing intrathoracic pressure. This associated increase leads to decreased venous return by the jugular venous system, increasing intracranial pressure (ICP). The rise in ICP is mitigated by reverse Trendelenburg and exacerbated by steep Trendelenburg [39,40]. In a study evaluating the effect of pneumoperitoneum and reverse Trendelenburg position, Kurukhavecioglu et al. found that cerebral oxygenation did not change significantly despite initiation of CO_2 pneumoperitoneum during laparoscopic cholecystectomy (LC) with use of reverse Trendelenburg position [35]. In addition, the use of intermittent sequential compression devices on legs increased cerebral oxygenation when compared with a control group [41]. Closhen et al. similarly measured cerebral oxygenation during robotic surgery using two different near-infrared spectroscopy monitors [40]. Neither initiation of pneumoperitoneum nor steep Trendelenburg position was found to alter cerebral oxygenation greater than 5 percent, the accepted threshold for clinical significance [40].

While measurable changes in cerebral perfusion and oxygenation occur during robotic abdominal surgery, these changes do not appear to be clinically relevant in healthy patients. Jo et al. studied cerebral oxygenation and postprocedural cognitive function after laparoscopic and open gastrectomies [42]. In their study, patients undergoing minimally invasive gastrectomy had similar cerebral oxygen saturation as compared to open surgery, and there was no difference in Mini Mental Status Exam pre- or postoperatively [42]. These data appear to demonstrate that cerebral autoregulation is able to overcome the physiologic demands of RS and LS in majority of patients.

Renal Effects

Increased IAP causes compression of renal vasculature and parenchyma [18]. This has direct and indirect effects on the kidney. Directly, there is an immediate decrease in glomerular filtration rate and urine output [43,44]. This can be exacerbated in the setting of hypovolemia associated with preoperative mechanical bowel preparation. The oliguria associated with renal compression has been linked to the degree of elevation of IAP and resolves quickly after release of pneumoperitoneum [27,43].

In a rat model, Bishara et al. found that while IAP of 7 mmHg did not alter urine output, glomerular filtration rate (GFR), or fractional excretion of sodium, all of these parameters were significantly changed by IAP of 14 mmHg. All values returned to normal 1 hour after desufflation [43]. Renal compression also has secondary neurohormonal effects [27,43,45]. Impaired renal blood flow leads to the release of vasopressin, endothelin, and activation of the renin–angiotensin–aldosterone axis [27]. Excretion of aldosterone leads to the excretion of potassium and may contribute to mild postoperative hypokalemia. While the hormonal effects continue throughout pneumoperitoneum, these resolve within hours postoperatively due to the short half-lives of associated hormones. While caution should be exercised in patients with underlying renal dysfunction, chronic kidney disease (CKD) is not a contraindication to robotic surgery. Dolkart et al. investigated the effect of pneumoperitoneum in a previously validated rat model of CKD and in rats with acute kidney injury [44]. While creatinine and blood urea nitrogen levels did not change significantly, the CKD in rats did experience a slight decrease in creatinine clearance after pneumoperitoneum of 8 mmHg, while the acute kidney injury rats saw a small decrease in creatinine clearance following pneumoperitoneum of 5 and 8 mmHg. The authors concluded that pneumoperitoneum does not cause further dysfunction in the setting of CKD [44].

Intraoperatively, the anesthesiologist should expect mild oliguria associated with robotic surgery and avoid overcompensation with fluid administration. Insensible losses are significantly lower in robotic surgery versus open abdominal surgery, and long-term renal impairment is rare in minimally invasive surgery [27].

A rare complication associated with robot-assisted radical prostectomy with extended pelvic LN dissection is position-related rhabdomyolysis leading to renal failure. Rhabdomyolysis is defined as elevated serum creatine kinase (CK) of >5000 IU/L. It is hypothesized that hypoperfusion of the lower extremities occurs from the radical Trendelenburg positioning, causing tissue injury. The pathophysiologic mechanism of renal insufficiency from rhabdomyolysis is renal vasoconstriction, intraluminal cast formation, and direct myoglobin toxicity. Multiple risk factors contribute to the development of rhabdomyolysis, including high BMI, long operative times, extreme Trendelenburg in the perineolithotomy position, medications, pulmonary and cardiovascular disease. Rhabdomyolysis is associated with muscular pain, functional failure, skin lesions, and is diagnosed by elevated CK. Approximately 4% of patients developed rhabdomyolysis, requiring hypervolemic/diuretic therapy, and none developed renal failure [24,46].

Complications of Pneumoperitoneum

CO_2 Embolism

CO_2 embolism is a rare but potentially devastating consequence of pneumoperitoneum. Most CO_2 emboli are subclinical and of little consequence; the reported incidence ranges from 0.001 percent to 37.5 percent in the literature. Despite its rarity, mortality from clinically identifiable CO_2 embolism is as high as 28 percent [47]. The two primary causes of CO_2 embolism are direct insufflation of CO_2 into a blood vessel or vascularized parenchyma such as the liver during entry into the abdomen, or embolization through injury or transection of a major blood vessel during surgery. In a Cochrane review of laparoscopic entry techniques, zero gas emboli were recorded among twenty-two studies evaluated, suggesting that there is no observable difference in gas embolus among abdominal entry techniques [48].

CO_2 embolism should be suspected in the setting of sudden onset of hypotension or decrease in end-tidal CO_2 during insufflation, or during transection of either vascularized parenchyma or major vessels. The diagnosis can be confirmed by either auscultation of the characteristic "mill-wheel" murmur or through transesophageal echocardiography. If gas embolism is suspected, the robot should be rapidly undocked if necessary, and the patient should be placed in the left lateral decubitus position to facilitate trapping of the gas in the apex of the right ventricle [31]. In severe cases, rapid placement of a central venous catheter can allow aspiration of the gas. In most cases, the continued beating of the ventricle will break up the gas into small bubbles, and the solubility of CO_2 will lead to absorption.

Subcutaneous Emphysema

Insufflation of CO_2 requires intraabdominal placement of robotic ports to maintain pneumoperitoneum.

Displacement of the port or increased size of the incision can lead to subcutaneous tracking of gas. In a computed tomography study of laparoscopic patients, 56 percent demonstrated subcutaneous emphysema following surgery [48]. The majority of cases of subcutaneous emphysema are clinically insignificant, but the subcutaneous space can store additional CO_2, leading to retention and hypercarbia.

Pneumomediastinum and Pneumothorax

Dissection of naturally occurring planes can lead to gas tracking. In addition, upper abdominal surgery frequently calls for mobilization of the intrathoracic esophagus [29,31]. Violation of planes can lead to pneumomediastinum, which is usually asymptomatic, or pneumothorax in the case of violation of endothoracic fascia [27]. In lower abdominal surgery, gas dissection along natural myofascial planes can lead to pleural rupture and pneumothorax.

Pneumothorax can be diagnosed by unilateral decreased breath sounds, with or without changes in spirometry [29]. Tension pneumothorax will manifest as hemodynamic instability. Communication with the surgeon for prompt management via transabdominal surgical decompression of the thoracic cavity, desufflation of pneumoperitoneum, or tube thoracostomy is critical, as untreated tension pneumothorax can lead to complete cardiovascular collapse.

Facial, Laryngeal, and Pharyngeal Edema

Robotic surgery with prolonged pneumoperitoneum decreases venous return from the upper extremities, head, and neck. This can lead to migration of fluid into the extravascular compartment of head and neck, particularly when combined with steep Trendelenburg condition. While facial edema is common and may be bothersome to patients, laryngeal edema is of much more significant clinical concern [23,29]. Laryngopharyngeal edema can manifest postoperatively as stridor or respiratory failure requiring reintubation. Patients should be clinically evaluated prior to extubation for significant facial edema that may be suggestive of laryngopharyngeal edema, and cuff leak should be evaluated. Judicious use of fluids may reduce or prevent edema and decrease the risk of reintubation [16,17,23,29].

Ocular Complications

Corneal abrasion remains the most common ocular complication of robotic abdominal surgery. In their series, Danic et al. observed corneal abrasion in 3% of patients after robotic prostatectomy despite the use of tape, but noted a decrease to 1% following routine use of eye patches [16]. Of greater concern, pneumoperitoneum can increase intraocular pressure (IOP), especially when combined with steep Trendelenburg position. This can result in ischemic optic neuropathy and postoperative vision loss, a rare but devastating complication. Molloy observed that in the setting of steep Trendelenburg position, IOP increased significantly [41]. IOP increases further with longer duration of steep Trendelenburg, suggesting a relationship between duration of Trendelenburg and increased IOP [49]. Additionally, in 10 of 37 patients, IOP rose to levels higher than the calculated ocular perfusion pressure, suggesting poor autoregulation [49]. Yoo et al. measured intraoperative IOP during robotic prostatectomy in a randomized group of patients in deep and moderate NMB and reported a significant rise in IOP with pneumoperitoneum and steep Trendelenburg position [12]. In addition, they observed that patients with pneumoperitoneum in steep Trendelenburg had significantly higher IOP when given moderate vs. deep NMB ($p = 0.0003$). Multivariable analysis demonstrated that increased IAP was the only significant predictor of increased IOP (slope coefficient 0.5178, $p < 0.0001$) [12].

Robotic Abdominal Surgical Procedures

Robotic Hepatobiliary Surgery

Cholecystectomy

Minimally invasive cholecystectomy is the gold standard operation for people with symptomatic gallstones and cholecystitis. Professor Erich Mühe performed the first LC on September 12, 1985, and then he went on to perform over ninety such procedures [50–52]. Since then, GS and CRS have been utilizing minimally invasive techniques for a wide spectrum of procedures in the abdomen and pelvis. It is well accepted that cholecystectomy was the principal operation to begin with utilizing the robotic approach for two reasons: gall stone disease is very common and has a long accepted basis for minimally invasive technique. The first robot-assisted cholecystectomy was performed in 1998. Since then, there have been many reports comparing laparoscopic versus robotic approach to cholecystectomy [24]. The published reports have proven the safety and feasibility of robotic platforms for cholecystectomy [53,54]. In a 2004 study utilizing surgical residents with average laparoscopic expertise, the authors compared conventional laparoscopic cholecystectomy (CLC) with robot-assisted cholecystectomy (RAC) utilizing the ZEUS-AESOP surgical system. They compared total times and number of grasping and dissection actions. This very early study did indicate that RAC was feasible, but there was a longer operative time compared with CLC [54]. Over the years, the multiport robotic platform has undergone revisions from umbilical to low abdominal placement of the ports [54]. Kim et al. (2013), utilizing the four-arm da Vinci robot system, placed the trocars below the umbilicus and the other two arms laterally 7 to 10 cm from the midline camera. A fourth arm was placed in the right anterior axillary line in the upper quadrant, for more difficult dissections due to severe inflammation. A total of 83 patients had a RAC with a mean operative time of 52.4±17.1 min with a setup time of 11.9±5.4 (4–43) min and console time of 15.1±8.0 (range 4–50) min. The conversion rate to laparoscopic or open was zero. There were no common bile duct (CBD) injuries and the overall morbidity was 0.6 percent (one patient had bleeding) [55].

In 2008, a Canadian publication examined the safety of RAC, a retrospective study of two general surgeons with advanced laparoscopic skills comparing LC with RAC, the authors indicated that there were no major complications in either group, and in the RAC group, there were no conversions to laparoscopic approach. However, in the RAC group, the operative surgical time including docking time was statistically greater than the LC group (91 vs. 48 min, $p < 0.001$). Also postprocedure cleaning of the operative suite was significantly longer in the RAC group (14 vs. 11 min, $p = 0.015$). In the RAC group, anesthesia was also longer (23 vs. 15 min), though not statistically significant. They also "suggested" that in the RAC group there was a longer operative time, during the learning curve of the earlier RAC performed [56]. The increase in intraoperative times of RAC procedures was supported by multiple early studies [57–59].

As LC became the gold standard, utilizing various multiport placements above or below the umbilicus, then in 1997, Navarra et al. introduced the single-incision laparoscopic cholecystectomy (SILC) [60,61]. The SILC was developed for cosmetic reasons and then evolved to SILS. The SILS approach was stimulated by natural orifice transluminal endoscopy surgery (NOTES) [62].

The Robotic Single Site Platform RSSP has a special feature – the Intraoperative Firefly™ – which is a fluorescence imaging system. This imaging system allows the surgeon to visualize the biliary system during the surgery by a preoperative intravenous injection of indocyanine green (ICG), and then the near-infrared fluorescence light would help the surgeon to perform a real-time fluorescent cholangiography [63].

Initial experience with RSSP was published in 2011; all patients underwent surgery by two experienced surgeons with single-site surgery (>50 cases) and robotic surgery (>100 cases) for symptomatic cholelithiasis, excluding acute cholecystitis, a suspicion of CBD stones, pregnant patients, or severe systemic comorbidities. There were 28 patients who underwent RSSC: 22 were female, 6 men, mean age was 48 years, BMI of 26 kg/m^2 (18–30), and median ASA score of 2 (range 1–3). The most significant results were a median OR time of 80 min (range 45–195), a median port placement time of 3 min (range 1–8), a median docking time of 8 min (range 1–18), and a median console time of 53 min (range 23–134). There were no conversions to laparoscopic or major complications. There was a decrease in the median operative and docking time as the study progressed. The authors indicated that RSSC was safe and feasible [64].

In 2012, the first European experience with single-site robotic cholecystectomy (SSRC) versus SILC looked at and compared learning curves. It was a retrospective review of the first 25 patients who underwent SSRC for symptomatic biliary gallstones or polyposis. They excluded patients with BMI >33, acute cholecystitis, previous upper abdominal surgery, ASA >2, and age >80 years. These cases were then compared to the authors' first 25 SILC and with the literature. Both groups were similar in gender, age, and BMI. There were no major complications in either group. The results did show that operative time was longer in the SILC group compared to the SSRC group (83.2 vs. 62.7 min, $p = 0.0006$), and the SSRC did not change throughout the series. Average LOS was not statistically different in either group. The authors felt they proved the feasibility and safety of SSRC [65].

In a comparative study of first experience with RSSC versus single-site laparoscopic cholecystectomy (SSLC) in Asia, the authors found that there was no significant differences in operative outcomes regarding intraoperative blood loss, bile spillage, postoperative pain scale values, postoperative complications, and length of hospital stay between the two groups (p= 0.05). However, the actual dissection time (p = 0.003) and total operative time (p= 0.001) were significantly longer in the RSSC group than the SSLC group. This team utilized the Intraoperative Firefly™ fluorescence imaging for real-time fluorescent cholangiography [66].

The ICG fluorescence imaging system was first used for sentinel LN biopsies in patients with breast and colon cancers. ICG is a vital fluorescent dye with few side effects and low toxicity and allergic reactions. It has been used for visualization of vascular anatomy, anastomotic perfusion, hepatobiliary anatomy, tattooing of gastrointestinal lesions, sentinel LN biopsy, and LN road mapping. Currently in robotic surgery, it combines a surgical endoscope capable of visible light and near-infrared imaging, a three-dimensional high-definition stereoscopic camera head that provides visible light, and near-infrared illumination through the surgical endoscope via a flexible light guide. Since ICG is exclusively excreted in the bile, this fluorescence technique allows better visualization of the liver and the extrahepatic biliary tree during open, laparoscopic, and robotic surgery [67,68]. Utilizing intraoperative fluorescence imaging can facilitate better understanding of bile duct anatomy and help in avoiding injury [68].

Even with the utilization of intraoperative fluorescence imaging, robotic surgical exploration of the CBD has had minimal acceptance. Only 15% of patients with cholelithiasis have CBD stones. The standard of care of choledocholithiasis is endoscopic retrograde cholangiopancreatography (ERCP), preceded by cholecystectomy. However, when ERCP fails, surgical exploration of the CBD is necessary. Laparoscopic CBD exploration with sphincterotomy has been shown to be superior over open CBD exploration with sphincterotomy; however, it is utilized in highly selective cases [69]. The advantage of robotic CBDE is that it combines treatment of cholelithiasis and choledocholithiasis in a one-stage minimally invasive approach, eliminating the utilization of ERCP. The utilization of robotic CBDE in patients with refractory choledocholithiasis to ERCP has been shown to be a safe and effective alternative over open CBDE. Alkhamesi et al. compared 19 robotic CBDE with 39 open CBDE for refractory choledocholithiasis to ERCP; the patient demographics and comorbidities did not differ, nor in presenting symptoms. The mean operating times for robotic CBDE were longer (220±41.26 min) than for open CBDE (169±65.81 min) and were statistically significant (p = 0.01). The robotic CBDE mean LOS was shorter as compared to open CBDE (4 vs. 11 days; p= 0.02). There was no difference in T-tube utilization (74 vs. 61%; p = 0.414) or postoperative complications (p = 0.402) for robotic vs. open CBDE. There is benefit for robotic CBDE when ERCP fails in highly selected patients [70,71].

Minimally invasive surgery for cholecystectomy is the "standard of care" after almost 30 years of clinical application. One of the major issues of the application of robotic platforms for cholecystectomy is the overall cost of the procedure as compared to LC. A recent study compared cost of care and reimbursement between RC and LC based on several data points: hospital charges (amount requested for reimbursement), hospital cost (dollars spent on episode of care), net revenue (money received, regardless of cost), and earnings before depreciation, interest, and taxes (EBDIT). EBDIT is defined as the net income before considerations for depreciation, interest, and income taxes. It is used to compare profitability because it excludes the effects of financing and accounting decisions. Net income is the value after hospital cost has been applied to net revenue.

The authors further subdivided the hospital costs into variable costs, fixed costs, supply costs, drug costs, equipment costs, and facility costs. Fixed costs are expenses that are not dependent on the level of care provided (e.g., employee salaries and rents per month). Variable costs are usually volume-related and unique to any episode of care, which includes many resources (e.g., some drugs not included in drug costs, CT scans, laboratory tests) and services provided or consumed (e.g., components of nursing time, recovery room time, etc.) in the episode of care of an individual patient. Facility costs are inclusive of hospital costs (e.g., maintaining the hospital, utilities used to run the hospital, etc.); these costs are allocated to all patients and adjusted for severity of intervention and illness. An analysis of operative duration (defined as the time from when the patient entered the operating room until the time he or she was transported from the operating room) was done for each patient.

Thirty-one RCs were compared to 201 LCs from June 2012 to June 2013. The operative duration for RCs was 140 min (141±25.38) as compared to 93 min (102± 32.7) for LCs (p <0.01). Hospital charges for RCs were $33,238.42 ($34,178.10±6,023.66) as compared $25,055.85 ($27,020.69±8,624.90) for LCs (p<0.01). Variable costs for RCs were $1714.30 ($1,786.00±449.45), while for LCs, they were $1,449.54 ($1,555.53±527.52) (p<0.022) but only for a cost of $264.76 per case. There was no difference between either procedures as far as net revenue, EBDIT, net income, fixed costs, supply costs, drug costs, equipment costs, facility costs, and total costs [72].

This was the first study that compared RC to LC with multiple data points, and it appears to state that the only cost difference was the variable cost of $264.76 per case.

Robotic Liver Surgery

Minimally invasive surgery of the liver has been slow to develop because of the technical challenges of liver surgery, including access to the vena cava, major hepatic veins, and difficulty in dissections of the hilum and control of bleeding. So early liver procedures were limited to staging procedures and unroofing of hepatic cysts, then progressed to easily accessible parts for wedge resection, then to major hepatectomies with increasing experience. As the technology to control bleeding and advanced robot platforms have developed, robotic liver surgery has become more common [73]. Patient positioning for robotic liver resections has also developed depending on the segment being resected, for example, the left lateral position for lesions in segment 7 or 8.

Minor hepatectomy is the most common procedure performed robotically 58% of the time, including wedge resection, segmentectomy, bisegmentectomy, and left lateral sectionectomy. A review article of 217 patients with benign and malignant disease of the liver undergoing minor hepatectomy showed that wedge resection and segmentectomy had a conversion to open rate of 4.6% and a complication rate of 20.3%. Postoperative intraabdominal fluid collection of bile or abscess was the most common complication. Reasons for conversion to open were unclear tumor margin, bleeding control, obesity, or anatomical distortion of hilum from adhesions. Operative mean times ranged from 200 to 507 min with mean operative blood loss of 60–660 ml. The mean postoperative LOS ranged from 5.5 to 11.7 days, with a mean follow-up time of 36 months for colorectal liver metastasis and 25.1 months for hepatocellular carcinoma. The studies did support that robotic liver resection was safe and feasible for experienced surgeons with advanced laparoscopic skills [74,75].

Major hepatectomy is an advanced robotic surgical procedure that requires advanced laparoscopic skills and techniques. In one of the major series of robotic liver resections, Giulianotti et al. performed 70 procedures, including 33 major resections for both benign and malignant disease: 24 right hepatectomies, 5 left hepatectomies, 2 right trisectionectomies, and 1 extended right hepatectomy and 1 right lobe donor hepatectomy. Twenty-three of the 33 major resections were for malignancy, with 13 for colorectal metastasis. The mean operative time was 313 min (range 220–480) with a mean blood loss of 300 ml (range 100–2,000). These authors did discuss the advantages of the robotic approach, especially for dissection of the hilum and hepatocaval dissection. The robotic platform with its three-dimensional magnification and endowrist functions allows for microsurgical dissection of bile ducts and major blood vessels and was especially advantageous for biliary reconstruction during liver resection [74,75].

Overall, the utilization of the robot for minor and major hepatic resections has been slow to develop but has proven feasibility, safety, and acceptable complication rate when compared to laparoscopic hepatic resections. There is not enough data to compare a cost–benefit ratio for utilization of the robot for hepatic resections, nor is there any data on long-term oncologic outcomes [76].

Robotic Pancreatic Surgery

Pancreatic surgery, both open and minimally invasive, is both technically demanding because it is a retroperitoneal organ embedded in visceral organs. The minimal invasive approach is still developing, and because the anatomic location of pancreas positioning of the patient is still in development, the standard supine position is most common, but there is an early feasibility and safety study to approach from the posterior and lateral positions and perform a retroperitoneoscopic pancreatectomy (RP). These authors utilized minimally invasive techniques for the RP procedure on 19 patients with benign and malignant disease of the pancreas. Patients had enucleations (n = 8), distal panreatectomy (n = 4), pancreatic cyst resection (n = 2), and no pancreatic lesions (n = 5). Intraoperative complications occurred in 12.5%, including the peritoneum and splenic vein. Six cases developed pancreatic fistulas postoperatively [77].

The difficulty of laparoscopic pancreatic resection has prevented wider acceptance because of the complexity of the procedure, the accuracy required, and the steep learning curve to become proficient with the procedure. The robotic pancreatic resection has increased the acceptance of minimally invasive surgery on the pancreas, but it is also considered advanced robotic surgery. There is a retrospective review of one surgeon's experience of 134 patients in the United States and Italy from 2000 to 2007, utilizing the robot for benign (70 cases) and malignant (64) disease of the pancreas. The patient is placed in the low lithotomy position with the robot over the patient's head. The procedures were pancreaticoduodenectomy (PD) (50), distal pancreactectomy (DP) spleen preserving (23), distal splenopancreactectomy (23), cystogastrostomy (14), middle/total pancreactectomies (4), longmire procedure (10), cystoduodenstomy (1), cystojejunestomy (3), pancreaticogastrostomy (2), pancreaticojejunostomy (1), and enuculation (3). For the Italian group (77 patients), the results for all procedures were: mean operative time, 312 min (55–660); estimated blood loss, 261 cc (100–600); and LOS for patients with perioperative complications, 21.8 days (6–85), and those without perioperative complications, 10.2 days (4–15). In the US group (57 patients), the results for all procedures were: mean operative time, 351 min (73–630); estimated blood loss, 323 cc (5–2,000); and LOS for patients with perioperative complications, 9.3 days (3–30), and those without perioperative complications, 6.4 days (3–13).

The total conversion to open rate was 18.3% (11) in the PD group and 6.5% (3) in the DP group. The reasons for conversion in the Italian group were venous tangential infiltrations, hypercapnia, malfunction of robotic system, difficulty isolating anatomical structure, positive tumor margins, and infiltration of the superior mesenteric vein.

The most common postoperative complications in the combined groups were pancreatic fistula, which occurred in 31.3% (19 of 60 patients) in the PD group and 20.9% (9 of 43 patients) in the DP group. The 30-day total mortality was 1.5% [41].

The incidence of pancreatic fistula was high in this series than in other series utilizing minimally invasive techniques. The major question that has not been answered is whether the oncology outcome is better than or equal to open technique for pancreatic cancers [78,79].

Robotic Gastrectomy

The role of minimally invasive approaches (both laparoscopic and robotic) to gastrectomy has not been widely accepted in the United States or Europe. Laparoscopic gastrectomy (LG) was used for early gastric cancers that did not require extensive LN dissection. As the technology improved and with accumulation of surgical experience, the indications were broadened to later gastric cancers.

In 2009, a comparative study was carried out on 60 patients with gastric cancer: group 1 (initial robotic) of 20 patients underwent robot-assisted distal subtotal gastrectomy with gastroduodenostomy (RADG), group 2 (initial laparoscopic) of 20 patients underwent laparoscopic distal subtotal gastrectomy with gastroduodenostomy (LADG), and group 3 (recent laparoscopic) of 20 current patients underwent LADG. A single surgeon who had performed 177 laparoscopic gastrectomies and 100 open gastrectomies before starting robotic surgery performed all procedures. All patients were placed in supine position and reverse Trendelenburg with the surgical cart above the right side of the patients' head.

The demographics of the patients were all similar based on sex, age, BMI, and comorbidities. Operative time of the initial RADG was significantly shorter than the initial LADG group ($p = 0.003$); however, in comparison the initial RADG had a significantly longer operative time than the recent LADG group ($p < 0.001$). The initial LADG had the longest operating times (289.5±59.3 min) followed by the initial RADG (230±34.9 min). There was a trend in the initial RADG of decreasing time with increasing experience.

There were no significant difference in tumor characteristics ($p = 0.399$) or difference in LN retrieval ($p = 0.080$). Stage IA was the most common for all groups. There was no statistical difference in LOS, tolerance of diet, and only four postoperative complications with zero mortality [80].

In a recent meta-analysis comparing robot-assisted gastrectomy (RAG) and laparoscopy-assisted gastrectomy (LAG), it found that RAG was acceptable than LAG when performing radical gastrectomy. The study compared 1,875 patients in eight studies.

There was no difference between RAG and LAG in LOS ($p > 0.5$), no difference in postoperative complications ($p > 0.1$), proximal margin was similar in RAG and LAG ($p > 0.05$), but the distal margin was longer in RAG then LAG ($p > 0.05$), and harvested LNs were similar in both groups ($p > 0.05$). However, in the RAG group the operative time was longer because of setting and docking. Three of the studies indicated that the operative time did decrease as the surgeons' experience increased. The da Vinci allowed for intracorporeal anastomosis in all cases. The authors concluded that long-term studies of clinical outcomes should be evaluated before final conclusions can be drawn [81].

In a retrospective review comparing RAG to LAG in short-term surgical outcomes, there were 423 patients from October 2011 to August 2014 with gastric cancer. Ninety-three patients had RAG and 330 had LAG; a comparative analysis was performed for clinicopathological characteristics and short-term surgical outcomes.

There was no significant difference in age, BMI, tumor location, TNM staging, and medical comorbidities ($p > 0.05$). The extent of resection (subtotal or total gastrectomy or distal gastrectomy) and the extent of LN dissection to achieve R0 resection was the decision of the operating surgeon. Reconstruction was either gastroduodenostomy, or gastrojejunostomy for distal gastrectomy, Roux-en-Y esophagojejunostomy for total gastrectomy, and esophagogastric anastomosis for proximal gastrectomy, and most were performed extracorporeally. Operating time was longer for RAG (257.1±74.5 min) than LAG (226.2±61.3 min), which was significant ($p < 0.001$). RAG (176.6±212.2 ml) had less intraoperative blood loss than LAG (212.5±198.8 ml), which was significant ($p = 0.001$). There was no difference between types of resections performed ($p = 0.686$). The proximal and distal margins were not significantly different in either group ($p = 0.092$ and 0.486, respectively). The short-term outcomes – days to first flatus and days to tolerating diet – were similar in RAG and LAG groups ($p > 0.05$). Postoperative complication rates were not statistically different between RAG (9.8%) and LAG (10%) with $p = 0.927$. Hospital LOS was also similar with a $p = 0.41$.

In summary, the RAG requires a longer operative time, but over time the mean operative time does reduce. This study did demonstrate that RAG is acceptable over LAG in terms of surgical and oncologic outcomes in the short term [82].

Robotic Splenectomy

The use of minimally invasive surgery for splenectomy is an established procedure and is the standard of care for diseases of the spleen. The minimal invasive approaches are multiport laparoscopic splenectomy, hand-assisted laparoscopic splenectomy (for very large spleens), robotic splenectomy, natural orifice transluminal endoscopy, and single-port access splenectomy. LS is performed for idiopathic thrombocytopenic purpura, hereditary spherocytosis, autoimmune hemolytic anemia, thrombocytopenic purpura, Hodgkin's and non-Hodgkin's lymphoma, chronic lymphocytic leukemia, hemangiomas, idiopathic myelofibrosis myelodysplastic syndrome, hairy cell leukemia, splenic abscess, or cyst and tuberculosis. The utilization of RS has not surpassed the level of LS. The position of the patient is the right lateral decubitus, with reverse Trendelenburg inclination and the table is flexed [83].

The use of the robot for either total or partial splenectomy has been very slow to evolve because of very few studies. In a comparative study in 2012 of 32 consecutive subtotal splenectomies, only 10 cases were performed with the robotic platform. The authors felt that the robot was superior in dissection of splenic vessels, but the effective cost–benefit ratio was not acceptable. They felt that only difficult cases be referred for robotic surgery [84]. In a review in 2015 of minimally invasive surgery comparing LPS and RPS, out of 195 publications only 33 articles were included with a total of 187 patients: the mean total operative time for LPS was between 70 and 216 min and between 108 and 120 min for RPS. The complication rate with similar: LPS 5.36% and RPS 5.56%. The authors felt that the robotic approach needed more research to prove efficacy over LS or LPS [85]. The current data for the utilization of robotic platform for diseases of the spleen is limited and indications for it are evolving. It does require a high degree of robotic and advanced laparoscopic skills before attempting to treat diseases of the spleen.

Robotic CRS

Since the first reported LC in 1991, the use of minimally invasive approaches to diseases of the colon and rectum had begun [86]. The first robot-assisted CRS in 2001 for ileocolic resections and sigmoid resections for benign disease was published [87]. Since that time, LC has become more widely utilized for benign and malignant diseases of the colon and rectum with significant short-term benefits over open colectomy, for example, reduction of postoperative pain, shorter hospital LOS, and earlier return to work. Studies have also shown no difference in LC versus open colectomy for colon cancer for short- and long-term oncologic outcomes [88–90].

The more common robotic platform utilized today is the da Vinci Si series, and the approach to the colon or rectum involves "hybrid" procedures, including laparoscopic–robotic procedures. For all left-sided colon or rectal procedures, the patient is in the perineolithotomy position with radical Trendelenburg position, with radical tilt to the right. Many sigmoid resections or low anterior resections with low pelvic anastomoses include laparoscopic mobilization (either pure laparoscopic or hand-assisted laparoscopic) of the splenic flexure and/or ligation of the inferior mesenteric artery. When performed, the inferior mesenteric vein then robotic mobilization of the rectum, with a hybrid hand-assisted colorectal anastomosis. With greater experience, there has been mobilization of the splenic flexure with one docking of the robot, then redocking in order to perform the resection of sigmoid or rectum with an intracorporeal colorectal anastomosis. Now the only disadvantage of multiple docking methods is increased operative time.

The majority of right colectomy resections are performed in the supine position tilted to the left in the Trendelenburg (some surgeons prefer the reverse Trendelenburg) utilizing robotic mobilization of the ileum and colon with extracorporeal anastomosis, while other surgeons perform robotic high vascular ligation, with intracorporeal resection of the ileum and transverse colon, then utilizing either intracorporeal or extracorporeal anastomosis [91]. With the recent release of the da Vinci Xi platform, the entire abdominal and rectal procedure can be performed with the robotic platform.

A systematic review of articles compared robot-assisted CRS with laparoscopic and open surgery in 2014. For robot-assisted CRS studies in 69 publications, there were a total of 2,644 operations performed, and in 62 sex-reported studies, there were 1,445 males (54.7%) and 1,092 females (45.3%). In 60 age-reported studies, the average age was 60.1±6.2 for 2,478 patients. In 46 BMI-reported studies, the mean BMI was 25±1.8 kg/m^2 for 2,269 patients. There were 499 (19.3%) procedures for benign disease and 2,089 (80.7%) for malignant diseases in 65 studies. The types of procedure reported in 66 studies were: 966 low anterior resections (37.8%), 387 (15.2%) right colectomies, 385 (15.1%) anterior resection, 170 (6.7%) sigmoid colectomies, 168 (6.6%) abdominoperineal resections, 104 (4.1%) rectopexies, 70 (2.7%) left colectomies, and 36 (1.4%) total or subtotal proctocolectomies.

In 66 studies involving RC, the mean operative time (OT) was 253.3±65.8 min. When compared to laparoscopic surgery (LS) and open surgery (OS), the mean OT was significantly greater than the LS time, while RS and LS times were significantly greater than OS times. Interestingly, the average LOS, was inconsistent in the RS and LS procedures, which were statistically similar but less than OS.

Intraoperative complications in 2,391 patients (61 studies) reported a 0.8% complications, which included associated bowel or vascular injuries, intraoperative bleeding, and two ureteral injuries. There were 504 (21.1%) postoperative complications, of which 21.4% anastomotic leaks, 20.4% ileus, 10.5% wound infection, 9.9% urinary or sexual dysfunction, 7.1% pelvic abscess, 6.9% medical problems, 4.8% bleeding, and 3.2% neurologic problems (positioning injury). Conversion from RS to OS was 2.4% (0–40%) and to LS was 0.7% (0–33%), and the most common reason was obesity (15.3%), followed by technical problems (13.9%) and difficult dissections or anatomy (9.7%). Regarding oncology pathologic outcomes when comparing RS to LS and/or OS, there was no statistical difference in harvested LN, distal resection margins (DRM), circumferential resection margins (CRM), total mesorectal excisions (TME), or mortality. With regard to oncologic outcomes comparing RS to LS and/or OS, there was no statistical significance ($p = 0.873$). This systematic review of RS as compared to LS and OS did determine that RS is safe and feasible in diseases of the colon and rectum and not inferior to LS or OS. They also stated that there is a longer OT, steeper learning curve, and a higher cost [92]. Minimally invasive rectal surgery is an advanced laparoscopic technique, and robotic platform has just started to be utilized, and weather the procedure is performed minimally invasive or by open surgery, the gold standard for rectal cancer (RC) is a TME. A 2015 meta-analysis compared outcomes in robotic TME (RTME) versus laparoscopic TME (LTME) in randomized controlled trials (RCTs) and nonrandomized controlled trials (NRCTs) to evaluate whether RTME was as safe and efficacious as LTME. Utilizing a strict inclusion and exclusion criteria, the authors were able to find eight studies (7 NRCTs and 1 RCT) out of 192 studies. There were 1,229 patients with RC, of which 554 (45.08%) were RTME versus 675 (54.92%) who underwent LTME. When comparing the two groups, there was no statistical difference in the pooled data for LOS ($p = 0.43$), overall complications ($p = 0.23$), anastomotic leaks ($p = 0.66$), wound infection rates ($p = 0.52$), or overall pathologic data (LN $p = 0.84$, DRM $p = 0.36$, PRM $p = 0.32$, CRM $p = 0.50$). The complication of urinary and sexual function was mixed, but when looking at the pooled data, there was no statistical difference ($p = 0.72$). And there was no difference in OS or DFS in either group ($p = 0.404$ and 0.914, respectively).

Overall, the total hospital costs for RTME ($14,080) was higher than LTME ($9,120) and OS ($8,386) with $p < 0.01$. The conversion to open in the RTME (6/554) was significantly lower than the LTME (35/675), the reasons being obesity with thick mesentery, inability to identify important vascular structures, vascular injury, adhesion, and narrow pelvis. The mean operative time was longer in RTME versus LTME in most of the studies. In some of the studies with the addition of neoadjuvant chemoradiotherapy (NCRT), there was a higher anastomotic leak rate in the lower RC patients. The authors admitted that the meta-analysis has limitations; the most important issues were that the primary studies determine the quality of meta-analysis, which indicated methodological problems; only one study was RCT; and there was always heterogeneity in the patients. Overall this study did suggest that RTME is safe and feasible with lower conversion rates than LTME, but the disadvantage was higher cost [93]. The ACOSOG Z6051 randomized clinical trial determined that among patients with stage II and stage III RC, the use of laparoscopic resection as compared to open resection failed to meet the criteria for noninferiority of pathologic outcomes. The authors recommended, pending clinical oncologic outcomes, that the findings do not support the use of laparoscopic resection in these patients [94]. In the Australasian Laparoscopic Cancer of the Rectum (ALaCaRT) randomized non-inferiority phase III trial with a total of 475 patients (237 open rectal resection/238 laparoscopic resections), T1–T3 RCs 15 cm from the anal verge showed that laparoscopic resection did not reach noninferiority versus open resection. The authors did not recommend a routine use of LS for RC [95].

Postoperative Management

Enhanced Recovery after Surgery

The advent of ERAS programs for perioperative care of the surgery patient has done more to foster the modern multiteam approach to patient-centered management pathways. It has been through the collective development of protocols and multidisciplinary team, including nursing and other ancillary care givers under the leadership of surgeons and anesthesia providers, that evidence-based perioperative protocols have been implemented in the management of the surgical patient, which have led to improved outcomes.

These perioperative protocols contain facets that focus on preoperative, intraoperative, and postoperative management techniques that require multidisciplinary team cooperation. These ERAS protocols developed to reduce the surgical stress response and thereby improve patient's outcomes, reduce complications, and shorten postoperative hospitalization. The proliferation of ERAS studies and resultant protocols have spawned an Enhanced Recovery After Surgery Society, which serves as a valuable databank available at www.erassociety.org.

The predominance of medical literature on postoperative recovery pathways has been centered on the CRS patient, but there is growing evidence that other postoperative procedures, particularly other abdominal pelvic procedures, are amenable to ERAS protocols as well. The majority of this literature demonstrates a reduction in hospital stay coupled with a lack of an increase in readmission rates or mortality [96]. These advantages are not relegated to only younger, healthier patients as ERAS protocols have been safely applied to elderly patients and have been demonstrated to reduce complications and shorten length of hospital stay in those patients as well [97].

While the initial studies were actually performed on open colectomy patients by Kehlet et al., LS has predominated recently and robotic surgery is ideally suited for incorporation into these pathways as well [98]. The minimally invasive approach has been demonstrated to better preserve the immune response and enhance faster postoperative recovery [99,100]. The utilization of ERAS is obviously not unique to RS or LS, but it is particularly germane to these operative techniques and is a critical component of perioperative management of these patients. It really is not a question of whether ERAS should be done, but rather how best to develop and implement an ERAS protocol for robotic surgical patients [4].

It is critical when embarking on ERAS pathways that it is done with a multidisciplinary team and is patient-centered. Initially, it is very labor-intensive and is a significant allocation of resources [101]. There are current systems based on practice pathways and cultural barriers that can be impediments to implementing ERSA protocols. These barriers must be overcome in order to standardize care through education of staff to overcome cultural and organizational roadblocks. If an ERAS protocol is developed and instituted and the nursing personnel have not embraced it or the surgeons and anesthesiologists are not committed, then it is doomed to fail.

Protocol compliance and clinical outcomes must be continually monitored, updated, and even modified. An initial pilot study conducted by a dedicated team was able to maintain a compliance of the protocol 93% of the time with a median length of hospital stay (LOS) of 3 days and a 30-day readmission rate of 4%. However, when the protocol was implemented hospital wide, compliance fell to 74% and median LOS rose to 6 days. These results demonstrate a quicker postoperative recovery and shorter LOS compared to historical controls, but also emphasize the importance of constant vigilance and monitoring of the protocol [102].

Just as there are multiple methods for performing a given operation or providing anesthesia for a surgery, no two ERAS pathways are identical. The tenets of the protocol that is developed and instituted must be incorporated into the individual institution and eventually through the healthcare system. Since the predominance of studies involve multiple separate parameters, it is often difficult to pinpoint and then separate out the most critical components. The longstanding question of which ERAS component is the most critical for the patient with respect to postoperative recovery remains unanswered.

What follows is not an exhaustive review of literature, but rather an attempt to coalesce some of the pertinent data on ERAS and allow the practitioners to build a protocol that can be incorporated into the cultural goals of their own institution. The goal is to allow the multidisciplinary ERAS teams to examine the evidence and to use the data to develop optimal perioperative management for their robotic surgical patients.

ERAS Protocol Overview

Since the advent of ERAS or fast-track protocols almost 20 years ago, a voluminous number of studies have been performed. The initial studies in Europe have spread to North America and throughout the world [103]. Studies demonstrate that these protocols are safe and effective and can be inculcated into any size and makeup of hospital – in both academic and private institutions [104]. There have been multiple meta-analyses studies addressing colorectal ERAS programs and a Cochrane review that has indicated enhanced patient outcomes. As with meta-analysis studies, heterogeneity of patient populations, as well as disparate protocols, there is difficulty in combining these studies to evaluate patient outcomes. In addition, most studies are compared to historical controls, which makes the outcomes even more problematic. Despite these methodology problems, all studies have demonstrated a decreased hospital LOS, without compromising patient safety. These studies uniformly indicate that complications and readmission rates are equivalent. The data on complications is less clear, with some studies showing a reduction in complications as well as some showing a savings in healthcare costs [105–112].

Applicable Robotic Surgical Procedures

Although the predominance of literature, especially the initial studies on ERAS protocols, mainly involved CRS, there are multiple other procedures that are amenable to a robotic ERAS protocol, for example, the bariatric and obstetric patients who are commonly operated using robotic technology have incorporated ERAS protocols. Due to the fact that these patients have already shorter length of hospital stays than CRS patients, it has been somewhat difficult to demonstrate improvement in LOS and less readmission rates utilizing ERAS protocols, but overall these have been shown to benefit patients [113–116].

ERAS Protocol Components

The ERAS protocols are typically divided into three components for conceptualization, but it is critical to realize that these are an organizational division only and there is significant overlap such that all the providers are involved in one aspect or another in each phase of the protocol. Anesthesiologists play perhaps the most critical role in facilitating the recovery of patients, as many of the ERAS elements are under their direct control. At least one author contends that for successful implementation of an ERAS program, anesthesiologists must become more involved in perioperative care and be more aware of the impact of anesthetic techniques on surgical outcomes and recovery [117].

The multidisciplinary protocol and team must transition the patient from one provider to the next in a smooth and consistent manner. Communication between team members during protocol development and implementation is crucial to enhance patient experience and outcomes. The three components are roughly divided into preoperative, intraoperative, and postoperative care of the surgical patient [118,119].

Preoperative ERAS Component

The preoperative care component is identifying patients who will benefit from the protocol. While most patients can garner some benefit, some may not be adequate candidates, so the ERAS protocol should not be "instituted" on every patient unless the team believes that the patient will benefit. Patients with significant comorbidities or those who cannot ambulate without assistance or lack cognitive abilities to follow instructions may be poor candidates for inclusion in the protocol. Following patient selection there is a designated team member who gives extensive preoperative counseling and coaching. It is important to understand patient's expectations and provide counseling on the protocol and allow ample amount of time for the patient and their family members to understand the goals of the protocol and also encourage them to ask questions. Both surgical and anesthesia providers should ideally be involved in preoperative counseling, highlighting their own respective areas. This team approach further enhances the patients "buying in" the protocol and its goals.

At preoperative assessment and testing, in addition to the standard assessment of comorbidities, nutritional concerns and smoking cessation, if applicable, should be addressed. The patients are also provided instructions on any preoperative bathing requirements and Chlorhexidine sponges or wipes, if indicated.

When a mechanical bowel preparation is to be used, a review of the prep protocol should be performed along with assurance that the patient has the necessary prescription for the mechanical prep. Instructions should be given during preoperative assessment on the amount of time the patient is not to take any liquids or solids by mouth (NPO). A decrease in traditional NPO time is preferable, allowing clear liquids up to 2 hours prior to surgery. In addition, carbohydrate drink recommendations are supplied for carbohydrate loading on the morning of surgery.

Intraoperative ERAS Component

On the day of the procedure, it is important to identify and document any patient who will be included in the protocol. As per the protocol, initiate antibiotic prophylaxis and antithrombotic medications and apply pneumatic leg compression devices. Additional medications for the prevention of postoperative ileus such as alvimopan are also administered at this time.

The intraoperative anesthesia management of the ERAS protocol centers on not using sedative medications prior to the surgery. Typically, an epidural catheter is placed and epidural analgesia is used throughout the operative procedure, and opioids are avoided if possible. Goal-directed perioperative fluid management is also employed in an attempt to avoid giving the patient excessive crystalloid fluid, as this can contribute to postoperative ileus. In addition, antiemetic prophylaxis is typically given at the conclusion of the case in order to facilitate early resumption of oral intake.

The surgical portion of the protocol concentrates on minimally invasive surgery, with laparoscopy or robotic surgery. When laparoscopic operative principals are combined with ERAS, 60% of CRS patients can be discharged within 72 hours [120]. The incisions should be infiltrated with local anesthesia prior to making the incision. Drains should not be used routinely and any gastric tube should be removed at the conclusion of the case.

Postoperative ERAS Component

The postoperative care centers on early mobilization of the patient in an attempt to return them to a more functional status. The epidural catheter is used for postoperative analgesia, typically for at least the first 48 hours following the surgery. Intravenous ketorolac or acetaminophen is commonly used while the patient is transitioned to oral nonsteroidal antiinflammatory medications as soon as possible, again trying to avoid narcotics, in an effort to reduce postoperative ileus and postoperative nausea and vomiting (PONV).

The postoperative care includes early initiation of oral feeding in conjunction with the discontinuation of routine intravenous fluids a few hours after the surgery. The patient is allowed liquids shortly after the surgery, often with protein supplementation. The IV fluids are discontinued in the recovery room or shortly after arrival to the patient floor.

Early mobilization and assisted ambulation is encouraged within 2 to 4 hours postoperatively. The first postoperative day the patient is encouraged to spend 8 hours out of bed and to begin take meals, consisting of light semisolid food seated out of bed.

The Foley catheter is typically discontinued on the first postoperative day, except in the case of low pelvic operations, when it is left in place for an additional few days. The discharge criteria are unchanged from any other operative procedure. Patients can be safely discharged to home when they are taking oral food without nausea and their pain is controlled with oral medication.

ERSA Protocol Failure

It is obvious that whatever components make up the protocol, it may not work in every patient. Due to the number of variables, it is impossible to determine the contribution of each individual facet to either ultimate success or failure. It is possible to determine which facets are less likely to be followed and which are more likely to result in failure of the protocol.

One study looking at almost 20 facets of different ERAS protocols found that none of the published studies used the same variables. This obviously makes it difficult to establish superiority of one over another. What was found, not surprisingly, was that compliance was poorest during the postoperative period [120]. The postoperative component is the longest period and is the period that is subject to most variability, emphasizing the need for multidisciplinary team management and monitoring of protocol compliance. In a randomized trial comparing colectomy coupled with or without ERAS, the combination of LS with ERAS protocols resulted in superior results with a shorter hospital stay [121].

A study of patient postoperative needs assessment following discharge to home utilizing ERAS guidelines indicated that receiving this information was vital as patients attempted to regain control over their life after surgery during transition from hospital to home. These variables varied from hospital to site of transition. This suggests an even greater need for patients to receive information preoperatively but also reinforcement of the goals of the protocol throughout their hospital stay and the importance of monitoring their understanding of those goals [122].

Muller et al. in 2009 found that fluid administration greater than the restricted limits and a nonfunctioning epidural analgesia were independent predictors of postoperative complications and fast-track failure [123]. In fact, failure to follow the established protocol rather than any patient factors was the predictor of ERAS protocol failure. Deviations of the protocol at the end of the first postoperative day – for example, continuing intravenous fluid infusion, lack of functioning epidural, inadequate mobilization and ambulation, vomiting, and/or reinsertion of a Foley catheter – are all strongly associated with a delay in discharge and an increase in LOS in several studies [124–126].

ERSA protocols are successful when adequate patient education is given, minimally invasive surgical techniques are used, postoperative nausea is prevented, and excessive intravenous fluid administration is avoided.

ERAS Prevention of Ileus and PONV

Several of the ERAS facets are designed to minimize ileus and subsequent PONV. Refraining from the routine use of nasogastric tubes, early ambulation, and avoiding narcotic analgesia are all used in an attempt to facilitate normal intestinal function. Initiation of antiemetic premedication and continued use in ERAS protocols has become standard at many institutions because of their efficacy of prevention of PONV. Despite these measures, postoperative ileus and PONV continues to be a significant problem in postoperative abdominal surgery patients [127–130].

Alvimopan

The ERAS protocols were begun well before the introduction of Alvimopan, which was approved for use in the United States in 2008. Since that time, the medication has been commonly adopted into ERAS protocols with some positive results [131]. Alvimopan is a mu-opioid receptor antagonist, which blocks the constipating effects of narcotic medication without compromising any analgesic effect. Alvimopan has been demonstrated to lower the incidence of postoperative ileus following gastrointestinal surgery. Several studies have demonstrated that Alvimopan is useful in accelerating GI recovery and hospital discharge after laparoscopic and open abdominal surgery and may be effective in lowering hospital costs [132].

A 2015 meta-analysis of five studies indicated that the use of Alvimopan in the perioperative period showed a relative risk reduction (>75%) in postoperative ileus when compared to placebo [133]. Twelve milligrams of Alvimopan is administered to patients throughout the perioperative recovery until discharge, a component of an ERAS protocol for patients undergoing abdominal surgery [131–133].

ERAS Fluid Management

The administration of excessive amounts of crystalloid fluid both during intraoperative and postoperative periods is common in the management of patients undergoing elective abdominal surgery. Intraoperative and postoperative oliguria is common, especially in LS, and the traditionally employed monitoring of urine output has been demonstrated to be an inaccurate measurement of overall fluid status [134–136]. The goal is to have a hydrated, euvolemic patient at the beginning of the surgery in order to achieve a zero fluid balance by the end of surgery. The postoperative goal of a balanced oral intake without the addition of intravenous fluid infusions will achieve the end result of euvolemia of the patient throughout the perioperative period.

Through the use of ERAS protocols, it has been demonstrated that patients do better clinically if the goal of directed fluid management is utilized and maintained throughout the perioperative period. Fluid management begins in decreasing the time a patient is required to be NPO prior to the surgery. Most ERAS protocols decrease the time that a patient must refrain from oral intake and actually encourage patients to drink clear liquids up to 2 hours prior to the induction of anesthesia. In addition, patients are given or instructed to consume carbohydrate drinks the morning of surgery.

Carbohydrate Drinks

The addition of carbohydrate or protein supplementation on the morning of surgery has become a common component of ERAS protocols. Initial studies involving patients who were given a carbohydrate drink prior to elective surgery demonstrated a reduction in insulin sensitivity [137]. The utilization of patients taking carbohydrate drinks preoperatively led to better glucose homeostasis as well as grip strength during the postoperative period [138].

In a systemic review of 17 RCTs involving 1,445 patients, preoperative carbohydrate drinks significantly improved insulin resistance and some indices of patient comfort following surgery, including hunger, thirst, malaise, anxiety, and nausea [139]. A Cochrane review of RCTs of preoperative carbohydrate treatment did find that despite a high risk of bias due to inadequate blinding in most of the studies, there was a small reduction in hospital LOS. It also indicated that preoperative carbohydrate treatment did not increase complication rates, especially of aspiration pneumonitis [140].

Goal-Directed Fluid Therapy

There are numerous methods of perioperative fluid management and one approach is fluid-restrictive therapy. A 1 L crystalloid bolus is administered in the preoperative holding area and continues to be infused during induction. After induction the bolus injection is stopped.. The remainder of the operation uses a rate of 3 mL/kg/h, using the patient's lean body weight, to a maximum of 240 mL/h.

If an esophageal Doppler is to be used, it is placed after induction, and an initial SV is calculated. After pneumoperitoneum is established, a 250 mL colloid bolus is given over 15 min. If the SV increases by >10%, then the patient is intravascularly depleted and a repeat bolus should be given. If the SV is unchanged or actually decreases, then the patient should be considered to be euvolemic, as any additional fluid does not result in an improvement in CO. There are other methods of noninvasive monitoring during surgery, but no one method has proven superiority [141].

Analgesia Management

Adequate postoperative analgesia is another critical component of ERAS protocols. While the use of an epidural catheter has demonstrated effectiveness, they can at times be difficult to place, can be time-consuming, and have variable success. It is important for the team to be familiar with and include alternative pain management techniques within any ERAS pathway.

Liposomal Bupivacaine

The introduction of bupivacaine liposome injectable suspension has been used with some success as a component of a perioperative analgesia regimen. Patients who had liposomal bupivacaine infiltrated preoperatively in the operative sites had lower postoperative pain scores and a decreased use of opioid narcotics [142].

Transversus Adbominis Plane Block

The transversus adbominis plane (TAP) block is a peripheral nerve block, which functions to anaesthetize the abdominal wall. There is limited evidence that TAP block reduces opioid consumption and pain scores after abdominal surgery as compared to no intervention or placebo [143]. Nine studies (including published and unpublished data), containing a total of 413 patients, indicated that cumulative morphine utilization was significantly reduced following TAP block [143]. While there are no studies that compared TAP block with epidural analgesia directly, a meta-analysis of all relevant RCTs comparing the efficacy of TAP block with local infiltration of local anesthesia was performed. The patients in the TAP block group had lower pain scores 24 hours postoperatively when compared with the local anesthesia infiltration group; at rest and with movement also, the TAP block group demonstrated better long-lasting effect [143].

Conclusion

This chapter has covered a broad topic on robotic surgery being utilized in the realm of abdominopelvic procedures in GS and CRS. The preoperative section discussed the importance of the physiologic effects of pneumoperitoneum and radical patient positioning that is required in order to perform complex surgical procedures. These are difficulties that our anesthesia colleagues have had to conform and learn under a much higher level of stress in order to manage our patients in an entirely different environment. And they have been performed at the highest level of patient management.

The chapter has pointed out the advantages of robotic platforms over laparoscopic platforms for very complex procedures. The development of a "wrist-like" motion and visual acuity of the robotic technology have stimulated surgeons to successfully incorporate complex abdominopelvic procedures into their armamentarium of techniques which has led to less complications and a comparable decrease in hospital stays in many cases as compared to other minimally invasive techniques. Then, incorporating the ERAS protocols in the postoperative management of their patients has enhanced early discharge and patient satisfaction. The ERAS protocols have shown benefit in patients undergoing abdominal surgery. These protocols can be labor-intensive, but they have a documented benefit with a reduced length of hospital stay without a concomitant increase in readmission or complications. Minimally invasive techniques such as robotic surgery play a key role in these protocols. While no two protocols will be identical as each is developed within the hospital and system in which they are to function, their development requires multidisciplinary input from both surgeons and anesthesiologists using evidence-based methods.

References

1. Kwoh YS, Hou J, Honckheere EA, Hayati S. A robot with improved absolute positioning accuracy for CT guided stereotactic brain surgery. *IEEE Trans Biomed Engineering* 1988; 35(2): 152–160.
2. Sackier JM, Wang Y. Robotically assisted laparoscopic surgery: from concept to development. *Surg Endosc* 1994; 8: 63–66.
3. Marescaux J, Rubino F. The ZEUS robotic system: experimental and clinical applications. *Surg Clin North Am* 2003; 83(6): 1305–1315.
4. Ballantyne GH, Moll F. The da Vinci telerobotic surgical system: the virtual operative field and telepresence surgery. *Surg Clin North Am* 2003; 83(6): 1293–1304.
5. Samarasekera D, Kaouk JH. Robotic single port surgery: current status and future considerations. *Indian J Urol* 2014; 30(3): 326–332.
6. Joseph RA, Goh AC, Cuevas SP, et al. Chopstick surgery: a novel technique improves surgeon performance and eliminates arm collision in robotic single-incision laparoscopic surgery. *Surg Endosc* 2010; 24.
7. Lasser MS, Patel CK, Elsamra SE, et al. Dedicated robotics team reduces pre-surgical preparation time. *Indian J Urol* 2012; 28(3): 263–266.
8. Mühlmann G, Klaus A, Kirchmayr W, et al. DaVinci robotic-assisted laparoscopic bariatric surgery: is it justified in a routine setting? *Obes Surg* 2003; 13(6): 848–854.
9. Delaney CP, Lynch AC, Senagore AJ, et al. Comparison of robotically performed and traditional laparoscopic colorectal surgery. *Dis Colon Rectum* 2003; 46(12): 1633–1639.
10. Danic MJ, Chow M, Alexander G, et al. Anesthesia considerations for robotic-assisted laparoscopic

prostatectomy: a review of 1,500 cases. *J Robotic Surg* 2007; 1(2): 119–123.

11. Gainsburg DM. Anesthetic concerns for robotic-assisted laparoscopic radical prostatectomy. *Minerva Anestesiol* 2012; 78(5): 596–604.
12. Yoo YC, Kim NY, Shin S, et al. The intraocular pressure under deep versus moderate neuromuscular blockade during low-pressure robotic assisted laparoscopic radical prostatectomy in a randomized trial. *PLoS ONE* 2015; 10(8): e0135412.
13. Madsen MV, Istre O, Staehr-Rye AK, et al. Postoperative shoulder pain after laparoscopic hysterectomy with deep neuromuscular blockage and low-pressure pneumoperitoneum. *Eur J Anaesthesiol* 2015; 32: 1–7.
14. Madsen MV, Gatke MR, Springborg HH, et al. Optimizing abdominal space with deep neuromuscular blockade in gynaecologic laparoscopy – a randomized, blinded crossover study. *Acta Anaesthesiologica Scandinavica* 2015; 59(4): 441–447.
15. Van Wijk RM, Watts RW, Ledowski T, et al. Deep neuromuscular block reduces intra-abdominal pressure requirements during laparoscopic cholecystectomy: a prospective observational study. *Acta Anaesthesiologica Scandinavica* 2015; 59(4): 434–440.
16. Hsu RL, Kaye AD, Urman RD Anesthetic challenges in robotic-assisted urologic surgery. *Rev Urol* 2013; 15(4): 178–184.
17. Lee, JR. Anesthetic considerations for robotic surgery. *Korean J Anesthesiol* 2014; 33(1): 3–11.
18. Rencuzogullari A, Gorgun E. Robotic rectal surgery. *J Surg Onc* 2015; 112(3): 326–331.
19. Song J, Kang WH, Oh SJ, et al. Role of robotic gastrectomy using da Vinci system compared with laparoscopic gastrectomy: initial experience of 20 consecutive cases. *Surg Endosc* 2009; 23(6): 1204–1211.
20. Koc G, Tazeh NN, Joudi FN, et al. Lower extremity neuropathies after robot-assisted laparoscopic prostatectomy on a split-leg table. *J Endourol* 2012; 26(8): 1026–1029.
21. Wexner SD, Bergamaschi R, Lacy A, et al. The current status of robotic pelvic surgery: results of a multinational interdisciplinary consensus conference. *Surg Endosc* 2009; 23(2): 438–443.
22. Awad H, Walker CM, Shaikh M, et al. Anesthetic considerations for robotic prostatectomy: a review of the literature. *J Clin Anes* 2012; 24(6): 494–504.
23. Zimmern A, Prasad L, deSouza A, et al. Robotic colon and rectal surgery: a series of 131 cases. *World J Surg* 2010; 34(8): 1954–1958.
24. Di Pierro GB, Wirth JG, Ferrai M, et al. Impact of a single-surgeon learning curve on complications, positioning injuries, and renal function in patients undergoing robot-assisted radical prostatectomy and extended pelvic lymph node dissection. *Urology* 2014; 84(5): 1106–1111.
25. Balick-Weber CC, Nicolas P, Hedreville-Montout M, et al. Respiratory and haemodynamic effects of volume-controlled vs. pressure-controlled ventilation during laparoscopy: a cross-over study with echocardiographic assessment. *Br J Anaesth* 2007; 99(3): 429–435.
26. Choi EM, Na S, Choi SH, et al. Comparison of volume-controlled and pressure-controlled ventilation in steep Trendelenburg position for robot-assisted laparoscopic radical prostatectomy. *J Clin Anesth* 2011; 23(3): 183–188.
27. Jobe BA, Hunter JG. Minimally invasive surgery: In *Schwartz's principles of surgery, eighth edition.* New York: McGraw-Hill, 2005, pp. 379–401.
28. Sood J. Advancing frontiers in anaesthesiology with laparoscopy. *World J Gastroenterol* 2014; 20(39): 14308–14314.
29. Neudecker J, Sauerland S, Neugebauer EAM, et al. The EAES clinical practice guidelines on the pneumoperitoneum for laparoscopic surgery. *Surg Endosc* 2002; 16(7): 1121–1143.
30. Meininger D, Byhahn C, Wolfram M, et al. Prolonged intraperitoneal versus extraperitoneal insufflation of carbon dioxide in patients undergoing totally endoscopic robot-assisted radical prostatectomy. *Surg Endosc* 2004; 18(5): 829–833.
31. Sumpf E, Crozier TA, Ahrens D, et al. Carbon dioxide absorption during extraperitoneal and transperitoneal endoscopic hernioplasty. *Anesth Analg* 2000; 91(3): 589–595.
32. Lestar M, Gunnarsson L, Lagerstrand L, et al. Hemodynamic perturbations during robot-assisted laparoscopic radical prostatectomy in 45° Trendelenburg position. *Anesth Analg* 2011; 113(5): 1069–1075.
33. Kearon C, Kahn SR, Agnelli G, et al. Antithrombotic therapy for venous thromboembolic disease: *American College of Chest Physicians Evidence-Based Clinical Practice Guidelines* (8th Edition). *Chest* 2008; 133(6 suppl): 454S–545S.
34. Moghadamyeghaneh Z, Hanna MH, Carmichael JC, et al. A nationwide analysis of postoperative deep vein thrombosis and pulmonary embolism in colon and rectal surgery. *J Gastrointest Surg* 2014; 18(12): 2169–2177.
35. Falabella A, Moore-Jeffries E, Sullivan MJ, et al. Cardiac function during steep Trendelenburg position

and CO2 pneumoperitoneum for robotic-assisted prostatectomy: a transoesophageal Doppler probe study. *Int J Med Robotics Comput Assist Surg* 2007; 3(4): 312–315.

36. Haas S, Haese A, Goetz AE, et al. Haemodynamics and cardiac function during robotic-assisted laparoscopic prostatectomy in steep Trendelenburg position. *Int J Med Robotics Comput Assist Surg* 2011; 7(4): 408–413.
37. Joris JL, Noirot DP, Legrand MJ, et al. Hemodynamic changes during laparoscopic cholecystectomy. *Anesth Analg* 1993; 76(5): 1067–1071.
38. Speicher PJ, Fanapathi AM, Englum BR, et al. Laparoscopy is safe among patients with congestive heart failure undergoing general surgery procedures. *Surgery* 2014; 156(2): 371–378.
39. Kalmar AF, Dewaele F, Foubert L, et al. Cerebral haemodynamic physiology during steep Trendelenburg position and CO_2 pneumoperitoneum. *Br J Anaesth* 2012; 108(3): 478–484.
40. Closhen D, Treiber AH, Berres M, et al. Robotic assisted prostatic surgery in the Trendelenburg position does not impair cerebral oxygenation measured using two different monitors: a clinical observational study. *Eur J Anaesthesiol* 2014; 31(2): 104–109.
41. Kukahvecioglu O, Sare M, Karamercan A, et al. Intermittent pneumatic sequential compression of the lower extremities restores cerebral oxygen saturation during laparoscopic cholecystectomy. *Surg Endosc* 2008; 22(4): 907–911.
42. Jo YY, Kim JY, Lee MG, et al. Changes in cerebral oxygen saturation and early postoperative cognitive function after laparoscopic gastrectomy: a comparison with conventional open surgery. *Korean J Anesthesiol* 2016; 69(1): 44–50.
43. Bishara B, Karram T, Khatib S, et al. Impact of pneumoperitoneum on renal perfusion and excretory function: beneficial effects of nitroglycerine. *Surg Endosc* 2009; 23(3): 568–576.
44. Dolkart O, Khoury W, Amar E, et al. Pneumoperitoneum in the presence of acute and chronic kidney injury: an experimental model in rats. *Urology* 2014; 192 (4): 1266–1271.
45. Wiesenthal JD, Fazio LM, Perks AE, et al. Effect of pneumoperitoneum on renal tissue oxygenation and blood flow in a rat model. *Urology* 2011; 77(6): 1508. e9–e15.
46. Mattei A, Di Pierro GB, Rafeld V et al. Positioning injury, rhbadomyolysis, and serum creatine kinase-concentration course in patients undergoing robot-assisted radical prostatectomy and extended pelvic lymph node dissection. *J Endo Urology* 2013; 27(1): 45–51.
47. Park EY, Kwon JY, Kim KJ. Carbon dioxide embolism during laparoscopic surgery. *Yonsei Med J* 2012; 53(3): 459–466.
48. Ahmad G, Gent D, Henderson D, et al. Laparoscopic entry techniques. *Cochrane Database of Systemic Reviews* 2015; 8.
49. Molloy BL. Implications for postoperative visual loss: steep Trendelenburg position and effects on intraocular pressure. *AANA J* 2011; 79(2): 115.
50. Reynolds Jr. W. The first laparoscopic cholecystectomy. *JSLS* 2001; 5: 89–94.
51. Litynski GS. Erich Mühe and the rejection of laparoscopic cholecystectomy (1985): a surgeon ahead of his time. *JSLS* 1998; 2: 341–346.
52. Himpens J, Leman G, Cadiere GB. Telesurgical laparoscopic cholecystectomy. *Surg Endosc* 1998; 12(8): 1091.
53. Kornprat P, Werkartner G, Cerwenka H, et al. Prospective study comparing standard and robotically assisted laparoscopic cholecystectomy. *Lagenbecks Arch Surg* 2006; 391: 216–221.
54. Nio D, Bemelman WA, Busch OR, et al. Robot-assisted laparoscopic cholecystectomy versus conventional laparoscopic cholecystectomy: a comparative study. *Surg Endosc* 2004; 18: 379–382.
55. Kim JH, Baek NH, Guangyl LI, et al. Robotic cholecystectomy with new port sites. *World J Gastroenterol* 2013; 19(20): 3077–3082.
56. Jayaraman S, Davies W, Schlachta C. Getting started with robotics in general surgery with cholecystectomy: the Canadian experience. *J Can Chir* 2009; 52(5): 374–378.
57. Cadiere GB, Himpens J, Germay O, et al. Feasibility of robotic laparoscopic surgery: 146 cases. *World J Surg* 2001: 16: 1187–1191.
58. Ruurda JP, Broeders IA, Simmermacher RP, et al. Feasibility of robotic-assisted laparoscopic surgery: an evaluation of 35 robotic-assisted laparoscopic cholecystectomies. *Surg Laprarosc Endosc Percutan Tech* 2002; 12: 41–45.
59. Giulianotte PC, Coratti A, Angelini M, et al. Robotics in general surgery: personal experience in a large community hospital. *Arch Surg* 2003; 138: 777–784.
60. Vidovszky TJ, Smith W, Ghosh J, et al. Robotic cholecystectomy: learning curve, advantages and limitations. *J Surg Res* 2006; 136: 172–178.
61. Navarra G, Pozza I, Occhionorelli S, Carcoforo P, Donini I. One-wound laparoscopic cholecystectomy. *Br J Surg* 1997; 84: 695.
62. Chamberlin RS, Sakpal SV. A comprehensive review of single-incision laparoscopic surgery (SILS) and

natural orifice transluminal endoscopic surgery (NOTES) techniques for cholecystectomy. *J Gastrointest Surg* 2009; 13: 1733–1740.

63. Spinoglio G, Priora F, Bianchi PP, et al. Real-time near-infrared (NIR) fluorescent cholangiography in single-site robotic cholecystectomy (SSRC): a single-institutional prospective study. *Surg Endosc* 2013; 27: 2156–2162.
64. Morel P, Hagan ME, Bucher P, Buchs NC, Pugin F. Robotic single-port cholecystectomy using a new platform: initial clinical experience. *J Gasrtoint Surg* 2011; 15: 2182–2186.
65. Spinoglio G, Lenti LM, Maglione V, et al. Single-site robotic cholecystectomy (SSRC) versus single-incision laparoscopic cholecystectomy (SILC): comparison of learning curves. First European experience. *Surg Endosc* 2012; 26: 1648–1655.
66. Lee SH, Jung MJ, Hwang HK et al. The first experiences of robotic single-site cholecystectomy in Asia: a potential way to expand minimally-invasive single-site surgery? *Yousei Med J* 2015; 56(1): 189–195.
67. Buschs NC, Hage ME, Pugin F, et al. Intra-operative fluorescent cholangiography using indocyanine green during robotic single site cholecystectomy. *Int J Med Robot* 2012; 8: 436–440.
68. Marano A, Priora F, Lenti LM et al. Application of fluorescence in robotic general surgery: review of the literature and state of the art. *World J Surg*. 2013; 37: 2800–2811.
69. Parra-Membrives P, Diaz-Gomez D, Vilegas-Portero R, et al. Appropriate management of common bile duct stones: a RAND Corporation/UCLA appropriateness method statistical analysis. *Surg Endosc* 2010; 24: 1187–1194.
70. Alkhamesi NA, Davies WT, Pinto RF, Schlachta CM. Robot-assisted common bile duct exploration as an option for complex choledocholithiasis. *Surg Endosc* 2013; 27: 263–266.
71. Milone L, Daskalaki D, Fernandes E, et al. State of art in robotic hepatobiliary surgery. *World J Surg* 2013; 37: 2747–2755.
72. Rosemurgy A, Ryan C, Klein R, et al. Does the cost of robotic cholecystectomy translate to a financial burden? *Surg Endosc* 2015; 29: 2115–2120.
73. Cheriqui D, Husson E, Hammond R, et al. Laparoscopic liver resections: a feasibility study in 30 patients. *Ann Surg* 2000; 232: 753–762.
74. Cheng-Maw H, Wakabayashi G, Nitta H, et al. Systematic review of robotic liver resection. *Surg Endosc* 2013; 27: 732–739.
75. Milone L, Daskalaki D, Fernandes, E et al. State of the art in robotic hepatobiliary surgery. *World J Surg* 2013; 37: 2747–2755.
76. Leung U, Fong Y. Robotic liver surgery. *Hepatobiliary Surg Nutr* 2014; 3(5): 288–294.
77. Giulianotte PC, Sbrana F, Bianco FM, et al. Robot-assisted laparoscopic pancreatic surgery: single-surgeon experience. *Surg Endosc* 2010; 24: 1646–1657.
78. Adachi Y, Shiraishi N, Shiromizu A, et al. Laparoscopy-assisted Billroth I gastrectomy compared with conventional open gastrectomy. *Arch Surg* 135: 806–810.
79. Song J, Kang WH, Oh SJ, et al. Role of robotic gastrectomy using da Vinci system compared with laparoscopic gastrectomy: initial experience of 20 consecutive cases. *Surg Endosc* 2009; 23: 1204–1211.
80. Shen WS, Xi HQ, Chen L, A meta-analysis of robotic versus laparoscopic gastrectomy for gastric cancer. *Surg Endosc* 2014; 28: 2795–2802.
81. Shen W, Xi H, Wei B, et al. Robotic versus laparoscopic gastrectomy for gastric cancer: comparison of short-term surgical outcomes. *Surg Endosc* 2016; 30: 574–580.
82. Gamme G, Birch DW, Karmali S, et al. Minimally invasive splenectomy: an update and review. *Can J of Surg* 2013: 56: 280–285.
83. Vasilescu C, Stanciulea O, Tudor S. Laparoscopic versus robotic subtotal splenectomy in hereditary spherocytosis. Potential advantages and limits of and expensive approach. *Surg Endosc* 2012; 26: 2802–2809.
84. Balaphas A, Buchs NC, Meyer J, et al. Partial splenectomy in the era of minimally invasive surgery: the current laparoscopic and robotic experiences. *Surg Endosc* 2015; 29: 3618–3627.
85. Jacobs M, Verdeja JC, Goldstein HS. Minimally invasive colon resection (laparoscopic colectomy). *Surgical Laparoscopy & Endoscopy* 1991; 1(3): 144–150.
86. Weber PA, Meorola S, Wasielewski A, et al. Telerobotic assisted laparoscopic right and sigmoid colectomies for benign disease. *Dis Colon Rectum* 2002; 45: 1689–1694.
87. Jayne DG, Guillou PJ, Thorpe H, et al. Randomized trial of laparoscopic-assisted versus open surgery for colorectal carcinoma: 3-year results of the UK MRC CLASICC Trial group. *J Clin Oncol* 2007; 25(21): 3061–3068.
88. Jayne DG, Thorpe HC, Copeland J, et al. Five-year follow-up of the Medical Research Council CLASSICC Trial of laparoscopically assisted versus open surgery for colorectal cancer. *Br J Surgery* 2010; 97(11): 1638–1645.

89. Fleishman JW, Nelson H, Peters AR, et al. Early results of laparoscopic surgery for colorectal cancer: retrospective analysis of 372 patients treated by Clinical Outcomes of Surgical Therapy (COST) study group. *Dis Colon Rectum* 1996; 39(10): 545–551.

90. Peterson C, Weiser MR, Robotic colorectal surgery. *J Gastrointest Surg* 2014; 18: 398–403.

91. Kim CW, Kim CH, Baik SH, Outcomes of robotic-assisted colorectal surgery compared with laparoscopic and open surgery: a systematic review. *J Gastrointest Surg* 2014; 18: 816–830.

92. Xiong B, Ma L, Huang W, et al. Robotic versus laparoscopic total mesorectal excision for rectal cancer: a meta-analysis of eight studies. *J Gastrointest Surg* 2015; 19: 516–526.

93. Fleishman J, Branda M, Sargent D, et al. Effect of laparoscopic-assisted resection vs. open resection of stage II or stage III rectal cancer on pathological outcomes. The ACOSOG Z6051 randomized clinical trial. *JAMA* 2015; 314(13): 1346–1355.

94. Stevenson ARL, Solomon MJ, Lumley JW, et al. Effect of laparoscopic-assisted resection vs. open resection on pathological outcomes in rectal cancer. The ALaCaRT randomized clinical trial. *JAMA* 2015; 314(13): 1356–1563.

95. McDonald R. Enhanced recovery clinical education program improves quality of post-operative care. *BMJ Qual Improv Rep*. 2015; 4(1).

96. Bagnall NM, Malietzis G, Kennedy RH, et al. A systematic review of enhanced recovery care after colorectal surgery in elderly patients. *Colorectal Dis* 2014; 16(12): 947–956.

97. Kehlet H, Mogensen T. Hospital stay of 2 days after open sigmoidectomy with a multimodal rehabilitation program. *Br J Surg* 1999; 86: 227–230.

98. Rawlinson A, Kang P, Evans J, Khanna A. A systematic review of enhanced recovery protocols in colorectal surgery. *Ann R. Coll Surg Engl* 2011; 93(8): 583–588.

99. Wang G, Jiang Z, Zhao K, Li G, Liu F, Pan H, Li J. Immunologic response after laparoscopic colon cancer operation within an enhanced recovery program. *J Gastrointest Surg* 2012; 16: 1379–1388.

100. Maessen J, Dejong CH, Hausel J, et al. A protocol is not enough to implement an enhanced recovery programs for colorectal resection. *Br J Surg* 2007; 94: 224–231.

101. Bona S, Molteni M, Rosati R, et al. Introducing an enhanced recovery after surgery program in colorectal surgery: a single center experience. *World J Gastroenterol* 2014; 20(46): 17578–17587.

102. Keane C, Savage S, McFarlane K, et al. Enhanced recovery after surgery versus conventional care in colonic and rectal surgery. *ANZ J Surg* 2012; 82(10): 697–703.

103. Zhuang CL, Ye XZ, Zhang XD, et al. Enhanced recovery after surgery programs versus traditional care for colorectal surgery: a meta-analysis of randomized controlled trials. *Dis Colon Rectum* 2013; 56(5): 667–678.

104. Miller TE, Thacker JK, White WD, et al. Enhanced Recovery Study Group. Reduced length of hospital stay in colorectal surgery after implementation of an enhanced recovery protocol. *Anesth Analg* 2014; 118(5): 966–975.

105. Varadhan KK, Neal KR, Dejong CH, et al. The enhanced recovery after surgery (ERAS) pathway for patients undergoing major elective open colorectal surgery: a meta-analysis of randomized controlled trials. *Clin Nutr* 2010; 29(4): 434–440.

106. Geltzeiler CB, Rotramel A, Wilson C, et al. Prospective study of colorectal enhanced recovery after surgery in a community hospital. *JAMA Surg* 2014; 149(9): 955–961.

107. Eskicioglu C, Forbes SS, Aarts MA, Okrainec A, McLeod RS. Enhanced recovery after surgery (ERAS) programs for patients having colorectal surgery: a meta-analysis of randomized trials. *J Gastrointest Surg* 2009; 13(12): 2321–2329.

108. Lv L, Shao YF, Zhou YB. The enhanced recovery after surgery (ERAS) pathway for patients undergoing colorectal surgery: an update of meta-analysis of randomized controlled trials. *Int J Colorectal Dis* 2012; 27(12): 1549–1554.

109. Greco M, Capretti G, Beretta L, et al. Enhanced recovery program in colorectal surgery: a meta-analysis of randomized controlled trials. *World J Surg* 2014; 38(6): 1531–1541.

110. Spanjersberg WR, Reurings J, Keus F, vanLaarhoven CJ. Fast track surgery versus conventional recovery strategies for colorectal surgery. *Cochrane Database Syst Rev* 2011; (2).

111. Barreca M, Renzi C, Tankel J, et al. Is there a role for enhanced recovery after laparoscopic bariatric surgery? Preliminary results from a specialist obesity treatment center. *Surg Obes Relat Dis* 2015; pii: S1550-7289(15)00063-5.

112. Miralpeix E, Nick AM, Cata J, et al. A call for new standard of care in perioperative gynecologic oncology practice: impact of enhanced recovery after surgery (ERAS) programs. *Gynecol Oncol* 2016.

113. Nelson G, Kalpgera E, Dowdy SC. Enhanced recovery pathways in gynecologic oncology. *Gynecol Oncol* 2014; 135(3): 586–594.

114. Hahl T, Peromaa-Haavisto P, Tarkiainen P, Knutar O, Victorzon M. Outcomes of laparoscopic gastric bypass (LRYGB) with a program for enhanced recovery after surgery (ERAS). *Obes Surg* 2016; 26(3): 505–511.

115. Baldini G, Fawcett WJ. Anesthesia for colorectal surgery. *Anesthesiol Clin* 2015; 33(1): 93–123.

116. Fearon KC, Ljungqvist O, VonMeyenfeldt M, et al. Enhanced recovery after surgery: a consensus review of clinical care for patients undergoing colonic resection. *Clin Nutr* 2005; 24(3): 466–477.

117. Lassen K, Soop M, Nygren J, et al; Enhanced Recovery After Surgery (ERAS) Group. Consensus review of optimal perioperative care in colorectal surgery: Enhanced Recovery After Surgery (ERAS) Group recommendations. *Arch Surg* 2009; 144(10): 961–969.

118. Chand M, DeAth HD, Rasheed S, et al. The influence of peri-operative factors for accelerated discharge following laparoscopic colorectal surgery when combined with an enhanced recovery after surgery (ERAS) pathway. *Int J Surg* 2015; 25: 59–63.

119. Ahmed J, Khan S, Lim M, et al. Enhanced recovery after surgery protocols – compliance and variations in practice during routine colorectal surgery. *Colorectal Dis* 2012; 14(9): 1045–1051.

120. Vlug MS, Wind J, Hollmann MW, et al. Laparoscopy in combination with fast track multimodal management is the best perioperative strategy in patients undergoing colonic surgery: a randomized clinical trial (LAFA-study). *Ann Surg* 2011; 254: 868–875.

121. Lithner M, Klefsgard R, Johansson J, Andersson E. The significance of information after discharge for colorectal cancer surgery-a qualitative study. *BMC Nurs* 2015; 14: 36.

122. Muller S, Zalunardo MP, Hubner M, et al. A fast-track program reduces complications and length of hospital stay after open colonic surgery. *Gastroenterology* 2009; 136: 842–847.

123. Smart NJ, White P, Allison AS, et al. Deviation and failure of enhanced recovery after surgery following laparoscopic colorectal surgery: early prediction model. *Colorectal Dis* 2012; 14(10): e727–734.

124. Aarts MA, Okrainec A, Glicksman A, et al. Adoption of enhanced recovery after surgery (ERAS) strategies for colorectal surgery at academic teaching hospitals and impact on total length of hospital stay. *Surg Endosc* 2012; 26(2): 442–450.

125. Erhan Y, Erhan E, Aydede H, Yumus O, Yentur A. Ondansetron, granisetron and dexamethasone compared for the prevention of postoperative nausea and vomiting in patients undergoing laparoscopic cholecystectomy: a randomized placebo-controlled study. *Surg Endosc* 2008; 22(6): 1487–1492.

126. Fujii Y, Itakura M. Reduction of postoperative nausea, vomiting and analgesic requirement with dexamethasone for patients undergoing laparoscopic cholecystectomy. *Surg Endosc* 2010; 24(3): 692.

127. Cox F. Systematic review of ondansetron for the prevention and treatment of postoperative nausea and vomiting in adults. *Br J Theatre Nurs* 1999; 9(12): 556–563.

128. Bragg D, El-Sharkaway AM, Psaltis E, Maxwell-Armstrong CA, Lobo DN. Poatoperative ileus: recent developments in pathophysiology and management. *Clin Nutr* 2015; 34(3): 367–376.

129. Vaughan-Shaw PG, Fecher IC, Harris S, Knight JS. A meta-analysis of the effectiveness of the opioid receptor antagonist alvimopan in reducing hospital length of stay and time to GI recovery in patients enrolled in a standardized accelerated recovery program after abdominal surgery. *Dis Colon Rectum* 2012; 55(5): 611–620.

130. Earnshaw SR, Kauf TL, McDade C, et al. Economic impact of Alvimopan considering varying definitions of postoperative ileus. *J Am Coll Surg* 2015; 221(5): 941–950.

131. Nguyen DL, Maithel S, Nguyen ET, Bechtold ML. Does alvimopan enhance return of bowel function in laparoscopic gastrointestinal surgery? A meta-analysis. *Ann Gastroenterol* 2015; 28(4): 475–480

132. Matot I, Paskaleva R, Eid L, et al. Effect of the volume of fluids administered on intraoperative oliguria in laparoscopic bariatric surgery: a randomized controlled trial. *Arch Surg* 2012; 147(3): 228–234.

133. Gupta R, Gan TJ. Peri-operative fluid management to enhance recovery. *Anaesthesia* 2016; 71 suppl 1: 40–45.

134. Wool DB, Lemmens HJ, Brodsky JB, et al. Intraoperative fluid replacement and postoperative creatine phosphokinase levels in laparoscopic bariatric patients. *Obes Surg.* 2010; 20(6): 698–701.

135. Smith MD, McCall J, Plank L, et al. Preoperative carbohydrate treatment for enhancing recovery after elective surgery. *Cochrane Database Syst Rev.* 2014; 14; 8.

136. Nygren J, Soop M, Thorrell A, et al. Preoperative oral carbohydrate and insulin resistance. *Clin Nutr* 1999; 18(2): 117–120.

137. Lidder P, Thomas S, Fleming S, et al. A randomized placebo controlled trial of preoperative carbohydrate drinks and early postoperative nutritional supplement drinks in colorectal surgery. *Colorectal Dis* 2013; 15(6): 737–745.

138. Bilku DK, Dennison AR, Hall TC, et al. Role of preoperative carbohydrate loading: a systematic review. *Ann R Coll Surg Engl* 2014; 96(1): 15–22.

139. Waldron NH, Miller TE, Thacker JK, et al. A prospective comparison of a noninvasive cardiac output monitor versus esophageal Doppler monitor for goal-directed fluid therapy in colorectal surgery patients. *Anesth Analg* 2014; 118(5): 966–975.

140. Beck DE, Margolin DA, Babin SF, Russo CT. Benefits of a multimodal regimen for postsurgical pain management in colorectal surgery. *Ochsner J* 2015; 15(4): 408–412.

141. Charlton S, Cyna AM, Middleton P, Griffiths JD. (TAP) blocks for analgesia after abdominal surgery. *Cochrane Database Syst Rev* 2010; (12).

142. Johns N, O'Neill S, Ventham NT, et al. Clinical effectiveness of transversus abdominis plane (TAP) block in abdominal surgery: a systematic review and meta-analysis. *Colorectal Dis* 2012; 14(10): e635–642.

143. Yu N, Long X, Lujan-Hernandez JR, et al. Transversus abdominis-plane block versus local anesthetic wound infiltration in lower abdominal surgery: a systematic review and meta-analysis of randomized controlled trials. *BMC Anesthesiol* 2014; 14: 121.

Chapter 8

Gynecology Robotic Surgery

Barry Hallner, Erin Dougher, and Lisa M. Peacock

Introduction

The introduction of robot assistance to the field of gynecologic surgery, specifically the da Vinci Surgical System, represents a remarkable breakthrough in minimally invasive surgery. Subsequent to the 2005 FDA approval of the da Vinci Surgical System, robotics for gynecologic surgery has been rapidly adopted nationwide as a means to improve access to minimally invasive surgery for surgeons and their patients. At centers where it is available, it has assumed an important role in the surgical armamentarium (1). The current application of robotic technology in gynecology includes hysterectomy, myomectomy, oophorectomy, ovarian cystectomy, resection of endometriosis, sacrocolpopexy, and lymphadenectomy with an increasing role of robotic surgery in gynecologic oncology. Known advantages of robotic surgery include three-dimensional visualization, improved ergonomics, reduced fatigue, decreased tension tremor, seven degrees of motion, and decreased blood loss (2).

This chapter will focus on the preoperative workup that pertains to gynecology, our surgical technique, and common intra- and postoperative complications related to the most commonly performed robotic procedures: hysterectomy, oophorectomy, ovarian cystectomy, myomectomy, and sacrocolpopexy.

Robotic-Assisted Total Hysterectomy with or without Bilateral Salpingo-Oophorectomy

In the United States, hysterectomy is the second most common surgical procedure and the most common gynecologic procedure. There has been a steadily increasing trend toward the minimally invasive approach of laparoscopic or robotically assisted hysterectomy (3,4). The number of benign hysterectomies performed via laparoscopy doubled from 14 percent in 2005 to 30.5 percent in 2010 (4), and robotic-assisted hysterectomy increased from 0.5 percent in 2007 to 9.5 percent in 2010 (5). The American College of Obstetrics and Gynecology (ACOG) and the Society of Gynecologic Surgeons recommend surgeons should be skilled at both abdominal and laparoscopic procedures prior to the use of robotics. The selection of cases should be based on available data and expert opinion. It is also recommended that use of this technique should be driven by patient benefit and satisfaction without external commercial pressure. Furthermore, didactic and hands-on training is in development at most centers and should take place at the institutional level. In keeping with the goal of performing the least invasive procedure, ACOG continues to recommend the transvaginal route of hysterectomy whenever possible (4).

Regardless of the route of hysterectomy, the preoperative evaluation is similar for all approaches. The indication for hysterectomy should be valid and the choice to use robotic assistance should be based upon operator experience and patient benefit and safety (4). The gynecologic preoperative evaluation includes obtaining a full gynecologic and obstetrical history. This includes, but not limited to, a history of gynecologic malignancies, STDs, menstrual history, obstetrical history, familial history of breast or gynecologic malignancies (cervix, uterus, ovaries, fallopian tubes), and previous gynecologic procedures. A thorough pelvic examination is important to assess uterine size and mobility as these attributes can significantly impact technical difficulty and ultimately the success of the procedure and potential complications. There is no agreed-upon size that precludes a minimally invasive approach. However, a wide bulky uterus with minimal mobility can be more difficult to adequately manipulate, thereby limiting exposure during surgery and significantly increasing tissue extraction time. Cervical cancer screening should be performed according to the currently published guidelines for any woman aged 21 or older, with the exception of those infected with HIV who warrant screening at the time of diagnosis (6). Abnormal uterine bleeding and postmenopausal bleeding should be evaluated per current guidelines with ultrasound and possible endometrial biopsy as well as any other indicated testing to exclude malignancy prior to hysterectomy (7,8). Preoperative lab work should include, but not limited to, CBC, type and screen, and a pregnancy test in reproductive-aged women.

Bilateral salpingo-oophorectomy (BSO), or salpingectomy, can be performed at the time of benign hysterectomy or as an isolated procedure for the purpose of risk reduction of ovarian cancer and the treatment of benign ovarian conditions such as neoplasm, endometriosis, and pelvic pain (9). Genetic susceptibility for ovarian carcinoma is based on family history and possibly genetic testing. The presence of bilateral ovarian neoplasms, severe endometriosis, pelvic inflammatory disease, bilateral tuboovarian abscesses, or postmenopausal status favor BSO over ovarian conservation (9). The benefits of ovarian conservation, e.g., a decreased risk of cardiovascular disease, osteoporosis, and cognitive impairment, were found to decrease after the age of 65 in the Nurses' Health Study and, as such, should favor BSO (10). It is appropriate for surgeons to offer risk-reducing salpingectomy with ovarian conservation to decrease the risk of ovarian cancer at time of benign hysterectomy without the risk of ovarian compromise (10). At the same time, women should be informed of the reduction in breast and ovarian cancer associated with bilateral oophorectomy (11). The decision for BSO versus salpingectomy should be individualized and fully discussed with each patient.

Supracervical hysterectomy may be chosen based on patient or physician preference, need to decrease operative time, or to use the cervix for pelvic organ prolapse (POP) reconstruction. If a decision is made to retain the cervix, the patient will need to continue pap screening per current guidelines. She will need to be informed of the risk of continued bleeding or potential need for later trachelectomy. Removal of the uterus may be done through a mini-laparotomy with or without an extraction system or through power morcellation. If power morcellation is the mode of extraction, patients should be informed of the potential for undiagnosed gynecologic malignancy and the risk of intraperitoneal dissemination of benign or malignant disease with secondary implantation (12). Power morcellation can be performed within a containment bag creating a pseudo-peritoneum; however, this technique is currently experimental. Nongynecologic preoperative work-up includes pulmonary, cardiovascular, and other indicated assessment similar to any operative procedure and not unique to robotic-assisted hysterectomy. This should include a thorough history and physical and pertinent diagnostic testing (13,14). Patient's at high risk of postoperative venous thromboembolism should be identified preoperatively and treated according to recommended guidelines. If longer operating times or conversion to laparotomy are anticipated or preexisting VTE risks are present, then prophylaxis is indicated (15).

Antibiotic prophylaxis is indicated for all routes of hysterectomy (3). First-generation cephalosporin is dosed appropriately for weight and considered first-line prophylaxis due to its effectiveness, low cost, and lower risk for stimulating a B-lactamase response (3). For penicillin-allergic patients, the recommendations include clindamycin or metronidazole plus gentamycin or a quinolone (16). Preoperatively the patient should also be treated for any known bacterial vaginitis or trichomoniasis to reduce the risk of vaginal cuff infection postoperatively (17).

Similar to an open approach, the possible risks of this procedure include blood loss and the need for transfusion, unplanned adnexectomy, and injury to other pelvic organs, especially bladder, ureter, and bowel. Complications related to robotic-assisted procedures include entry injury to the major vessels, bladder, and bowel. The ureters are also at greater risk during laparoscopic hysterectomy compared to other approaches (18); however, the use of ureteral catheterization to prevent such injury is of unproven benefit (19). The risk of conversion to an open procedure should also be discussed with the patient preoperatively.

Surgical Technique

Our typical setup for a robotic-assisted laparoscopic hysterectomy is the same regardless of whether we are doing a total or supracervical hysterectomy. We use monopolar scissors in the number 1 arm (right) and Maryland bipolpar grasper in the number 2 arm (left). In cases that may be more technically difficult, we use a prograsp or cadiere in the number 3 robotic arm.

In addition, a uterine manipulator that has a cupping device is helpful for making colpotomy and for tissue extraction prior to cuff closure. If a uterine manipulator with a cupping device is not available, alternative instruments such as right-angle retractors, ring forceps with or without a sponge, and a thin malleable retractor may be used to help delineate the anterior and posterior fornices for colpotomy.

The patient is maintained in the low dorsal lithotomy position on a Pink Pad (Xodus Medical, New Kensington, PA) with the arms tucked at the side using the draw sheet. All bony prominences are padded typically with foam, and a bimanual examination is completed to determine uterine size, shape, and mobility and to determine port placement. The abdomen and vagina are surgically prepared. To avoid stomach puncture by a trocar during primary abdominal entry, an orogastric or nasogastric tube is placed to decompress the stomach. The patient is then draped and a foley catheter is inserted via the urethra. A uterine manipulator with its attached cervical cup (VCare or KOH Cup with RUMI manipulator) is placed vaginally to assist uterine manipulation and delineate the cervicovaginal junction for colpotomy and the pneumo-occluding balloon is inflated.

Abdominal insufflation may be achieved using a Veress needle after "water drop testing" to confirm intraperitoneal entry or by direct visual entry using an optical trocar loaded with a laparoscope. The number of trocars and their caliber may vary, but in general, we use a 12-mm optical port, usually at the umbilicus, and two or three reusable robotic ports placed through the lower abdominal wall. Specifically, the two to three robotic ports are placed 9 cm from each other to avoid arm collisions during the procedure. A 5-mm assistant port is placed on the low right flank and, if necessary, a second 10-mm port is placed in the right upper quadrant to facilitate passage of sutures and other materials such as grafts, hemostatic agents, and clips. This port also allows the assistant to retract, irrigate, and suction effectively. The pelvis and abdomen are inspected and photodocumentation or videography is initiated. At this point, adhesiolysis is performed to restore normal anatomy, if needed, prior to docking.

Docking maneuvers are initiated once the patient is placed in steep Trendelenburg and the da Vinci system is guided into place. The robot is side-docked and the instruments are inserted into the abdomen under direct visualization. Prior to making any incisions, it is important to identify the ureters. In most cases the ureters can be visualized without difficulty peristalsing beneath the peritoneum on the pelvic side walls. However, it is sometimes necessary to open the peritoneum for identification. In such situations, the peritoneum medial to the infundibulopelvic (IP) ligament is grasped and tented using atraumatic forceps and incised with scissors. The opening in the peritoneum is then extended a short distance both caudally and cephalad along the length of the ureter. Through this peritoneal window, on the medial side the ureter is identified (20). The proximal round ligament is grasped and then divided. If preservation of the ovaries is planned, the proximal portions of the fallopian tube and uteroovarian ligament are then desiccated and transected.

With this, the tube and ovary are freed from the uterus and can be placed in the ovarian fossa. If removal of the ovaries is desired, the IP ligament is grasped and pulled up and away from retroperitoneal structures. The ureter's path is once again identified. The IP ligament is isolated and dissected away from the ureter. The pedicle is subsequently coagulated, desiccated, or stapled and divided. If the fallopian tubes are to be removed, the distal attachment of the tube to the ovary (fimbria ovarica) must be removed in its entirety and the mesosalpinx is coagulated and transected in a stepwise fashion moving toward the uterus.

Following round ligament transection, the leaves of the broad ligament peritoneum are separated and the loose connective tissue is localized between these leaves. The anterior leaf is incised with the monopolar scissors. This incision is made parallel to the border of the uterus and directed caudally to the midline above the vesicouterine fold. The posterior leaf is then taken down to the uterosacral ligaments. Opening the broad ligament allows the uterine vessels to be skeletonized and clearly visualized. Once the broad ligaments are opened bilaterally, the vesicouterine fold is grasped with atraumatic forceps, elevated away from the underlying bladder, and incised transversely.

The loosely attached connections can be bluntly divided by gently pushing against the cervix in a caudal direction. This displaces the bladder away from the cervix and upper vagina. Denser tissue in the vesicouterine space may be divided sharply with the aid of monopolar energy or sharp tissue dissection. Bipolar or monopolar electrosurgery may be utilized to coagulate small bleeding vessels. It is equally important to keep cephalad traction on the uterus with the uterine

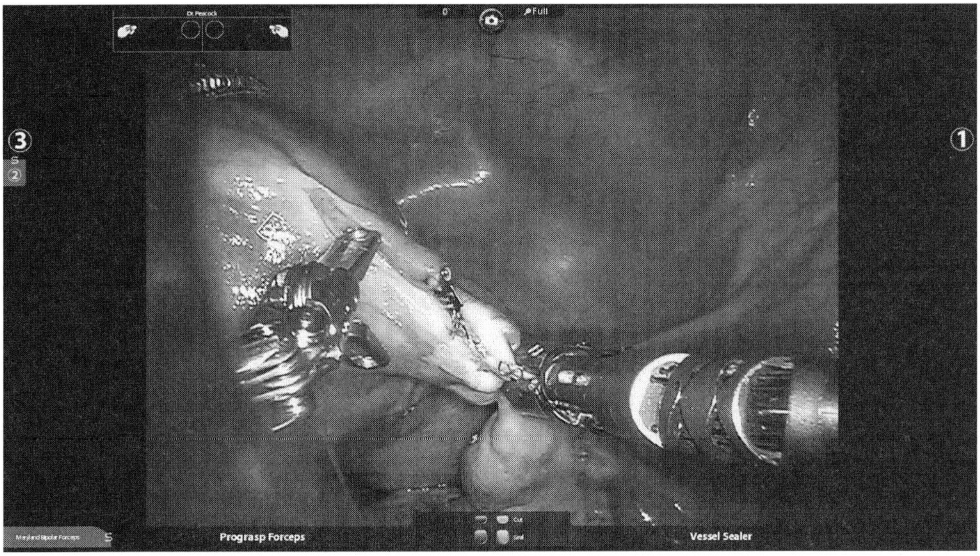

Figure 8.1 Desiccation of the uteroovarian ligament vessels. The uteroovarian ligament is desiccated with a bipolar grasper.

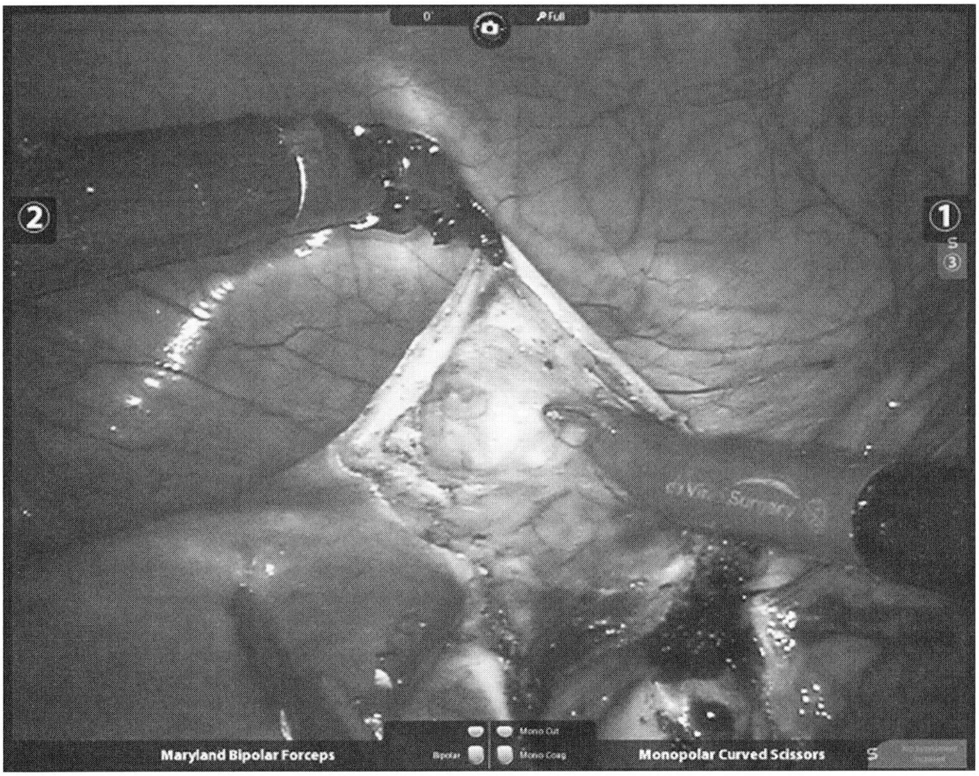

Figure 8.2 Creation of the bladder flap. The loosely attached connections can be bluntly divided by gently pushing against the cervix in a caudal direction. This displaces the bladder away from the cervix and upper vagina.

manipulator to assist with this dissection. Alternately, the prograsp or cadiere in the third arm of the surgical assistant can grasp the fundus to maintain cephalad traction on the uterus and improve visualization of the anterior and posterior surfaces. The mobilization of the bladder and sometimes the upper rectum is

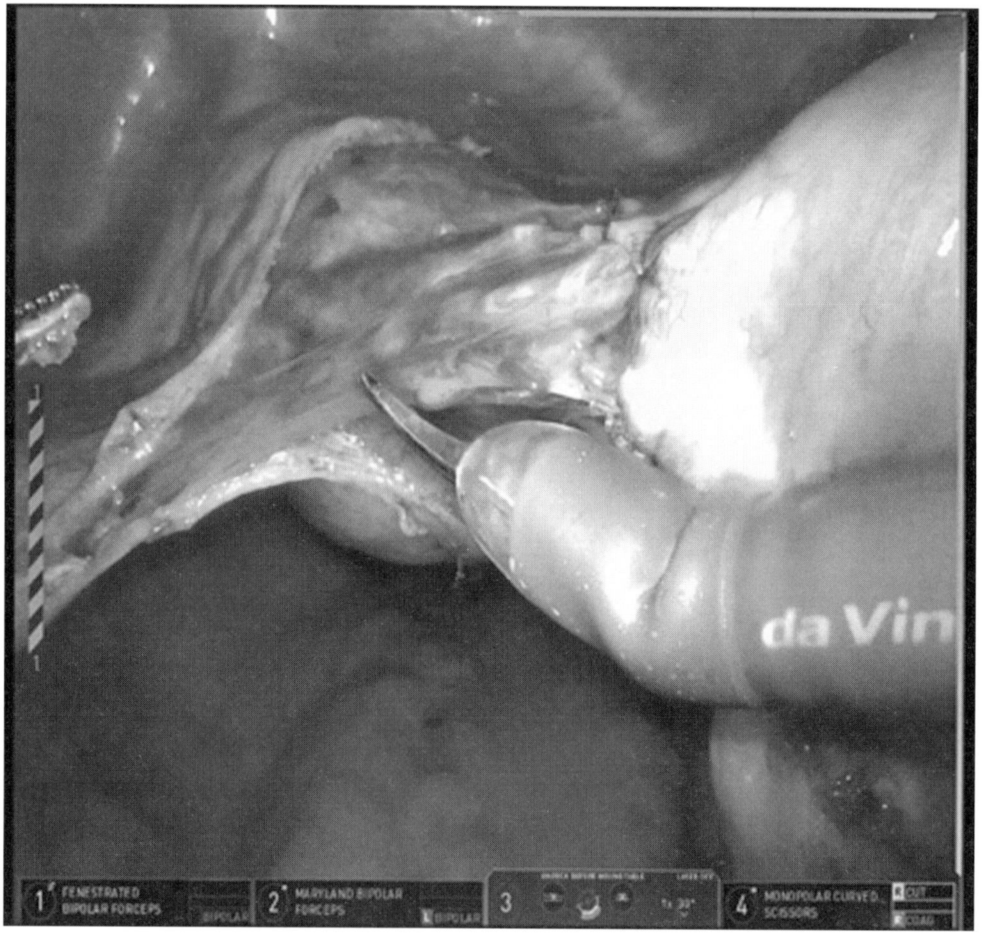

Figure 8.3 The uterine vessels are skeletonized. Skeletonizing of the vessels permits precise desiccation and transection of the uterine vessels.

necessary for the final colpotomy and removal of the uterus. Of all the hysterectomy approaches, the laparoscopic one has the highest risk of bladder injury, and when it occurs, its most frequent location is at the dome during this sharp or blunt dissection (21). The risk of bladder injury is increased when scarring from prior surgery such as cesarean delivery is present or when concomitant pelvic disease such as endometriosis exists.

After the uterine arteries are identified, the loose areolar connective tissue surrounding them is grasped and incised. This skeletonizing of vessels permits precise desiccation and transection of uterine vessels.

The lateral cardinal ligaments are then taken down to the level of uterosaccral ligaments bilaterally. Prior to colpotomy incision, the uterine manipulator is pushed cephalad to allow the colpotomy cup to displace the ureters laterally and expose the optimal location for the incision. The colpotomy can then be performed with monopolar scissors.

The colpotomy is initiated by placing the incising tool at the anterior cervicovaginal junction, which is delineated by the cervical cup. If a colpotomy cup is not used, a simple tool such as right-angle retractor or ring forcep is placed vaginally in the anterior or posterior fornix to assist with the identification of the cervicovaginal junction. The anterior vaginal wall is usually opened first followed by the posterior colpotomy. The uterosacral ligaments are then transected. To prevent thermal damage to vaginal tissues and potential later cuff dehiscence, surgeons should use the minimum amount of energy needed to incise vaginal tissues.

Intact uterine extraction is completed through vaginal colpotomy using a manipulator or alternatively with a transvaginally placed instrument such as a tenaculum. In cases involving large uteri, the uterus can also be transvaginally cored, bivalved, or morcellated. In some cases, the uterus can be placed in an Alexis contained extraction system (Applied Medical, Rancho Santa Margarita, CA) for intracorporeal morcellation through a slightly extended port incision.

Vaginal cuff closure can be achieved in numerous ways, including conventional laparoscopic, robotic, or vaginal suturing with or without a suture device, and laparoscopic or robotic suturing using barbed suture. We close the cuff robotically with interrupted delayed-absorbable sutures. Full-thickness closure with 1 cm depth is recommended to help prevent cuff dehiscence. To support the vaginal cuff long term, the uterosacral ligaments are incorporated into the closure as a separate step. After cuff closure, the pelvis is irrigated and hemostasis confirmed. Intraabdominal pressures are lowered to 5 mmHg during this inspection to reduce vascular compression and better identify sources of bleeding. Once completed, the robot is undocked and cystoscopy is performed to confirm ureteral patency and absence of bladder injury. The trocars are removed and the fascia is closed where trocar sites larger than 10 mm are present. The skin is closed with moncryl with or without supplemental skin adhesive.

Complications

Intraoperative and postoperative complications associated with robotic-assisted hysterectomy include genitourinary, gastrointestinal, vascular, and neurologic injury, as well as pelvic infection and vaginal cuff dehiscence.

Nerve injury during hysterectomy and BSO is rare but can occur at a rate of 0.2–2 percent during major pelvic surgery (22,23). The femoral nerve is the most common nerve injured during major pelvic surgery, usually on the anterior surface of the psoas muscle and inguinal canal. Although this injury occurs more commonly during abdominal hysterectomy due to compression from lateral retractors, it can also occur as an indirect stretch injury as it passes through the inguinal canal due to malpositioning of the legs in the stirrups. When placing patients in the dorsal lithotomy position, care must be taken not to hyperflex and externally rotate the hip to avoid this injury. The superficial branch of the peroneal nerve can also be easily injured by compression of the stirrup on the lateral edge of the fibular head during abdominopelvic procedures. The iliohypogastric and ilioinguinal nerves while rarely injured during laparoscopy can be injured during placement of lateral trocars at the location where the iliohypogastric nerve penetrates the fascia of the internal oblique and where the ilioinguinal nerve penetrates the fascia of the transverse abdominus muscles. Closure of fascial incisions and subsequent scarring are additional sources of nerve entrapment and injury (3).

Blood loss, in general, is lower in minimally invasive hysterectomy. The reported median blood loss during laparoscopic hysterectomy in randomized trials comparing two or more routes of hysterectomy is 156–660.5 mL (24). In a recent Cochrane Review, laparoscopic hysterectomy was found to have significantly lower estimated blood loss than abdominal hysterectomy but not when compared to vaginal hysterectomy (3). The loss of control of the uterine and ovarian blood supply is the most common reason for hemorrhage and increased blood loss during hysterectomy. Injury to any of the many vessels originating from the iliac arteries supplying the pelvis can significantly increase blood loss. The complex venous plexus, which is a collateral network of veins from the external and internal iliac veins, inferior mesenteric, and ovarian veins, is yet another possible major source of bleeding. Other risk factors for bleeding include pelvic adhesive disease and malignancy.

Genitourinary tract injury is an additional complication that can be incurred at the time of hysterectomy. The reported rate of genitourinary tract injury in major gynecologic surgery is approximately 1–2 percent (25). The occurrence of bladder injury during laparoscopic hysterectomy has been estimated at 2.1 percent compared to 1 percent and 1.2 percent in abdominal and vaginal routes, respectively, in a randomized trial of 1,300 hysterectomies (26). While it is reported that bladder injuries are more common than ureteral injuries, it is also noted that two-thirds of ureteral injuries are not identified at the time of injury (25,27). The occurrence of ureteral injury is highest for laparoscopic hysterectomy as compared to other routes, but the overall incidence of ureteral injury is low at 0.05–0.5 percent (27,28). Ureteral injury most commonly occurs during dissection and ligation of the infundibulo-pelvic ligament at the pelvic brim, followed by ligation of the cardinal and uterosacral ligaments and uterine arteries at the bladder base and lower uterine segment respectively (3). Hemorrhage, endometriosis, previous pelvic surgery, pelvic masses or fibroids, and obesity are associated with an increased risk of ureteral injury during hysterectomy and BSO (3). In addition, dissection of the prevesical plane during laparoscopic surgery is the most common source of bladder injury, especially in patients with previous cesarean delivery, endometriosis, pelvic adhesive disease, or cancer (3).

Gastrointestinal tract injury is yet another concern during robotic surgery. Injury to the vascular supply and tissues of the GI tract or bowel occurs by thermal, direct, or indirect etiologies. The reported rate of GI tract injury is 0.1–1 percent of all hysterectomies, with 0.2 percent occurring in association with the laparoscopic approach (29). The use of monopolar current during hysterectomy is a common cause of thermal bowel injury most often incurred during deep pelvic dissection in the posterior cul-de-sac when performing colpotomy. In addition, direct bowel injury can occur when placing laparoscopic trocars and when performing blunt or sharp adhesiolysis. Devascularization of the bowel is most likely to occur during dissection of the mesentery of the bowel, and is more common in surgical cancer staging procedures (3).

Surgical site infection is not an uncommon event after hysterectomy. The prevalence of infectious complications after laparoscopic hysterectomy has been estimated at 9.0 percent (29). Hysterectomy is considered to be a "clean-contaminated" procedure due to its entry into the vagina (3). Postoperative infection may occur in the form of infected pelvic hematoma, vaginal cuff abscess, wound infection, urinary tract infection, or respiratory infection. Symptoms or signs of infection should be evaluated with a thorough history and physical and indicated diagnostic laboratory and clinical tests to determine the source and differentiate infection from febrile morbidity (3).

The vaginal cuff is the primary source of postoperative complications that are unique to hysterectomy. Vaginal cuff cellulitis is found to occur in 0–8.3 percent of patients after hysterectomy (24). This typically presents within a few days after surgery with fever, purulent vaginal discharge, and pelvic pain. A pelvic examination usually confirms the diagnosis with demonstration of cuff tenderness or induration with or without purulent discharge (3). Cuff cellulitis is commonly polymicrobial (3,16), and the type and duration of treatment should be based on current standards of care.

Another potential complication specific to hysterectomy involving the vaginal cuff is dehiscence with or without evisceration. In a large retrospective review, Cronin et al. found the rate of dehiscence after all routes of hysterectomy to range from 0.14 to 4.1 percent. Reported rates of dehiscence after total laparoscopic and robotic hysterectomy are found to be the highest (1–4.1 percent) when compared to other routes of hysterectomy (0.14–0.27 percent) (30). The creation of colpotomy using electrocautery with the attendant thermal injury coupled with smaller tissue incorporation during cuff closure due to laparoscopic magnification has been implicated in the causation of this postoperative complication. Vaginal cuff dehiscence is a serious postoperative complication that more frequently follows laparoscopic hysterectomy as compared to vaginal or abdominal hysterectomy (30,31). In most cases, the precipitating event in premenopausal woman is sexual activity, and in postmenopausal women any increased intraabdominal pressure (e.g., constipation) exerted on a weak, atrophic vagina (32).

Robotic-Assisted Cystectomy

A robotic approach can be used to safely remove the adnexa and, in most cases, offers a faster recovery and less postoperative pain when compared to laparotomy. Indications for adnexectomy vary but may include mass, torsion, ovarian cyst rupture, suspicion of ovarian malignancy, and symptomatic ovarian remnant. Robotically assisted cystectomy accounted for 2.4 percent of minimally invasive cystectomies performed in 2009 and has increased annually thereafter to 12.9 percent currently. The minimally invasive approach can also be safely performed in pregnant women, preferably in the early second trimester (33).

Sonography is the primary perioperative tool used to evaluate ovarian pathology, and the sonographic characteristics of a cyst aid in determining the malignant potential of a given lesion. In cases in which the anatomy may be unclear, magnetic resonance imaging may add additional information. Tumor markers, such as serum cancer antigen 125 (CA125) levels, are typically drawn preoperatively in postmenopausal patients and in any woman whose tumor displays other signs consistent with ovarian epithelial cancer. In addition, serum alpha-fetoprotein (AFP), lactate dehydrogenase (LDH), inhibin, and β-hCG levels may be measured to exclude germ cell or sex cord-stromal ovarian neoplasms. As with any surgical procedure, patients should be informed of the unique complications associated with minimally invasive surgery. In particular with adnexal surgery, the risk of ureteral injury should be discussed. In some cases, unanticipated bilateral adnexectomy may be required, and the patient should be aware of the significance of hormonal deprivation. Lastly, many adnexa are removed due to concerns of potential malignancy, and the patient should be apprised of the additional procedures required for the surgical staging of ovarian cancer.

In general, robotic-assisted adnexal surgery does not require antibiotic prophylaxis. Bowel preparation is also not usually required, but may be considered in addition to antibiotic prophylaxis if extensive adhesions are suspected. Venous thromboembolism (VTE) prophylaxis is typically not recommended for robotic-assisted cystectomy. However, those with greater risk of malignancy, VTE, and conversion to laparotomy may benefit from those measures. Generally accepted guidelines for VTE prophylaxis should be applied.

Surgical Technique

For robotic-assisted ovarian cystectomy, we use monopolar scissors, a Maryland bipolar forcep, and if an additional robotic arm is required we use a prograsp or cadiere. We also typically use a suction irrigation system and additional laparoscopic graspers and retractors through the ancillary ports. The patient is prepared and positioned for robotic surgery as previously described. The abdomen is insufflated with CO_2 to a pressure of 15 mmHg and the camera port is inserted (34). Secondary trocars are then placed. Depending on the size of the adnexa, at least one trocar should be 10 mm or larger to allow for the use of an endoscopic retrieval bag to contain the specimen at the conclusion of surgery.

Once the abdomen is entered, inspection of the pelvis and upper abdomen for signs of malignancy such as ascites and peritoneal implants is performed. Pelvic washings are obtained if malignancy is a concern. Peritoneal implants should be biopsied and sent for intraoperative frozen section. If a malignant neoplasm is found, then the cystectomy is aborted and an intraoperative consult is obtained from a gynecologic oncologist.

Adhesions are divided to restore anatomy, and the anterior and posterior surface of the ovary is carefully inspected. The ovary is then stabilized and the monopolar scissor blade is used to make an incision along the antimesenteric surface of the ovary to minimize disruption of the extensive vascular supply located at the ovarian base. The incision is extended into the ovarian stroma to the level of the cyst wall but no deeper to avoid rupturing the cyst. A space between the ovary and cyst wall is created bluntly using Maryland forceps or scissors. The grasping forceps are then used to hold the ovarian tissue, while a prograsp can be used to separate the cyst wall from the ovarian capsule. Depending on the adherence of the cyst to its surrounding ovarian tissue, sharp dissection with monopolar scissors may be required to complete the cystectomy. Following cyst removal, bleeding sites and isolated vessels may be grasped and coagulated with the bipolar grasper. Not uncommonly, during the dissection of the cyst away from the ovary, the cyst may rupture. As a result, the grasping forceps can be used to strip the cyst wall away from the underlying ovarian stroma (35). To prevent damage to the underlying healthy ovary, the dissection plane between the cyst and stroma should be clearly delineated by traction on each side to prevent laceration.

Specimen retrieval is then performed. A small excised cyst wall can be removed directly through one of the laparoscopic ports. In some cases, a posterior vaginal colpotomy is used for removal of the intact cyst or cyst wall (36). Yet another option is to place the cyst in an endoscopic retrieval bag and decompress the cyst inside the bag. This procedure significantly decreases the possibility of spilling the cyst contents into the pelvic cavity, which is important given one study reported a 7.3–8.1 percent spillage rate for laparoscopic ovarian cystectomy (37). Contained rupture and extraction is possible with even larger cysts wherein the cannula is removed, and the pursestringed opening of the bag is drawn through the trocar incision and fanned out onto the skin surface. The open edges of the bag are pulled upward to lift and press the cyst up against the incision. A needle tip is then directed into the incision and pierces the cyst contained within the endoscopic bag. An attached syringe is used to aspirate the contents. Alternatively, the cyst may be ruptured by an instrument such as a Kocher clamp placed through the skin incision and into the sac. The endoscopic sac and decompressed cyst wall are then removed together through the incision. During removal, care is taken to ensure that the endoscopic bag is not inadvertently punctured or torn, and all measures are used to prevent spillage of cyst contents into the abdomen or port site.

Closure of the ovarian capsule is not required following cyst removal due to the risk of adhesion formation, technical difficulty, and additional operative time required for laparoscopic suturing. Several studies have shown that leaving the capsule open does not lead to an increase in adhesion formation (38,39). Application of an adhesion barrier such as oxidized regenerated cellulose (Interceed, Ethicon, Inc., Somerville, NJ) may be considered to reduce adhesion formation (40,41). However, no substantial evidence documents that their use improves fertility, decreases pain, or prevents subsequent bowel obstruction (42).

As previously recommended, intraabdominal pressures are lowered to 5 mmHg during final pelvic inspection to identify sources of bleeding. The addition of hemostatic agents such as Surgicel Fibrillar, Evicel, Surgiflo (Ethicon Inc., Somerville, NJ), Tisseel, Floseal and Gelfoam (Baxter International, Inc., Deerfield, IL) can be used when indicated. After conclusion of the laparoscopic portion of the procedure, the robot is undocked and cystoscopy and skin closure is completed as previously described.

Complications

In women undergoing robotic-assisted cystectomy, the overall complication rate is reported to be 3.7 percent (95 percent CI, −0.8 to 8.2 percent) (33). Complications include bleeding and inadvertent cyst rupture. Bleeding can usually be controlled with a judicious use of electrocautery with or without the application of hemostatic agents previously described. Another potential complication is injury to the ovary itself, resulting in impaired function. Ovarian preservation is crucial for patients desiring future fertility, and methods of obtaining hemostasis should not be overly destructive of the ovarian parenchyma. It has been shown in some studies that ovarian cystectomy can have a negative impact on ovarian reserve as measured by serum antimullerian hormone (AMH) (43,44).

Another crucial concern regards rupture of the cyst during resection and removal. The frequency of intraoperative cyst rupture at laparoscopic cystectomy ranges from 6 to 27 percent and occurs more frequently than when performed through a laparotomy (36,37). Depending on the type of cyst, e.g., endometrioma, teratoma, or malignancy, inadvertent spillage of the contents may result in subsequent spread to other areas of the abdomen and pelvis or severe peritoneal irritation. The rupture of a malignant cyst is more serious as it may result in tumor dissemination, advancing stage of disease, and adverse impact to patient survival (36). If spillage occurs during any cystectomy, the pelvis should be copiously irrigated.

Robotic-Assisted Myomectomy

Myomectomy involves the surgical excision of leiomyomata from the surrounding normal myometrium in an attempt to resolve abnormal uterine bleeding, pelvic pain, mass effect, and infertility. The surgical technique of abdominal myomectomy was first developed by Bonney in 1931 as a procedure for women who wish to preserve their uterus or who declined hysterectomy (45). In 1979, Semm demonstrated that this operation could be performed with laparoscopic techniques (46). Robotic myomectomy followed on the successes of endoscopic surgery with specific advantages, especially to those surgeons with limited or no laparoscopic experience. The popularity and rapid adoption of robotic technique for myomectomy is predominantly due to the ease of suturing robotically compared to laparoscopic technique. The fact that myomectomy is a suture-intensive surgery requiring a multilayered closure only further drives the conversion to the robotic approach (1). Robotic myomectomy has been reported to be as effective as classic open myomectomy with comparable safety and acceptance (47). The pregnancy outcomes following robotic-assisted myomectomy are also comparable to open surgery (48).

Preoperative planning requires delineation of leiomyoma size, number, and location. Sonography, magnetic resonance imaging, or hysteroscopy may all be utilized to evaluate the tumors (49). Abnormal uterine bleeding commonly occurs with leiomyomata, such that the presence of anemia should be assessed preoperatively. Numerous studies have shown the benefit of the administration of a GNRH agonist preoperatively to significantly reduce uterine volume and concurrently improve blood counts (50). When myomectomy is performed for fertility, antibiotic prophylaxis is advocated to reduce the risk of tubal adhesions that can be associated with pelvic infection (49) and typically consists of a first- or second-generation cephalosporin unless penicillin-allergic (51,52). Preoperative bowel preparation has not been shown to improve visualization but may be given in patients at increased risk of bowel injury as previously described.

Surgical Technique

The patient is positioned, prepped, and draped as previously described. A kronner uterine manipulator (Cooper Surgical, Trumbull, CT) and foley are placed. Port placement, docking, instrumentation, and positioning of assistants were as previously described but can vary by physician preference. In particular, a robotic tenaculum and monopolar spatula are useful for the dissection and enucleation of leiomyomata. The subserosa of the myomata can be injected with dilute vasopressin to decrease bleeding. A vertical incision is made over the leiomyoma using monopolar scissors. The myoma is grasped with a single tooth tenaculum and placed on tension, while sharp and blunt dissection of the pseudocapsule surrounding the leiomyoma frees the tumor from normal myometrium. The risk of excessive bleeding correlates with uterine size, total weight of leiomyomas removed, and operative time (53). Sequential fulguration of the vascular supply to the tumors prior to transection is preferable to reduce bleeding. Smaller internal incisions into the myometrium may be required to excise all the tumors. If the endometrial cavity is entered, it should be closed by running a 3-0 or 4-0 delayed-absorbable suture (49). The surgeon should minimize the number of incisions on the uterus to reduce the risk of postoperative adhesion formation. In addition, care must be taken to avoid disrupting the fallopian tubes during the course of dissection and enucleation.

Once all the leiomyomas have been excised, the internal myometrial incisions are closed first with 0 delayed-absorbable suture. The myometrium is then sutured in layers to prevent hematoma formation and to secure hemostasis. Closure of serosal incisions is performed with 3-0 or 4-0 delayed-absorbable suture using a locking or baseball stitch. The pneumoperitoneum is transiently reduced to 5 mmHg to check for hemostasis prior to the placement of Interceed (Ethicon, West Somerville, NJ) adhesion barrier over the hysterotomy sites. Due to the recent FDA safety communication, we no longer use power morcellation for tissue extraction (54). Alternatively, we use the Alexis Contained Extraction System (Applied Medical, Rancho Santa Margarita, CA). The large containment bag carrying leiomyomas is inserted through the 10-mm trocar and placed in the pelvis near the uterus. The robot is undocked and the Alexis Contained Extraction System (Applied Medical, Rancho Santa Margarita, CA) is then deployed through the umbilical port for contained tissue morcellation. Alternatively, tumors may be removed through a posterior colpotomy or mini-laparotomy. Fascial and skin closure proceeds as previously described.

Complications

Bleeding complications are the most commonly encountered during myomectomy. Uncontrolled hemorrhage or massive myometrial injury during tumor removal can precipitate the need for hysterectomy. If significant adhesiolysis is required during the procedure, it is important to inspect the bowel for injury. Serosal injuries can be oversewn. An incidental or intentional enterotomy should be repaired by a qualified surgeon. Other operative complications include delayed bowel or bladder injury, fistula, hematoma, and adhesion formation.

While myomectomy is often performed to preserve fertility, postoperative adhesions can jeopardize the success of the procedure. Single, vertical, anterior, and midline uterine incisions induce adhesions that are less likely to compromise fertility (55). While several adhesion barriers are available or are under development, none of them have been shown to be completely effective in preventing postoperative adhesions (56,57). It is equally important to counsel patients regarding the risk of uterine rupture during pregnancy after myomectomy. Fortunately, this risk is low at 0.75 percent but can be associated with significant fetal and maternal mortality when it does occur (58).

Robotic-Assisted Sacrocolpopexy

Pelvic organ prolapse (POP) is a common problem among women with an increasing incidence in the aging population. It is estimated that by 2050, 43.8 million women will be affected by at least one bothersome pelvic floor disorder, including prolapse (59). Sacrocolpopexy is one of several operations for the resuspension of the vaginal apex. It is preferred over other approaches when restoration of normal vaginal anatomy and durability of the repair are primary concerns (60). Long-term success rates for sacrocolpopexy range from 78 to 100 percent when success is defined as no postoperative apical prolapse, and from 58 to 100 percent when defined as no prolapse in any compartment (60).

Sacrocolpopexy provides durable support by attaching the vaginal apex and the anterior and posterior vaginal walls to the anterior longitudinal ligament of the spine at the level of sacrum using a bridging graft. Although grafts of autologous, cadaveric, or synthetic materials may be used, permanent synthetic mesh has the best success rate and should be used unless otherwise contraindicated (61). Prior to sacrocolpopexy, patients with symptoms of urinary incontinence may undergo simple or complex urodynamic testing to determine the need for an antiincontinence procedure (62). Similarly, women without incontinence should also undergo testing with reduction of the prolapse to assess whether the repair will unmask occult incontinence. Alternatively, an anti-incontinence procedure can be performed routinely at the time of sacrocolpopexy; however, the patient needs to be counseled regarding the risks and benefits of this approach prior to surgery.

When determining the appropriate surgical intervention for a specific patient, factors that influence the decision regarding approach include overall health, body habitus, presence of intraabdominal adhesions, and surgeon preference. Minimally invasive transabdominal sacrocolpopexy may be indicated for patients who have advanced prolapse, a large anterior defect, or those with a history of failed prolapse repair. Patients with a foreshortened vagina may also benefit from this approach, as transvaginal repair can result in further decrease in vaginal length (63). It is important to counsel the patient that even if a sacrocolpopexy is performed, concomitant vaginal prolapse repair for persistent cystocele or rectocele may be required, especially in cases of advanced prolapse (60).

The preoperative evaluation includes a history that assesses the degree of prolapse symptoms, the presence of urinary incontinence, as well as any past history of urologic or gynecologic surgery. If she has not had a hysterectomy, a discussion should be held as to whether she wishes to keep her uterus in situ or undergo a supracervical hysterectomy while retaining the cervix. Cervical cancer screening should be performed according to the currently published guidelines, for any woman aged 21 or older, with the exception of those infected with HIV who warrant screening at the time of diagnosis (6). Abnormal uterine bleeding and postmenopausal bleeding should be worked up per current guidelines to exclude malignancy (7,8). A complete physical examination, including a pelvic exam with a defined measurement of the prolapse (POP-Q), should be performed. As with any surgical procedure, a preoperative risk assessment should be conducted.

Different methods for minimally invasive sacrocolpopexy have been described in the literature. However, there is no consensus on how these procedures should be performed to have optimized outcome (64). Here we describe our technique as an option for performing robotic sacrocolpopexy.

Surgical Technique

The patient is positioned, prepped, draped, and instrumented as described previously. Side or parallel docking is preferred to allow access to the vagina, bladder, and rectum intraoperatively if needed. Port placement and conduct of the initial setup for the procedure are as previously described with variations relative to surgeon preference and clinical scenario.

After any necessary adhesiolysis, the procedure starts with the dissection of sacral promontory since the completion of this portion is essential to complete the surgery. The bowel is gently swept out of the pelvis to the left and above the pelvic brim. Not infrequently, the congenital attachments of the sigmoid colon on the left must be taken down to mobilize the bowel out of the pelvis. The aortic bifurcation and iliac vessels are identified, and the sacral promontory is visualized and delineated at the midline. We identify the ureters coursing along the pelvic side wall, especially the right ureter, which is closest to the field of dissection. Once the promontory has been identified, the peritoneum overlying it is grasped and incised vertically with monopolar scissors.

It is important to be aware of the left common iliac vein, as this structure is frequently located more medial than the artery and can be injured during exposure of the promontory. The incision is extended caudally into the cul-de-sac, creating peritoneal leaves that are later used to cover the graft.

The anterior longitudinal ligament at sacral promontory is then identified and carefully cleared, taking care to avoid any sacral vessels as these may be difficult to control if interrupted. If bleeding is encountered, it may be controlled by applying direct pressure to the area of bleeding, increasing insufflation pressures to 20 mmHg, by bipolar coagulation of discreet vessels, or oversewing the source of bleeding with absorbable sutures. Laparoscopic thumbtacks may also be used to control bleeding from the presacral region (65). Ultimately, if hemostasis cannot be controlled

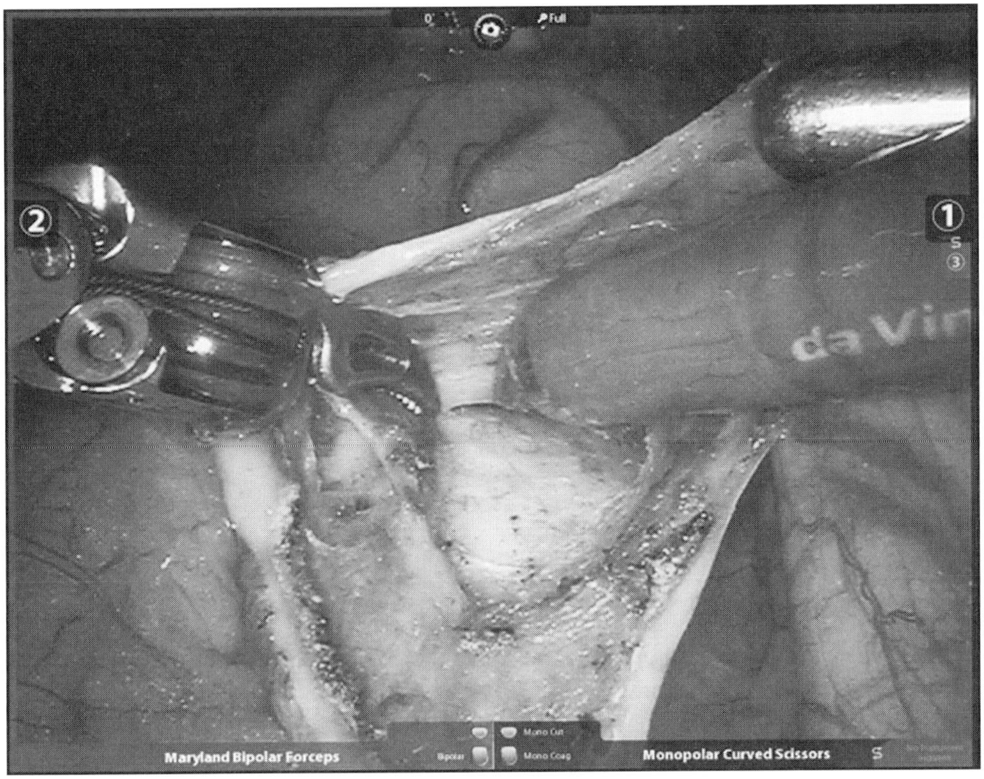

Figure 8.4 Dissecting the anterior longitudinal ligament. The anterior longitudinal ligament at sacral promontory is then identified and carefully cleared, taking care to avoid any sacral vessels.

laparoscopically, then the robotic procedure should be abandoned, laparotomy performed and bleeding controlled in the traditional open fashion.

The upper vagina and vaginal apex must be elevated and distended with a vaginal stent. This permits adequate dissection and visualization of fibromuscular layers of the vaginal wall and aids graft placement. The vaginal stent may be a large end-to-end anastomosis sizer, which is present in most operating rooms, a cylindrical Lucite rod, or the Colpassist Vaginal Positioning Device (Boston Scientific, Marlborough, MA). The vaginal stent is used to elevate the vaginal apex, and the peritoneum covering it is incised transversely. Sharp and blunt dissection is used to separate the peritoneum and bladder from the anterior vaginal wall. This anterior dissection extends approximately 5 to 6 cm caudally to create an adequate surface for graft fixation. Dissection should progress at a depth above the fibromuscular layer of the vaginal wall. Entry into the proper plane above the fibromuscular layer will decrease the risk of incidental entry into the vagina. Accidental opening of the vaginal wall increases the risk of future graft exposure especially when using synthetic mesh. If the vaginal wall is opened, it should be irrigated copiously followed by a two-layered closure with 2-0 or 3-0 delayed-absorbable suture. The vaginal apex is redirected anteriorly, and the peritoneum covering the posterior vaginal wall is opened. The rectovaginal space is identified and blunt dissection further opens this space to the level of rectal reflection for a distance of about 6 cm.

The selection of sacrocolpopexy graft is at the preference of the surgeon. In general, if using synthetic mesh it should be lightweight, flexible, and porous (66). At our institution, a prefabricated Y-shaped mesh is employed. The mesh is placed into the peritoneal cavity through the assistant's 10-mm cannula and guided into place. The graft may be secured to the anterior and posterior vaginal walls with delayed-absorbable or permanent suture or a combination of both.

Some studies have shown equivalent long-term outcomes with the use of absorbable suture compared with permanent suture for sacrocolpopexy mesh fixation (67).

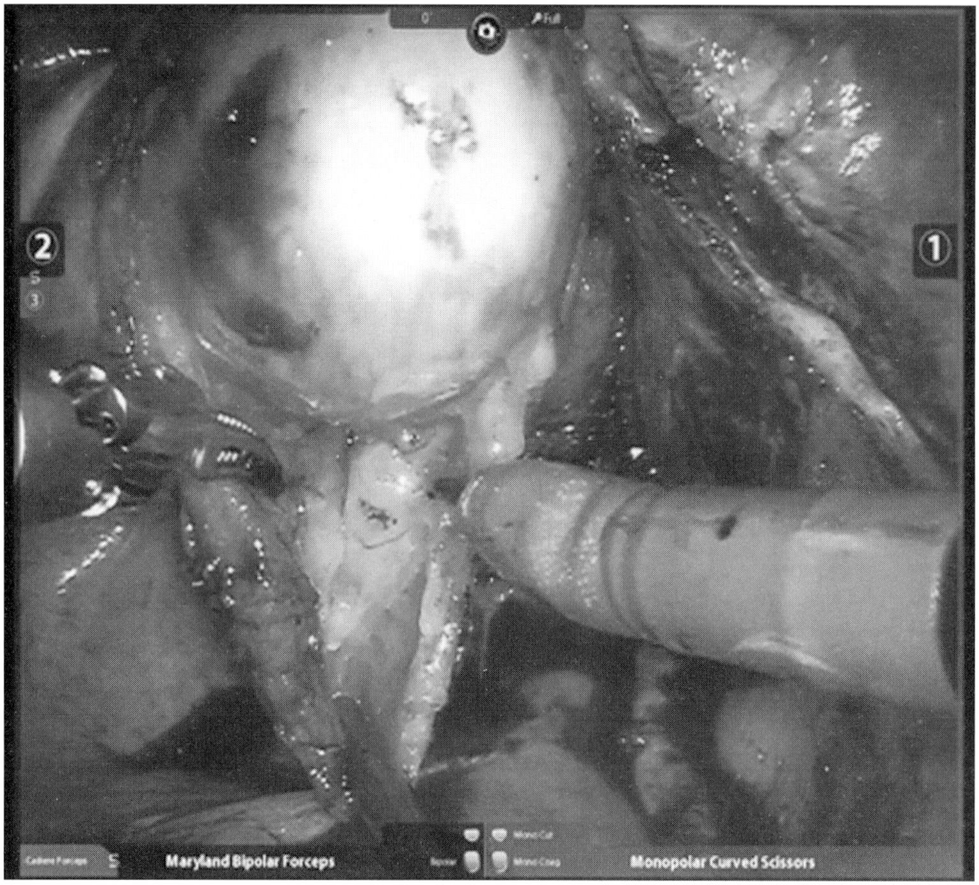

Figure 8.5 Dissecting the rectovaginal space. The avascular space may be bluntly dissected.

Once the anterior and posterior arms of the mesh have been secured to the vagina, the tail is extended toward the promontory. The graft is then tensioned to replicate normal vaginal compliance, as excessive tension can result in pain or de novo stress urinary incontinence (60). Tensioning can be performed through visual or direct vaginal examination techniques depending on surgeon preference and experience. The apical suspension should reduce prolapse of the apex as well as the apical segments of the anterior and posterior vaginal walls.

The apical tail of the graft is sutured to the anterior longitudinal ligament at the level selected by the surgeon. Traditionally suture placement is at S3 or S4 to recreate the normal axis of vagina; however, that approach increases the risk of injury to presacral venous plexus. Alternatively, placement of sutures at S1 or sacral promontory risks laceration of the middle sacral vessels or the left common iliac vein (68). The middle sacral vessels, however, are readily visible and can be isolated and avoided. Additionally, at S1 the anterior longitudinal ligament is thicker, which minimizes the risk of suture avulsion. For these reasons, many surgeons currently choose to fix the graft at S1, the level of sacral promontory (60).

The peritoneum is closed over the vaginal apex with 2-0 delayed-absorbable suture in a running fashion.

Cystoscopy is performed to rule out thermal or mechanical bladder injury, intravesical suture or mesh perforation, and to confirm ureteral patency. The robot is then undocked and port sites are closed as previously described.

Complications

Several important perioperative complications are inherent to both minimally invasive as well as open sacrocolpopexy. These include the risk of vaginotomy, cystostomy, ureteral injury, enterotomy, as well as

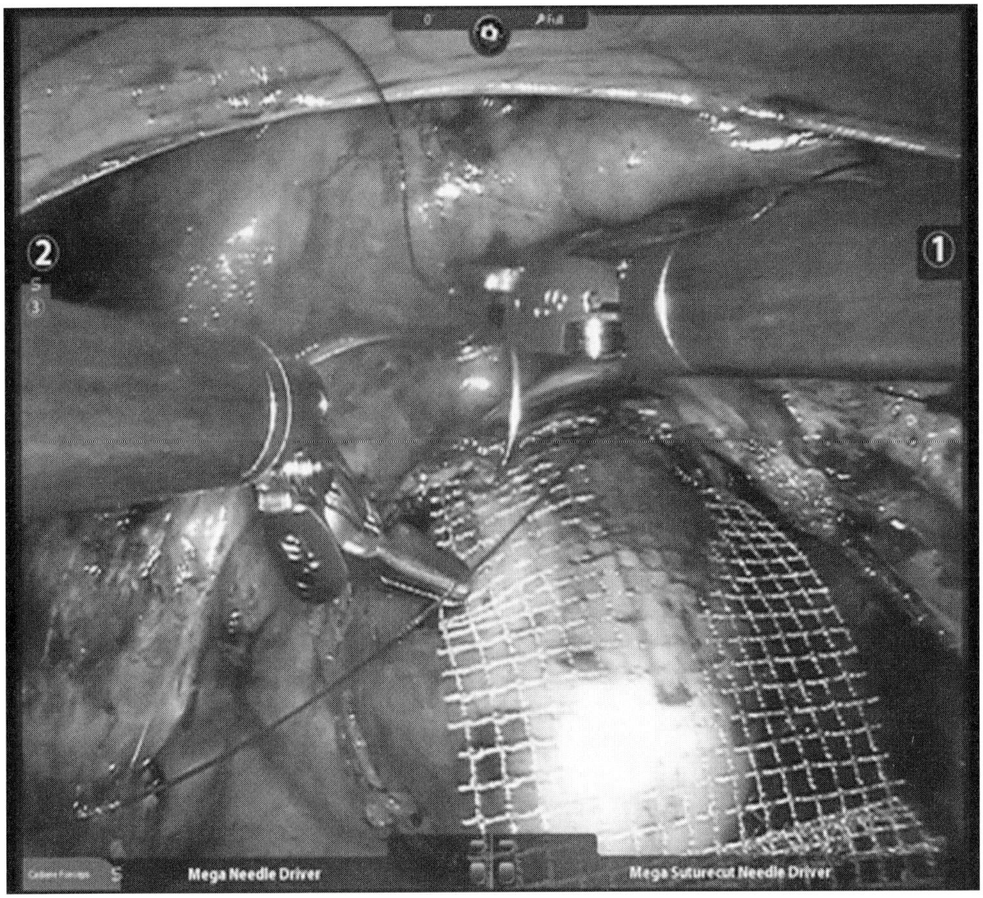

Figure 8.6 Suturing the graft to the anterior vagina. The mesh is sutured to the vagina with 2-0 delayed-absorbable suture.

mesh extrusion or perforation (69). Significant hemorrhage can develop during dissection and suture placement at the anterior longitudinal ligament. A thorough knowledge of pelvic anatomy is essential to prevent and manage intraoperative hemorrhage. The most common vessels lacerated during sacrocolpopexy are presacral venous plexus and middle sacral vessels. To control acute hemorrhage, several steps are critical. First, pressure is applied immediately and held for several minutes. This is particularly effective for venous bleeding. Sutures and clips may be employed, but injury of small veins traversing the sacrum frequently worsens with suturing. Additionally, as vessels retract into the foramena, isolation and ligation become difficult if not impossible. Although no studies have compared these agents for use in urogynecologic procedures, animal and vascular studies have shown FloSeal Matrix (Baxter International, Inc., Deerfield, IL) to be very effective (70–72).

Other complications include discitis after sacrocolpopexy, likely from suture placement into the vertebral disk at the time of surgery (73).

Following sacrocolpopexy, the graft material or its attaching sutures can expose through the vaginal muscularis and mucosa. This is a frequently cited complication of the procedure, but fortunately is uncommon and only develops in 2–5 percent of cases (74,60). Symptoms of exposure can develop on an average of 14 months following surgery and classically consist of vaginal bleeding and discharge (75). During speculum examination, mesh or sutures can usually be directly visualized.

Failure of the procedure to cure prolapse is an additional concern. A meta-analysis of data from 21 studies noted that the overall recurrence rate of prolapse after sacrocolpopexy was 6.4 percent (3.4, 0.4, and 2.6 percent for anterior, apical, and posterior compartments, respectively) (76). The reoperation

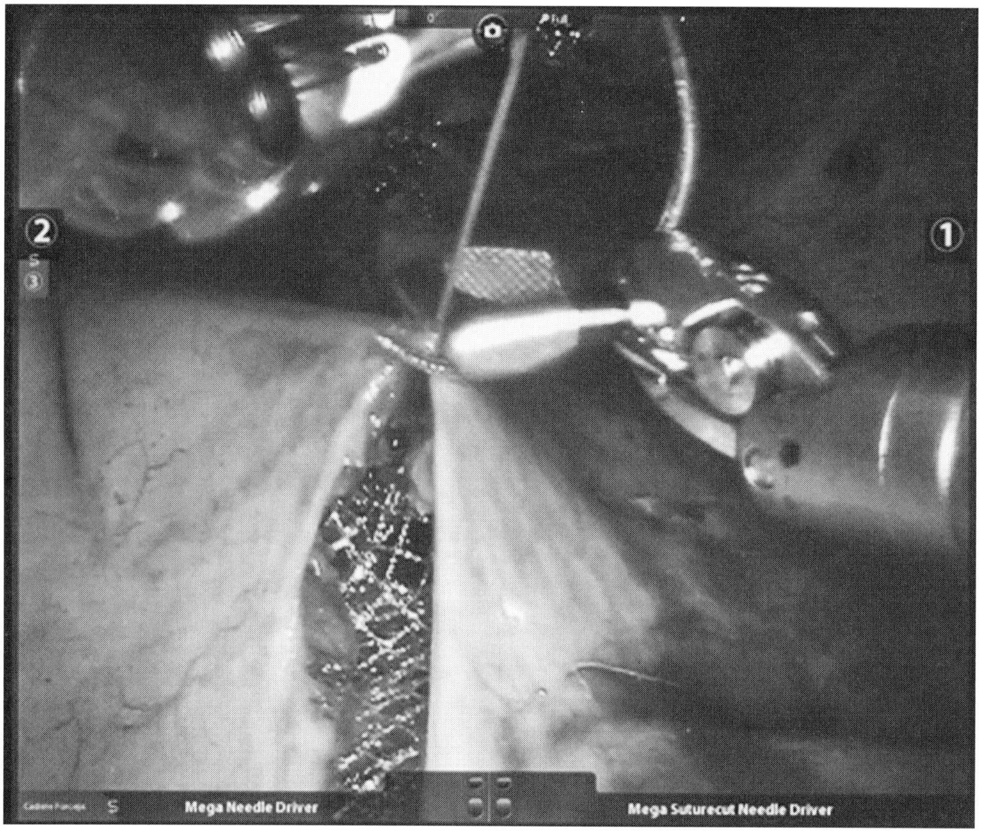

Figure 8.7 Closing the peritoneum. The peritoneum is closed from the vaginal apex to the sacral promontory with 2-0 delayed-absorbable suture in a running fashion.

rate was approximately 3 percent with 63.6 percent of those being posterior colporrhaphies (77). Overall, sacrocolpopexy is considered to be a durable and highly successful procedure.

In order to increase minimally invasive procedures for the repair of POP, the robotic-assisted and laparoscopic surgical approaches have been demonstrated to be feasible and are gaining popularity among pelvic floor reconstructive surgeons. Although outcome data for robotic-assisted sacrocolpopexy is only just emerging, several small series have demonstrated anatomic and functional outcomes, as well as complication rates, comparable to those reported for open surgery (78).

References

1. R. Sinha, M. Sanjay, B. Rupa, S. Kumari. Robotic surgery in gynecology. *J Minim Access Surg.* 2015; 11(1): 50–9.
2. S. Mesogitis, G. Daskalakis, A. Pilalis, N. Papantoniou, N. Thomakos, N. Dessipris. Management of ovarian cysts with aspiration and methotrexate injection. *Radiology* 2005; 235(2): 668–73.
3. D. L. Pearson-Clarke, E. Geller. Complications of hysterectomy. *Obstetrics & Gynecology* 2013; 121: 654–73.
4. American College of Obstetricians and Gynecologists. Robotic surgery in genecology. *Obstet Gynecol.* 2015; 125: 760–7.
5. J. D. Wright, T. J. Herzog, J. Tsui, et al. Nationwide trends in the performance of inpatient hysterectomy in the United States. *Obstet Gynecol.* 2013; 122: 233–41.
6. American College of Obstetricians and Gynecologists. Cervical cancer screening and prevention. *Obstet Gynecol.* 2016; 127: 1–20.
7. American College of Obstetricians and Gynecologists. Diagnosis of abnormal uterine bleeding in reproductive-aged women. *Obstet Gynecol.* 2012; 120: 197–206.
8. American College of Obstetricians and Gynecologists. Management of abnormal uterine bleeding associated with ovulatory dysfunction. *Obstet Gynecol.* 2016; 122: 176–85.

9. American College of Obstetricians and Gynecologists. Elective and risk-reducing salpingoophorectomy. *Obstet Gynecol.* 2008; 111: 231.

10. American College of Obstetricians and Gynecologists. Salpingectomy for ovarian cancer prevention. *Obstet Gynecol.* 2015; 127: 450.

11. W. H. Parker, M. S. Broder, E. Chang, et al. Ovarian conservation at the time of hysterectomy and long-term health outcomes in the nurses' health study. *Obstet Gynecol.* 2009; 113: 1027–37.

12. American College of Obstetricians and Gynecologists. Executive summary: Power morcellation and occult malignancy in gynecologic surgery. May 2014.

13. D. T. Mangano, L. Goldman. Preoperative assessment of patients with known or suspected coronary disease. *NEJM* 1995; 333(26): 1750–6.

14. G. W. Smetana. Preoperative pulmonary evaluation. *NEJM* 1999; 340(12): 937–44.

15. D. Rahn, M. M. Mamta, T. V. Sanses, et al. Venous thromboembolism prophylaxis in gynecologic surgery. *Obstet Gynecol.* 2011; 118(5): 1111–25.

16. American College of Obstetricians and Gynecologists. Antibiotic prophylaxis for gynecologic procedures. *Obstet Gynecol.* 2009; 113: 1180–9.

17. D. E. Soper, R. C. Bump, W. G. Hurt. Bacterial vaginosis and trichomoniasis vaginitis are risk factors for cuff cellulitis after abdominal hysterectomy. *Am J Obstetrics Gynecol.* 1990; 163: 1016–21.

18. P. Harkki-Siren, J. Sjoberg, A. Tiitinen. Urinary tract injuries after hysterectomy. *Obstet Gynecol.* 1998; 92: 113.

19. K. Kuno, A. Menzin, H. H. Kauder, et al. Prophylactic ureteral catheterization in gynecologic surgery. *Urology* 1998; 52: 1004.

20. W. H. Parker. Total laparoscopic hysterectomy and laparoscopic supracervical hysterectomy. *Obstet Gynecol Clin North Am.* 2004; 31: 523.

21. P. Harkki, T. Kurki, J. Sjoberg, et al. Safety aspects of laparoscopic hysterectomy. *Acta Obstet Gynaecol Scand.* 2001; 80: 383.

22. W. Irvin, W. Andersen, P. Taylor, L. Rice. Minimizing the risk of neurologic injury in gynecologic surgery. *Obstet Gynecol.* 2004; 103: 374–82.

23. R. J. Cardosi, C. S. Cox, M. S. Hoffman. Postoperative neuropathies after major pelvic surgery. *Obstet Gynecol.* 2002; 100: 240–4.

24. T. E. Nieboer, N. Johnson, A. Lethaby, et al. Surgical approach to hysterectomy for benign gynaecological disease. *The Cochrane Database of Systematic Reviews* 2009; issue 3.

25. D. T. Gilmour, P. L. Dwyer, M. P. Carey. Lower urinary tract injury during gynecologic surgery and its detection by intraoperative cystoscopy. *Obstet Gynecol.* 1999; 94: 883–9.

26. N. Johnson, D. Barlow, A. Lethaby, et al. Surgical approach to hysterectomy for benign genaecological disease. *The Cochrane Database of Systemic Reviews* 2006; issue 2.

27. D. T. Gilmour, S. Das, G. Flowerdew. Rates of urinary tract injury from gynecologic surgery and the role of intraoperative cystoscopy. *Obstet Gynecol.* 2006; 107: 1366–72.

28. M. E. Carley, D. McIntire, J. M. Carley, J. Schaffer. Incidence, risk factors and morbidity of unintended bladder or ureter injury during hysterectomy. *Int Urogynecol J Pelvic Floor Dysfunc.* 2002; 13: 18–21.

29. J. Makinen, J. Johansson, C. Tomas, et al. Morbidity of 10 110 hysterectomies by type and approach. *Hum Reprod.* 2001; 16: 1473–8.

30. B. Cronin, V. W. Sung, K. Matteson. Vaginal cuff dehiscence: risk factors and management. *Am J Obstet Genecol.* 2012; 206(4): 284–8.

31. M. Agdi, W. Al-Ghafri, R. Antolin, et al. Vaginal vault dehiscence after hysterectomy. *J Minim Invasive Gynecol.* 2009; 16(3): 313.

32. C. K. Lee, S. L. Hansen. Management of acute wounds. *Surg Clin North Am.* 2009; 89(3): 659.

33. J. D. Wright, A. Kostolias, C. V. Ananth, et al. Comparative effectiveness of robotically assisted compared with laparoscopic adnexal surgery for benign gynecologic disease. *Obstet Gynecol.* 2014; 124(5): 886–96.

34. C. Chapron, J. B. Dubuisson, X. Fritel, D. Rambaud. Diagnosis and management of organic ovarian cysts: indications and procedures for laparoscopy. *Hum Reprod Update* 1996; 2(5): 435–46.

35. A. Mahdavi, B. Berker, C. Nezhat, et al. Laparoscopic management of ovarian remnant. *Obstet Gynecol Clin North Am.* 2004; 31: 593.

36. N. Smorgick, O. Barel, R. Halperin, et al. Laparoscopic removal of adnexal cysts: is it possible to decrease inadvertent intraoperative rupture rate? *Am J Obstet Gynecol.* 2009; 200(3): 237.e1–3.

37. C. Nezhat, N. S. Saberi, B. Shahmohamady, F. Nezhat. Robotic-assisted laparoscopy in gynecological surgery. *JSLS* 2006; 10(3): 317–20.

38. R. Marana, A. A. Luciano, L. Muzii, et al. Reproductive outcome after ovarian surgery: suturing versus nonsuturing of the ovarian cortex. *J Gynecol Surg.* 1991; 7: 155.

39. A. K. Wiskind, A. A. Toledo, A. G. Dudley, et al. Adhesion formation after ovarian wound repair in

New Zealand white rabbits: a comparison of ovarian microsurgical closure with ovarian non-closure. *Am J Obstet Gynecol.* 1990; 163: 1674.

40. R. R. Franklin. Reduction of ovarian adhesions by the use of Interceed. Ovarian Adhesion Study Group. *Obstet Gynecol.* 1995; 86(3): 335.
41. D. M. Wiseman, J. R. Trout, R. R. Franklin, et al. Metaanalysis of the safety and efficacy of an adhesion barrier (Interceed TC7) in laparotomy. *J Reprod Med.* 1999; 44(4): 325.
42. American Society for Reproductive Medicine, Society of Reproductive Surgeons. Pathogenesis, consequences, and control of peritoneal adhesions in gynecologic surgery. *Fertil Steril.* 2008; 90(5 suppl): S144.
43. P. Litta, G. D'Agostino, L. Conte, et al. Anti-Mullerian hormone trend after laparoscopic surgery in women with ovarian endometrioma. *Gynecol Endocrinol.* 2013; 29(5): 452–4.
44. C. Yuqing, P. Huihui, C. Yajie, et al. The impact of endometrioma and laparoscopic cystectomy on ovarian reserve and the exploration of related factors assessed by serum anti-Mullerian hormone: a prospective cohort study. *J Ovarian Res.* 2014; 7: 108.
45. V. Bonney. The techniques and results of myomectomy. *Lancet* 1931; 220: 171–7.
46. K. Semm. New methods of pelviscopy (gynecologic laparoscopy) for myomectomy, ovariectomy, tubectomy and adnectomy. *Endoscopy* 1979; 11: 85–93.
47. S. Bocca, L. Stadtmauer, S. Oehninger. Uncomplicated full term pregnancy after da Vinci-assisted laparoscopic myomectomy. *Reprod Biomed Online* 2007; 14: 246–9.
48. M. C. Pitter, A. R. Gargiulo, L. M. Bonaventura, et al. Pregnancy outcomes following robot-assisted myomectomy. *Hum Reprod.* 2013; 28: 99–108.
49. J. W. Williams, B. L. Hoffman. *Williams gynecology* (2nd ed.). New York, NY: McGraw-Hill, 2012; 900–2.
50. American College of Obstetricians and Gynecologists. Alternatives to hysterectomy in the management of leiomyomas. *Practice Bulletin* 96, August 2008.
51. R. E. Iverson, Jr, D. Chelmow, K. Strohbehn, et al. Relative morbidity of abdominal hysterectomy and myomectomy for management of uterine leiomyomas. *Obstet Gynecol.* 1996; 88: 415.
52. S. W. Sawin, N. D. Pilevsky, J. A. Berlin, et al. Comparability of perioperative morbidity between abdominal myomectomy and hysterectomy for women with uterine leiomyomas. *Am J Obstet Gynecol.* 2000; 183: 1448.
53. E. S. Ginsburg, C. B. Benson, J. M. Garfield, et al. The effect of operative technique and uterine size on blood loss during myomectomy: a prospective, randomized study. *Fertil Steril.* 1993;60: 956.
54. Food and Drug Administration. Quantitative assessment of the prevalence of unsuspected uterine sarcoma in women undergoing treatment of uterine fibroids. 2014. Available at www.fda.gov/downloads/MedicalDevices/Safety/AlertsandNotices/UCM393589.pdf
55. V. C. Buttram, R. C. Reiter. Uterine leiomyomata: etiology, symptomatology, and management. *Fertil Steril.* 1981; 36: 433.
56. W. J. Harris. Uterine dehiscence following laparoscopic myomectomy. *Obstet Gynecol.* 1992; 80: 545.
57. S. P. Bayers, D. Jansen. Gore-Tex surgical membrane. In: DeCherney A, Diamond MP, eds. *Treatment of post-surgical adhesions.* Wiley-Liss, 1990.
58. J. Claeys, I. Hellendoorn, T. Hamerlynck, et al. The risk of uterine rupture after myomectomy: a systematic review of the literature and meta-analysis. *Gynecological Surgery* 2014; 11(3): 197–206.
59. J. M. Wu, A. F. Hundley, R. G. Fulton, et al. Forecasting the prevalence of pelvic floor disorders in U.S. women: 2010 to 2050. *Obstet Gynecol.* 2009; 114: 1278–83.
60. I. E. Nygaard, R. McCreery, L. Brubaker, et al. Abdominal sacrocolpopexy: a comprehensive review. *Obstet Gynecol.* 2004; 104: 805–23.
61. P. J. Culligan, L. Blackwell, L. J. Goldsmith, et al. A randomized controlled trial comparing fascia lata and synthetic mesh for sacral colpopexy. *Obstet Gynecol.* 2005; 106: 29.
62. J. C. Winters, R. R. Dmochowski, H. B. Goldman, et al. Urodynamics studies in adults: AUA/SUFU guideline. *J Urology* 2012; 188: 2464–72.
63. J. S. Tan, E. S. Lukacz, S. A. Menefee, et al. Determinants of vaginal length. *Am J Obstet Gynecol.* 2006; 195: 1846–50.
64. M. van IJsselmuiden, M. H. Kerkhof, R. P. Schellart, et al. Variation in the practice of laparoscopic sacrohysteropexy and laparoscopic sacrocolpopexy for the treatment of pelvic organ prolapse: a Dutch survey. *Int Urogynecol J* 2015; 26: 757–64.
65. S. D. Fox, S. L. Stanton. Vault prolapse and rectocele: assessment of repair using sacrocolpopexy with mesh interposition. *BJOG* 2000; 107: 1371–5.
66. B. N. Brown, D. Mani, A. L. Nolfi, et al. Characterization of the host inflammatory response following implantation of prolapse mesh in rhesus macaque. *Am J Obstet Gynecol.* 2015; 213: 668e1–10.
67. J. P. Shepherd, H. L. Higdon III, E. J. Stanford, et al. Effect of suture selection on the rate of suture or

mesh erosion and surgery failure in abdominal sacrocolpopexy. *Female Pelvic Med Reconstr Surg.* 2012; 16: 229–33.

68. C. K. Wieslander, D. D. Rahn, D. D. McIntire, et al. Vascular anatomy of the presacral space in unembalmed female cadavers. *Am J Obstet Gynecol.* 2006; 195: 1736.

69. M. Anand, J. L. Woelk, A. L. Weaver, et al. Perioperative complications of robotic sacrocolpopexy for post-hysterectomy vaginal vault prolapse *Int Urogynecol J* 2014; 25: 1193–200.

70. B. S. Kheirabadi, A. Field-Ridley, R. Pearson, et al. Comparative study of the efficacy of the common topical hemostatic agents with fibrin sealant in a rabbit aortic anastomosis model. *J Surg Res.* 2002; 106: 99.

71. M. C. Oz, D. M. Cosgrove III, B. R. Badduke, et al. Controlled clinical trial of a novel hemostatic agent in cardiac surgery. The Fusion Matrix Study Group. *Ann Thorac Surg.* 2000; 69: 1376.

72. F. A. Weaver, D. B. Hood, M. Zatina, et al. Gelatin-thrombin-based hemostatic sealant for intraoperative bleeding in vascular surgery. *Ann Vasc Surg.* 2002; 16: 286.

73. K. Propst, E. Tunitsky-Bitton, M. O. Schimpf, et al. Pyogenic spondylodiscitis associated with sacral colpopexy and rectopexy: report of two cases and evaluation of the literature. *Int Urogynecol J* 2014; 25: 21–31.

74. M. Beer, A. Kuhn. Surgical techniques for vault prolapse: a review of the literature. *Eur J Obstet Gynecol Reprod Biol.* 2005; 119: 144.

75. N. Kohli, P. M. Walsh, T. W. Roat, et al. Mesh erosion after abdominal sacrocolpopexy. *Obstet Gynecol.* 1998; 92: 999.

76. M. Serati, G. Bogani, P. Sorice, et al. Robot-assisted sacrocolpopexy for pelvic organ prolapse: a systematic review and meta-analysis of comparative studies. *Eur Urol.* 2014; 66: 303–18.

77. M. F. Paraiso, J. E. JJelovsek, A. Frick, et al. Laparoscopic compared with robotic sacral colpopexy for vaginal prolapse. *Obstet Gynecol.* 2011; 118: 1005–13.

78. J. P. Gilleran, M. Johnson, A. Hundley. Robotic-assisted laparoscopic mesh sacrocolpopexy. *Ther Adv Urol.* 2010; 2(5–6): 195–208.

Chapter 9

Robotic Urological Surgery

Danica N. May, Amanda F. Saltzman, and Ryan R. Krlin

Urologists have been at the forefront of the development and use of robotic technology. The first robot-assisted laparoscopic prostatectomy was performed in 2000. The FDA approved the da Vinci Robotic Surgical System in 2000. Its use has increased dramatically over the years, notably among urologists. Current residents and recently graduated urologists are almost universally exposed to robotic surgery. The field of robotics is ever changing. Advances are being made in the fields of telementoring and telerobotics as well as design changes making robotic surgery in combination with imaging such as MRI or CT more feasible. The field of urology has been quick to embrace technology and robotic surgical assistance, utilizing this technology for oncologic, urogynecologic, reconstructive, and pediatric urological cases.

Assistance during these operations is critical. Bedside assistants help with retraction, suction of the surgical field, placement of clips, passage of suture, use of a stapler, manipulation of the Foley catheter, removal of surgical specimen, etc. Clear communication between surgeon and assistant and surgeon and anesthesiologist is crucial for patient safety, operative technique, and patient outcomes.

Prostatectomy – Radical and Simple

In 2015, 220,800 men were diagnosed with prostate cancer, and 27,540 men died of the disease. Over 2.7 million men are living with prostate cancer in the United States currently (Howlader et al., n.d.). Overall, it is one of the most common conditions treated by urologists and is the most common urologic malignancy. In 2011, more than 80% of radical prostatectomies were performed with the assistance of a robot. While the cost of the robotic approach leads to criticisms, there are clear benefits (Skolarus et al., 2010). Further studies are ongoing, but with the widespread dissemination of robots into hospitals and ever-increasing number of urologists trained on the robot, robotic-assisted laparoscopic prostatectomies will likely remain the surgery of choice for prostate cancer treatment.

Radical Prostatectomy

This operation involves removal of the entire prostate gland and seminal vesicles, with reconnection of the urethra directly to the bladder to restore continuity of the genitourinary tract. This is typically done for prostate cancer. It is one of the most common procedures utilizing robotic assistance, across all specialties. The original radical prostatectomy was performed in 1905 via a perineal approach, which was then modified to the lower abdominal extraperitoneal approach (McDougal et al., 2011). Standard laparoscopy was tried for prostatectomy, but proved to be extremely difficult secondary to the lack of articulating instruments, which makes working in a deep, small space, such as the pelvis, difficult. While oncologic outcomes have not been proven to be superior to the standard open approach, blood loss, transfusion rates, and hospital length of stay have been improved with the robot. Incontinence and erectile dysfunction, two of the most common and significant complications of prostatectomy, are similar between open and robotic approaches (McDougal et al., 2011).

Most surgeons elect for a light bowel prep preoperatively as the anatomy of the prostate is in very close proximity to the rectum, and rectal injury is possible. We routinely instruct our patients to drink clear liquids the day before surgery, along with a bottle of magnesium citrate. This allows for a cleaner field if rectal injury occurs. Anticoagulation is left to the discretion of the surgeon, but most elect to hold all anticoagulants preoperatively. Unlike open radical prostatectomy, the rates of transfusion are low and many surgeons do not routinely type and screen patients. However, for simple prostatectomy, most surgeons will have blood readily available due to the risk of significant hemorrhage.

The operating suite is generally set up as shown in Figure 9.1. We do not administer pharmacologic DVT prophylaxis, but all patients have thromboembolic stockings and sequential compression devices for mechanical DVT prophylaxis. The patient is placed under general anesthesia with paralysis. It is our practice to have two large bore IVs with no need for arterial or central lines. An orogastric tube is placed for stomach decompression. The arms are tucked and the patient is placed in the low lithotomy position. Care is taken to ensure that the legs are well supported to avoid nerve injury, usually using Yellowfins® stirrups. A strap is placed across the chest to secure the patient to the table on nonskid padding, such as the Pink Pad®, which limits patient shifting with bed movement. The patient is placed in maximal Trendelenburg position to allow the bowels to move cranially out of the pelvis (Figure 9.2). The abdomen, upper thighs, and genitalia are prepped using chlorhexidine. A Foley catheter is placed after draping, which will be changed prior to the end of the procedure.

Entry into the abdomen is established just superior to the umbilicus, either using a Veress needle or the open Hasson technique. This location will be the camera port. As with any procedure involving the establishment of pneumoperitoneum, the anesthesiologist should watch for hypercarbia and oliguria. Communication between surgeon and anesthesiologist is key should pneumoperitoneum pressures need adjustment. If inguinal hernias are present, the scrotum may enlarge and fill with a significant amount of air, which should be manually decompressed at the conclusion of the procedure.

Once the 12-mm camera port is inserted just above the umbilicus, three 8-mm robotic trocars and a 12-mm assistant trocar are placed. The robot is docked between the patient's legs. Monopolar scissors are placed in the right hand, bipolar Maryland forceps in the left hand, and a ProGrasp™ in the fourth arm (located on the left). The assistant sits on the patient's right.

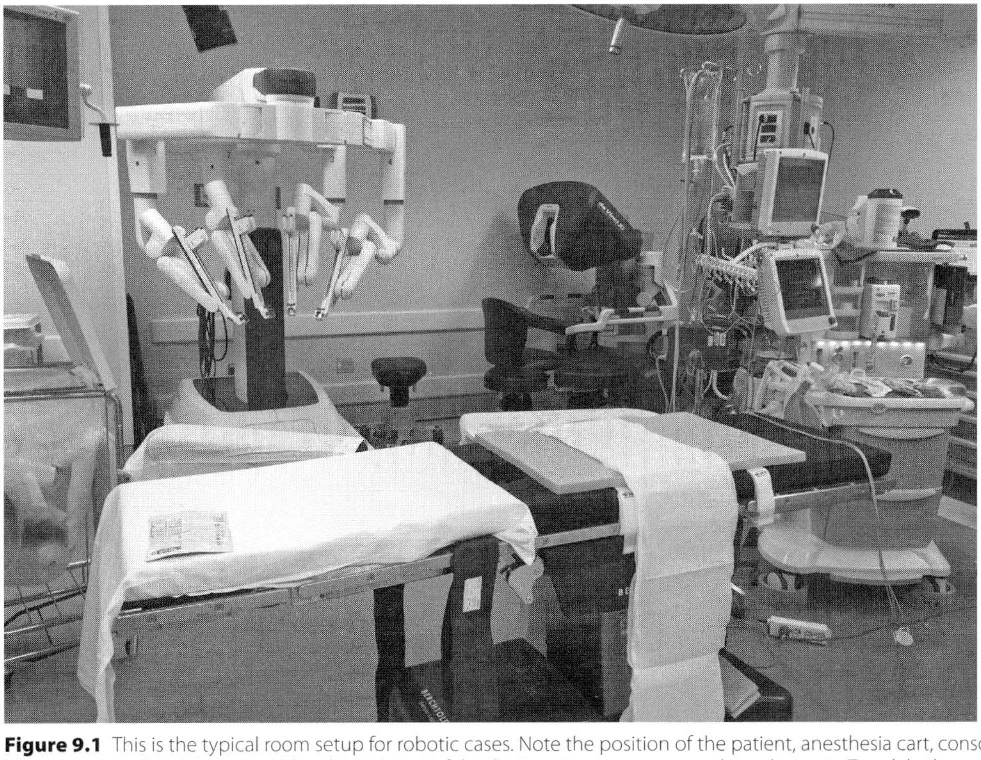

Figure 9.1 This is the typical room setup for robotic cases. Note the position of the patient, anesthesia cart, console, and robot. This is an example of the non-skid pad which is useful to limit patient movement when placing in Trendelenburg.

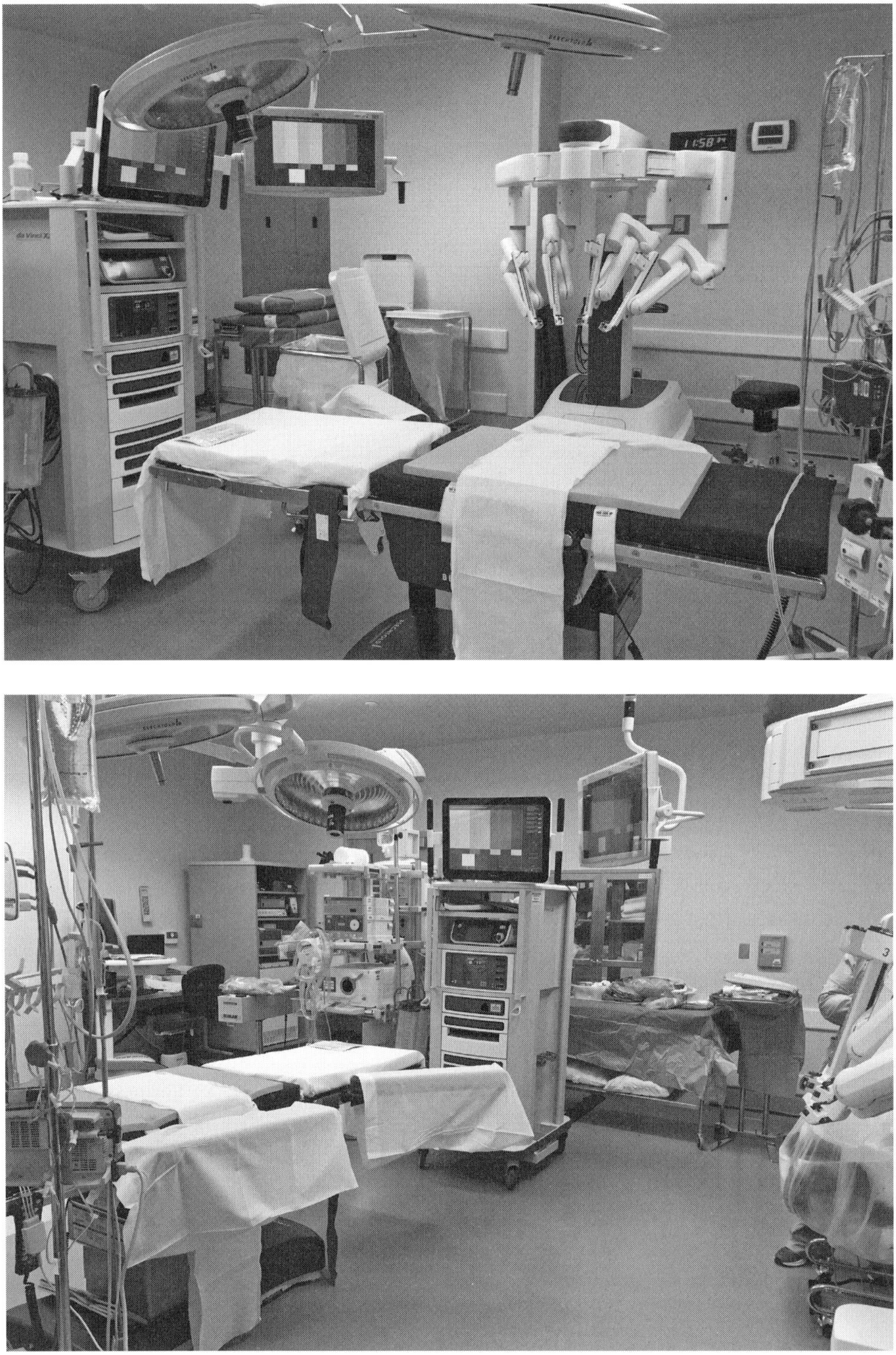

Figure 9.1 *(continued)*

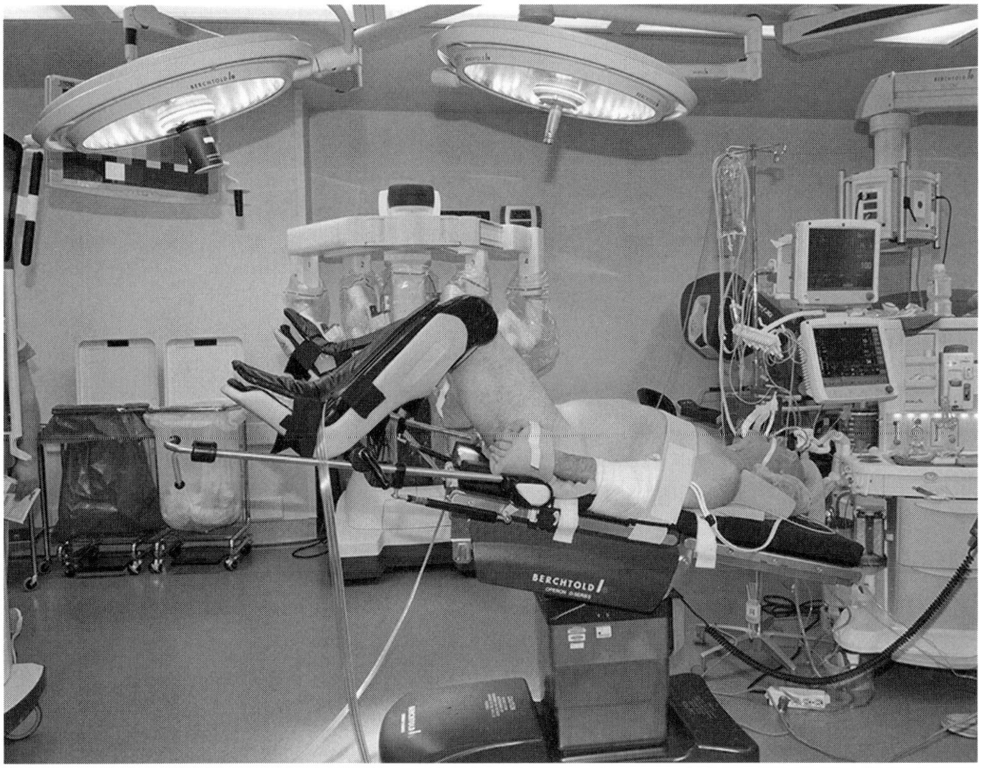

Figure 9.2 This is typical positioning for a RALP. The patient is in Trendelenburg. All pressure points are padded including padding around any pressure points on the legs. The arms are tucked and a chest strap is in place. A non-skid pad limits the patient from sliding towards the head.

Upon entering the abdomen, adhesions are lysed. The sigmoid colon is freed and retracted out of the pelvis using the fourth arm. The procedure can then be accomplished working first anterior then posterior, or posterior then anterior. We typically perform a posterior approach and will describe this here. The peritoneum overlying the seminal vesicles and vasa deferentia is incised. The vas and seminal vesicles are dissected free bilaterally. The vasa are clipped and amputated. The posterior prostate is then dissected from the rectum moving caudally, along Denonvillier's fascia. Care is taken during this step to avoid rectal injury. This completes the posterior dissection.

We then move anteriorly and drop the bladder from the anterior abdominal wall between the medial umbilical ligaments. This opens the potential space of Retzius and is a filmy alveolar layer with minimal bleeding. This allows entry into the pelvis. Care is taken during these steps to ensure no injury to the inferior epigastric vessels. The lateral endopelvic fascia is then incised and the levator ani muscles are dissected laterally, exposing the lateral edges of the prostate. Anteriorly, care is taken to maintain the musculature as much as possible as these muscles control continence. If clinically indicated, the external, internal, and obturator lymph nodes are dissected and sent to pathology to complete staging. Care is taken during these steps to ensure no damage to the iliac vessels, which may result in significant hemorrhage. Additionally, avoiding electrocautery around the obturator nerves is crucial to avoid stimulating an obturator reflex (adduction of the ipsilateral leg). Some surgeons use clips to control lymphatics to minimize postoperative lymphocele formation.

The dorsal venous complex is controlled. We use suture ligation tacked up to the posterior pubic rami to ensure adequate tensioning. This step is crucial as the dorsal venous complex can be a significant source of bleeding, which makes visualization during the remainder of the operation difficult. The junction between the bladder and prostate is then identified and then opened horizontally until the catheter is identified. It is important to ensure the bladder neck opening is small to improve continence rates and to avoid tailoring prior to anastomosis. It is also important to avoid ureteral injury. Once the bladder is opened, hematuria and/or decreased urine output is expected as urine drains into the abdominal cavity. The Foley catheter bag may fill with air as the pneumoperitoneum equalizes pressure via the exposed Foley catheter. The Foley catheter is then manipulated to alter exposure and the posterior bladder neck is transected. Dissection through the bladder neck has now reached our previous posterior dissection.

The prostatic pedicles are then controlled using clips or electrocautery. The dissection is then taken laterally and caudally releasing the prostate from its posterior and lateral attachments. This dissection is very important for the preservation of erectile function, and the nerve plexus responsible for erections lies in very close proximity. If possible, these nerves are spared, minimizing electrocautery in this plane. The apex of the prostate is then transected, the Foley removed, and the prostate is tucked into the lower abdomen near the assistant port. At this point, all major bleeding has ceased.

The pelvis is irrigated. Insufflation pressures are lowered to assess for hemostasis. The posterior urethrovesical anastomosis is then performed using an absorbable suture. Once the posterior plate of the anastomosis is completed, the Foley is replaced with a larger one, typically 18 Fr, under direct vision to ensure proper position of the catheter in the bladder. The anastomosis is completed and tied. It is then leak-tested with retrograde filling of the bladder with water or saline via the Foley catheter. Surgeons may leave a drain in the pelvis if the anastomosis is not watertight. The prostate is placed in a specimen bag and the robot is undocked. The specimen is extracted through the camera port site. Only the fascia at the extraction site is closed. The trocar sites are then closed using absorbable sutures.

The Foley catheter typically remains in place for one week postoperatively. If there is concern over healing of the anastomosis, the catheter may be left longer and a cystogram may be performed to evaluate for leakage.

Certain patient characteristics must be taken into consideration by both the surgeon and anesthesia team:

Obesity – Extra tissue and the steep Trendelenburg position may compromise the patient's respirations and may allow for shifting with extreme positioning. Obese patients are at high risk for compression nerve injury. Standard open prostatectomy is technically more difficult in the obese patient due to difficulty reaching the deep pelvis, thus a robotic approach may be preferred for these patients. If necessary, bariatric instruments are available and trocars can be moved caudally to improve access to the pelvis with the robotic arms. In addition, obese patients are more likely to suffer from a deep venous thrombosis, and the decision to utilize both mechanical and chemical prophylaxis must be weighed preoperatively (Su, 2011).

Salvage procedures – These include patients who have undergone prior treatment of the pelvis, typically radiation and/or radioactive seed placement. This increases the level of difficulty of the operation and increases the chance of complications such as rectal injury and hemorrhage.

Prior abdominal surgery – This may increase operative times due to adhesions or difficulty entering the abdominal cavity if mesh was used for hernia repairs. Open Hasson technique should be utilized to gain access into the abdomen in patients at risk for adhesions. One can also perform a minilaparotomy with open adhesiolysis to safely place ports prior to RALP. The incision can then be closed around the camera port. Hernia repair surgery can distort pelvic anatomy. Care must be taken to identify landmarks early on and throughout the case. The urachus and medial umbilical ligaments are common starting points to allow entry into the retropubic space. Care must be taken to dissect deep to any mesh that was previously placed during the hernia repair (Su, 2011).

Large prostate or median lobe – Large prostates may limit surgical advancement by limiting space in the pelvis for dissection and retraction. Early control of the dorsal venous complex is utilized to attempt to limit bleeding into the surgical field. Large prostates also often have increased vascularity, which can complicate dissection. Medan lobes distort anatomy of the bladder neck dissection. Care must be taken to ensure all prostate tissue is resected while preserving the ureteral orifices as they are closer to the prostatic base than in patients without a large median lobe (Su, 2011).

Simple Prostatectomy

This procedure treats benign urinary obstruction of the prostate, with glands that are too large to be efficiently treated by more traditional methods, i.e., transurethral resection. The posterior zone (where cancer typically develops) is left during subtotal resection; only the anterior and transition zones are removed. This procedure is very similar to the radical prostatectomy with respect to preparation and positioning. Only the obstructing glands of the prostate are removed; thus, the urethra and bladder are not cut and the urinary tract remains in continuity.

An important difference between the radical and simple robotic prostatectomy is an increased risk of hemorrhage with simple prostatectomy. Measures are utilized to mitigate this risk such as arterial line use and readily available blood products. Additionally, the patient typically is placed on continuous bladder irrigation at the conclusion of the case due to significant hematuria.

Port placement and access to the abdomen are similar to the technique used for radical prostatectomy. The bladder is mobilized and the space of Retzius is entered. The anterior prostatic capsule is identified and the dorsal venous complex is ligated as for a radical prostatectomy. The bladder is opened transversely on the anterior surface of the junction of the bladder and prostate. Care should be taken to identify the ureteral orifices as they are often very close to the enlarged prostatic tissue. Ureteral stents can be placed to have continuous identification of the ureteral orifices if indicated. Next, the prostatic adenoma is identified and retracted, allowing the adenoma excision beginning posteriorly. The plane between capsule and adenoma is identified and the adenoma is dissected from the capsule circumferentially, from base to apex. Careful attention is paid near the apex to avoid inadvertent damage to the urethral sphincter. Hemostasis is achieved with suture ligation, which is typically needed at the 4 and 8 o'clock positions where the vasculature is located. A large three-way Foley catheter is placed into the urethra and bladder and filled with approximately 30 cc of fluid. The cystotomy is closed in a two-layer manner to ensure that it is watertight. This can be tested by instilling fluid into the bladder retrograde via the catheter and watching for leakage. Finally, the specimen is removed and the port sites are closed after extraction of the trocars.

Nephrectomy – Radical, Simple, and Partial

The use of robotic assistance for renal surgery has become common. Traditional open renal surgery typically involves a large flank incision, which is very painful. Urologists are increasingly using laparoscopic and robotic assistance during renal surgery. Studies comparing robotic renal surgery to open renal surgery commonly find decreased blood loss, pain, postoperative hospitalization, and use of narcotics for the robotic group (Emtage et al., 2015). Patients also tend to prefer the superior cosmesis of a minimally invasive approach.

Renal surgery has shifted from removal of the entire kidney to removal of only the diseased part of the kidney, depending on tumor size and location. A radical nephrectomy includes removal of everything within Gerota's fascia, i.e., the entire kidney and adrenal gland, while simple nephrectomy implies removal of the entire kidney, but not everything else contained within Gerota's. A partial nephrectomy removes only a part of the kidney, leaving some remaining kidney in situ. As a group, urologists are performing more partial nephrectomies to spare nephrons and preserve as much renal function as possible. This is becoming increasingly important in patients with comorbidities that can affect renal function.

A formal lymph node dissection is rarely performed unless clinically indicated. Renal cell carcinoma may involve a tumor thrombus extending into the renal vein, inferior vena cava, or heart. Tumor thrombus does not preclude use of robotic technology, but makes resection significantly more challenging. Robotic resection involving tumor thrombus is usually used only at high-volume centers with highly experienced surgeons.

Radical and Simple Nephrectomy

Bowel prep is not typically used preoperatively unless there is concern about potential colon injury during resection. Anticoagulation is left to the discretion of the surgeon, but most elect to hold all anticoagulants preoperatively. Preoperatively, renal function is assessed and patients are counseled on the risk of postoperative renal impairment. We do not administer pharmacologic DVT prophylaxis, but all patients have thromboembolic stockings and sequential compression devices for mechanical DVT prophylaxis.

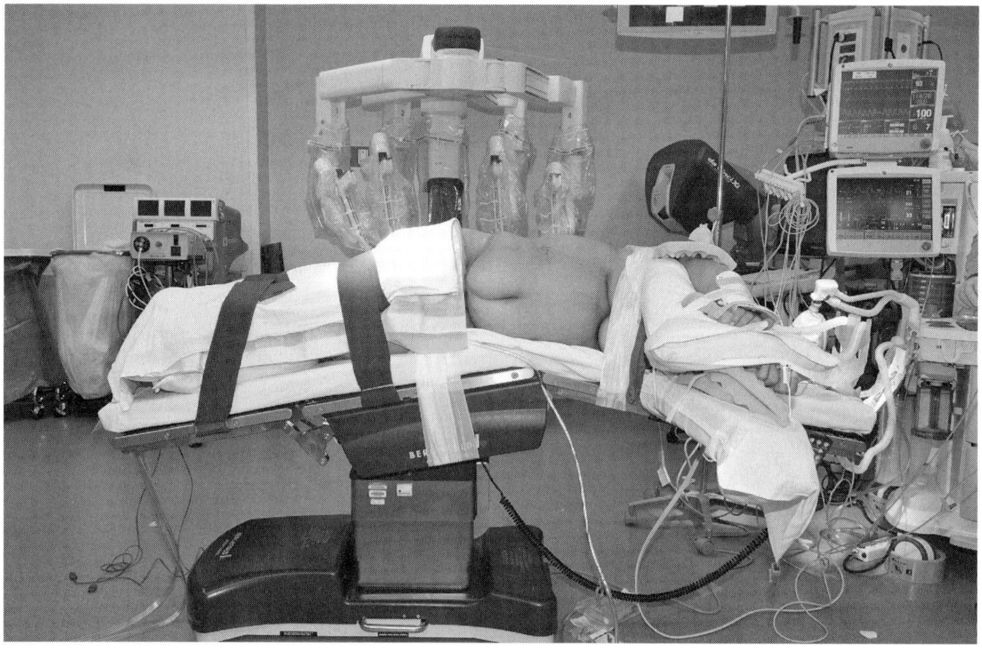

Figure 9.3 Flank positioning is frequently used for robotic surgery on the kidney. An axillary roll is placed and the lower leg is bent 90 degrees at the knee. Pillows are utilized to pad and position the arms. Silk tape secures the hips and chest to the table and the bed is then flexed to open the space below the ribs and above the iliac crest.

We advocate for preoperative imaging to be readily available in the operating suite, either on a large TV monitor or a nearby computer throughout the case, for reference if necessary.

The operating suite is generally set up as for prostatectomy, regardless of which side is being operated on. The patient is placed under general anesthesia with paralysis. It is our practice to have two large-bore IVs. Again, we do not routinely place arterial or central lines. An orogastric tube is placed for stomach decompression, and a Foley catheter is placed for bladder decompression. The patient is placed in the modified or full flank position with the affected kidney up toward the ceiling. This allows the bowels to fall away from the kidney. An axillary roll is placed along with a roll behind the patient's back for support. The lower leg is bent to 90 degrees. Numerous pillows are placed between the legs to support the top leg. The arms are carefully secured using pillows, ensuring no nerve injury and that the arms will not slip during the procedure. The hips and chest are secured to the table using silk tape. The bed is flexed to maximize working space between the costal margin and iliac crest (Figure 9.3). If necessary, the bed is then rotated, turning the patient's back toward the robot for docking. Communication between all members of the operating team is important during this step to ensure the endotracheal tube and lines remain in proper position. The patient is then prepped with chlorhexidine and draped.

Entry into the abdomen is established, either using a Veress needle or the open Hassan technique. The costal margin is palpated as the most cranial robotic port. The remaining ports are then chosen to allow adequate working space. Three or four arms may be used based on surgeon preference. The 12-mm camera port is placed first, and then 8-mm ports are placed under direct vision. Assistant port number and location is per surgeon preference, with many variations currently in use. The assistant sits on the patient's abdominal side. If working on the right side, a 5-mm trocar is placed just under the xyphoid process. A locking grasper is used to retract the liver cranially off the right kidney. The robot is docked from the patient's back. Monopolar scissors are placed in the right hand and bipolar Maryland forceps in the left hand. If the fourth arm is used, it is the most caudal arm, and usually a fenestrated bipolar instrument is used.

The colon is reflected medially along the white line of Toldt, from the iliac vessels to the diaphragm, exposing the retroperitoneum. Care is taken to avoid injury to the colon during this step. On the left, the splenorenal ligament is divided allowing the spleen to fall medially. The tail of the pancreas is in close proximity, and care is taken to avoid injury during the resection. On the right, the hepatorenal ligament is divided releasing the liver cranially. Also on the right, a Kocher maneuver is performed to release the duodenum medially.

Moving toward the inferior pole of the kidney, the ureter is identified and elevated off the psoas muscle. This dissection is carried cranially toward the lower pole of the kidney and then the renal hilum. On the left, the gonadal vein courses with the ureter and can be traced directly up to its insertion into the renal vein. On the right, the gonadal vein enters the IVC directly, and thus care is taken not to tear the gonadal vein from the IVC, which would lead to significant bleeding.

The renal hilum is identified. A window above and below the hilum is created and a stapler is usually employed to control and divide the hilum – this is done by the assistant through the assistant port. All personnel scrubbed for the case need to be well versed in loading, operation, and troubleshooting of the stapler. Additional loads must be readily available in case of hemorrhage.

The upper pole of the kidney is freed. Care must be taken near the adrenal vein as it can cause significant bleeding. The decision to remove or spare the adrenal gland depends on certain tumor and patient characteristics. This should not affect the hypothalamic–pituitary–adrenal axis as the patient has a remaining contralateral adrenal gland. The posterior and lateral renal attachments are freed leaving the ureter as the only remaining attachments. This is then clipped and amputated. The kidney is placed in a specimen bag and extracted, with the site of extraction being left to surgeon preference. Only the fascia at the extraction site is closed. Trocar sites are then closed using absorbable sutures. A drain is not typically placed unless there is concern for bleeding.

Partial Nephrectomy

Studies indicate that the adoption of robotic surgery by urologists has increased the rate of performing partial nephrectomies rather than a radical nephrectomy on small renal masses. The dexterity and visual detail provided by the robot have made this possible and more nephrons are spared as a result. Laparoscopic surgery decreases blood loss and length of stay for partial and radical nephrectomies as compared to open surgery (Skolarus et al., 2010).

Partial nephrectomy may be performed by one of two approaches, transperitoneal or retroperitoneal. The decision on which to employ is based on numerous factors, including tumor location, body habitus, surgical history, and surgeon experience. Retroperitoneal surgery avoids entry into the peritoneal cavity and would be preferable to avoid anticipated intraabdominal adhesions and decrease bowel manipulation. This has been shown to reduce postoperative ileus (Emtage et al., 2015). Posterior renal masses can be difficult to safely access transperitoneally and are thus best suited for the retroperitoneal approach.

Preoperative preparation for partial nephrectomy is similar to radical nephrectomy. Most surgeons will type and cross a patient and have blood readily available due to the increased risk of bleeding during this procedure, and anesthesia will often place an arterial line due to this risk. Mannitol and Lasix, if used by the surgeon, should be available and drawn up prior to induction of anesthesia. Some surgeons believe these diuretics help protect renal function through an osmotic diuresis and free radical scavenging, thus theoretically protecting against ischemic damage (Mir et al., 2015). Operating suite setup and patient positioning are similar to radical nephrectomy.

For the transperitoneal approach, access into the abdomen and initial steps to the operation are also similar to radical nephrectomy. The colon is reflected and the ureter elevated to allow dissection cranially toward the renal hilum. Once the hilum is identified, the artery is carefully dissected circumferentially if selective artery only clamping will be employed. Gerota's fat overlying the kidney is opened and the kidney is mobilized adequately to identify the renal mass and allow adequate exposure for excision and repair. Again, imaging must be readily available intraoperatively for constant reference. Intraoperative ultrasound, controlled by either the assistant or surgeon, is used to delineate the renal mass from its surrounding parenchyma. Mannitol and Lasix, if desired, are administered, ideally 10 minutes prior to vascular clamping. The renal capsule is scored around the tumor, leaving an adequate margin of normal renal tissue.

Prior to clamping, communication with all members of the operative team is imperative to ensure all supplies are readily available and that anesthesia is ready for potential blood loss. Personnel handoffs should be minimized during clamping. The hilum (or artery only) is clamped using a bulldog clamp introduced through the assistant port. A timer is started to monitor warm ischemia time. The tumor is then sharply excised. Some surgeons choose to control obvious vessels with clips during this dissection. The tumor is removed and tucked cranially under the diaphragm. The renal bed is then oversewn using an absorbable suture with a Lapra-ty® on the free end. Another Lapra-ty®, placed by the assistant, is used to tension this hemostatic stitch. The clamp is removed, the timer stopped, and hemostasis is assessed. Warm ischemia time less than 20 minutes is ideal to minimize ischemic damage to the remaining renal parenchyma. Another dose of Mannitol and Lasix is given, if desired. Additional vessels are oversewn as needed. The renorrhaphy – closure of the renal defect – is then performed using a larger absorbable suture with Hem-o-lock® and Lapra-ty® clips. These are cinched down and secured using more clips. The assistant passes all necessary sutures and clips.

Hemostatic agents may be placed over the renorrhaphy. Gerota's may be secured over the renal defect. A drain is left at the discretion of the surgeon, more often during partial nephrectomy than radical or simple nephrectomy. The kidney is placed in a specimen bag and extracted, with the site of extraction being left to surgeon preference, most commonly through the camera port site. Only the fascia at the extraction site is closed. All trocar sites are then closed using absorbable sutures.

For the retroperitoneal approach, positioning is the same as previously described. The camera port is placed above the iliac crest and lateral to the triangle of Petit. The lumbodorsal fascia is opened so that the finger can gently sweep away the peritoneum and create a small space within the retroperitoneum. A balloon dissector is inserted and inflated under direct vision to create a working space. The balloon is removed and the camera is replaced in this area. The rest of the ports are placed. The robot is docked over the patient's head and parallel to the patient's spine. It is essential that anesthesia prepare for this setup. Drapes are not secured during this case at the patient's head due to need for robotic arm mobility. Fat surrounding the kidney is dissected away until Gerota's fascia is identified and then opened. The kidney and perinephric fat is elevated until the hilar vessels are identified. The renal artery and vein are identified and dissected free to allow clamp placement. The remainder of the operation is similar to transperitoneal partial nephrectomy. Care must be taken during this operation to avoid entry into the peritoneum with port placement or during dissection (Ghani et al., 2014). Overall, the retroperitoneal approach is equivalent to the transperitoneal approach with respect to blood loss, alteration in renal function, and warm ischemia time. In one study, the retroperitoneal approach has been shown to decrease operative and hospital time compared to the transperitoneal approach (Stepanian et al., 2015).

The kidney is very vascular, receiving about 20 percent of total cardiac output. Bleeding is thus a challenge and concern for surgeons. This may be manifested as hemodynamic instability or hematuria intraoperatively, if the collecting system is entered. Immediately postoperatively, tight blood pressure control and bedrest can minimize the risk of bleeding. Blood counts are periodically checked. Should there be significant bleeding that does not respond to conservative measures such as transfusion or bedrest, embolization by interventional radiology is usually the next step.

Entry into the collecting system may occur during tumor excision. The collecting system is usually repaired with a running absorbable suture to prevent urine leak. A drain should be placed if the collecting system is entered to monitor for urine leak. Placement of a JJ ureteral stent in an antegrade fashion may also be employed.

Nephroureterectomy

Nephroureterectomy is utilized in the treatment of carcinoma of the ureter or renal pelvis, termed upper tract urothelial cell carcinoma (UTUC). Due to the rarity of UTUC, this procedure is not commonly performed and will not be described in great detail here. However, it is worth mentioning because of the recent Xi robotic system that has been developed.

This procedure involves removal of the entire kidney, entire ureter, and a cuff of bladder around the ipsilateral ureteral orifice. Thus, access to both the upper abdomen and lower pelvis is necessary to complete the operation. The kidney work can be done as described for a nephrectomy, but the bladder work cannot be done with ports in the described locations. With the previous S and Si models of the robot, the robot needed to be undocked, additional ports placed to work in the pelvis, and then redocked. One of the main advantages of the newest Xi system is the ability to manipulate the arms of the robot to perform multiquadrant surgery, such as that needed for nephroureterectomy.

Cystoprostatectomy with Reconstruction

The cystoprostatectomy for the treatment of bladder cancer involves removal of all organs of the anterior pelvis – bladder, prostate, seminal vesicles in men and bladder, vagina, uterus, fallopian tubes, ovaries in women. The procedure also calls for an aggressive lymph node dissection, removing the common, external, and internal iliac and obturator lymph nodes. Negative lymphadenectomy of at least 12 nodes is a positive prognostic indicator (McDougal et al., 2011). The rate of robotic cystectomies is increasing. Between 2004 and 2010, robotic cystectomy increased from 0.6 percent to 12.8 percent (Lau et al., 2015). This new approach has been proven to decrease transfusion rates and blood loss. Operative time may be longer than the traditional open approach, but hospital course tends to be shorter for surgeries undergoing robotic assistance (Skolarus et al., 2010; Lau et al., 2015).

Bladder cancer generally affects older men with significant comorbidities. Some surgeons elect for neoadjuvant chemotherapy for muscle-invasive bladder cancer, often consisting of regimens of methotrexate, vinblastine, doxorubicin, and cisplatin, or gemcitabine and cisplatin. There is clear data that neoadjuvant chemotherapy can achieve a complete pathologic node response in select patients (Zargar-Shoshtari et al., 2016). Chemotherapy has many obvious side effects, with two important ones being weight loss and malnutrition. These need to be minimized to allow patients to maintain adequate nutritional status.

Once the bladder and associated structures are removed, the ureters need to somehow be diverted so all urine can drain externally. This involves use of bowel to create either continent or incontinent diversions. Details of these different diversions are beyond the scope of this chapter, but suffice it to say that the creation of an ileal conduit is the most common diversion. It is an incontinent diversion and has the lowest complication rate of all diversion options but does require an external urostomy appliance for urine collection. Continent diversions have higher complication rates such as stones, incontinence, or inability to catheterize and are more complex to perform. Also, continent diversions require the patient to perform some type of catheterization program with irrigations (Farnham & Cookson, 2004).

Cystectomy surgery carries the highest rate of morbidity and mortality of all major urologic oncologic operations. The overall complication rate is 48 percent, with a 20 percent rehospitalization rate and 4.2 percent mortality rate (Lau et al., 2015). The need for mobilization and resection of bowel to create a urinary diversion makes patients at high risk for postoperative ileus and bowel obstruction. Prolonged hospital stays put patients at risk for urinary tract infections, venous thrombosis, pulmonary embolism, and pneumonia. Many studies look at the care of these patients intraoperatively and postoperatively to attempt to define pathways and decrease complications in this population.

Preoperatively, the patient meets with the ostomy nurse, who educates the patient on what to expect and marks the patient's future stoma site. This mark must persist until the operation is performed to allow for correct stoma localization when created. A formal bowel preparation is ordered preoperatively due to the harvesting of bowel to create the diversion as well as the risk of rectal injury. Some surgeons elect to check nutrition labs preoperatively to optimize wound healing after major surgery, as malnourishment increases perioperative morbidity and mortality (Cerantola et al., 2013). Anticoagulation is left to the discretion of the surgeon. Due to the high risk of thromboembolic events and the length of time of the procedure, most surgeons will administer some type of pharmacologic prophylaxis in addition to mechanical measures, prior to the induction of anesthesia. Like the radical prostatectomy, robotic cystectomy has decreased blood loss compared to the open version of the procedure, so patients are usually typed and screened preoperatively, but blood does not need to be readily available.

The operating suite is generally set up just as for a robotic prostatectomy. The patient is placed under general anesthesia with paralysis. It is our practice to have two large-bore IVs and an arterial line. An orogastric tube is placed for stomach decompression. The arms are tucked and the patient is placed in the low lithotomy position similar to a radical prostatectomy. The patient is again placed in maximal Trendelenburg position on nonskid padding, such as the Pink Pad®, and prepped and draped just as for prostatectomy. A Foley catheter is placed after draping, which will be removed prior to the end of the procedure.

Entry into the abdomen and port placement are performed the same as for a radical prostatectomy. We attempt to place the right hand port where the stoma is marked, if possible. The assistant sits on the patient's left. The robot is docked between the patient's legs. Monopolar scissors are placed in the right hand, bipolar Maryland forceps in the left hand, and a ProGrasp™ in the fourth arm located on the right. An additional suprapubic 12-mm port will be placed when the diversion portion of the procedure occurs.

We begin by reflecting the descending and sigmoid colon medially along the white line of Toldt. We then identify the ureter on the left, dissecting this free distally and proximally to allow significant mobility. The distal ureter is clipped and amputated. A margin is sent for frozen section to confirm no malignancy. On the left, it is imperative that the ureter is adequately freed as the ureter will pass under the sigmoid mesentery to the right side to be plugged into the ileal conduit. If the margin is positive, a more proximal margin is sent until a negative margin is achieved. We then proceed with the lymph node dissection, which removes the common, internal, and external iliac nodes along with the obturator nodes. Dissection around these large vessels has potential for significant bleeding should vascular injury occur. The posterior dissection is done as with a radical prostatectomy, clearing the prostate from the rectum posteriorly. The anterior dissection is also performed like a radical prostatectomy. This allows us to identify the lateral pedicle of the bladder and prostate, the only remaining attachments laterally, which is controlled with a stapler through the assistant port. These steps are repeated on the right side. The apex of the prostate is then transected and the specimen is freed. The specimen is placed in a bag and tucked deep into the pelvis. The urethra remains in place in a man. In a woman, the specimen contains the uterus, fallopian tubes, and ovaries, and the surgeon then performs a urethrectomy, due to the short length of the urethra, from a perineal approach. The vagina is then oversewn from this same approach to close the dependent portion of the pelvis.

A window is created bluntly behind the sigmoid mesentery and the left ureter is passed under the sigmoid, through this window, to the right side. Next the diversion is created. An ileal conduit will be described here, as it is the most common diversion and what we routinely perform. This may be done completely intracorporally or alternatively using a small lower midline laparotomy incision, per surgeon's preference. A 15–20-cm portion of ileum is isolated about 20 cm from the ileocecal valve using a stapler through an additional suprapubic 12-mm port. This allows the terminal ileum to remain in place, as this has important absorptive function of vitamin B12. The length of the conduit depends on the patient's body habitus and has important metabolic consequences as patients develop a hypokalemic, hyperchloremic metabolic acidosis with longer segments producing more profound derangements. The conduit, however, needs to reach from the peritoneal cavity to the patient's skin, which can be a great distance in the obese patient.

Bowel continuity is restored creating a side-to-side anastomosis, again with a stapler through the suprapubic port. The conduit segment is placed under the bowel anastomosis. The ureters are then connected to the conduit using an absorbable suture. Prior to finishing each anastomosis, the assistant introduces ureteral stents through the left lateral assistant port. These are placed up into the kidneys and into the conduit. These will be expelled on their own in the coming weeks, but may require cystoscopic removal if they remain in place. These stents protect the anastomosis while healing and ensuring adequate draining of the kidneys. We typically use a few additional sutures to reinforce our anastomosis as the majority of our patients are at risk for poor wound healing due to our aggressive use of neoadjuvant chemotherapy.

At this point, the robotic portion of the procedure is complete. The robot is undocked and the specimen is extracted through the midline camera port incision, which is extended as needed. The stoma end of the conduit is pulled to the skin at the marked location. The stoma is performed in the standard fashion using absorbable sutures. A drain is left to monitor for leaks. A Foley catheter may be left as a pelvic drain per surgeon's preference.

In conclusion, the robot has revolutionized surgery for many specialties, including urology. Initially embraced for robotic surgery, the uses and types of surgeries performed robotically have exploded over the past few years. Robots are utilized vastly for oncologic surgery but have also been embraced for reconstructive, pediatric, urogynecologic, and even stone surgery. The anesthesiologist must be well versed in laparoscopic and robotic surgery and familiarity with the basic surgical steps, and possible complications can only enhance the surgeon–anesthesiologist relationship and ultimately lead to improved patient outcomes.

References

Cerantola, Y., Valerio, M., Hubner, M., Iglesias, K., Vaucher, L., & Jichlinski, P. (2013). Are Patients at Nutritional Risk More Prone to Complications after Major Urological Surgery? *The Journal of Urology*, 190(6), 2126–2132. doi:10.1016/j.juro.2013.06.111.

Emtage, J. B., Agarwal, G., & Sexton, W. J. (2015). Robotic-Assisted Renal Surgery. *Cancer Control*, 22(3), 291–300.

Farnham, S. B., & Cookson, M. S. (2004). Surgical Complications of Urinary Diversion. *World J Urol*, 22(3), 157–167. doi:10.1007/s00345-004-0429-5

Ghani, K. R., Porter, J., Menon, M., & Rogers, C. (2014). Robotic Retroperitoneal Partial Nephrectomy: A Step-by-Step Guide. *BJU Int*, 114(2), 311–313. doi:10.1111/bju.12709.

Howlader N, Krapcho M, Garshell J, et al. (eds) (n.d.). SEER Cancer Statistics Factsheets: Prostate Cancer. National Cancer Institute. Retrieved from http://seer.cancer.gov/statfacts/html/prost.html. from National Cancer Institute

Lau, C. S., Blackwell, R. H., & Quek, M. L. (2015). Radical Cystectomy: Open vs Robotic Approach. *The Journal of Urology*, 193(2), 400–402. doi:10.1016/j.juro.2014.11.079

McDougal, W. S., Wein, A. J., Kavoussi, L. R., Novick, A. C., & Partin, A. W. (2011). *Campbell-Walsh Urology Tenth Edition Review*. Elsevier/Saunders.

Mir, M. C., Ercole, C., Takagi, T., et al. (2015). Decline in Renal Function after Partial Nephrectomy: Etiology and Prevention. *The Journal of Urology*, 193(6), 1889–1898. doi:10.1016/j.juro.2015.01.093

Skolarus, T. A., Zhang, Y., & Hollenbeck, B. K. (2010). Robotic Surgery in Urologic Oncology: Gathering the Evidence. *Expert Rev Pharmacoecon Outcomes Res*, 10(4), 421–432. doi:10.1586/erp.10.46

Stepanian, S., Haddad, A., Kowitz, J., Fuller, C., & Porter, J. (2015). Mp57-05 Matched Pair Analysis of Transperitoneal versus Retroperitoneal Robotic Partial Nephrectomy. *The Journal of Urology*, 193(4), e691. doi:10.1016/j.juro.2015.02.1993

Su, L.-M (ed.) (2011). *Atlas of Robotic Urologic Surgery* (1st edn). Humana Press.

Zargar-Shoshtari, K., Zargar, H., Lotan, Y., et al. (2016). A Multi-Institutional Analysis of Outcomes of Patients with Clinically Node Positive Urothelial Bladder Cancer Treated with Induction Chemotherapy and Radical Cystectomy. *The Journal of Urology*, 195(1), 53–59. doi:10.1016/j.juro.2015.07.085

Chapter

10 Anesthetic Considerations in Robotic Cardiac Anesthesia

Laurence Schachter and Robert Poston

Introduction

Robotic assistance enables cardiac surgery to be performed without a median sternotomy (rCABG). In the case of coronary artery bypass grafting (CABG), the robot is used to harvest one or both internal mammary arteries, and the distal anastomoses can then be performed by hand in a procedure called minimally invasive direct coronary artery bypass grafting (MIDCAB), or they can be performed with robotic instruments, known as totally endoscopic CABG (TECAB) (Poston 2008, Bonaros 2014). In the case of mitral valve surgery, it is used to gain visualization and dexterity around the valve in a way that improves the reliability of complex mitral repairs over what is possible using open techniques (Suri 2015). In both these operations, the avoidance of a sternotomy helps minimize blood loss and improve recovery time. Many patients report a quicker resolution of wound pain and cosmetically superior results.

Despite the demonstrated clear advantages of this novel procedure at a few expert centers, developing a successful robotic cardiac surgery program has not proven to be an easy task when it has been attempted across the broader cardiac surgery community. Success versus failure of these programs has primarily been about teamwork (Edmundson 2001). It takes a coordinated team effort to perform complex surgical procedures like robot-assisted surgery. An important characteristic of successful teams is that they become good at rapidly learning from and correcting mistakes. Expert teams develop implicit communication and coordination patterns, anticipate needs of the situation, and minimize interruptions. During a crisis, these teams illustrate their skill at "sensemaking," or the ability to quickly uncover the seriousness of a situation through action. Expert teams are able to quickly interpret the situation and act safely to resolve the current crisis and prevent any additional ones.

Coaching is the antidote to most problems that occur when trying to develop new programs. In robotic surgery, the value of coaching to get through the learning phase as quickly as possible has been underappreciated and largely overlooked. Computer simulation and cadaver dissection have been proposed as useful for team practice, but these only teach the basics (Valdis 2015). The fidelity of available models is not adequate to develop or test the types of skills that would influence patient outcome. Until simulation technology improves, actual clinical cases seem to be the only place for learning the more complex skills that are needed for proficiency. Since doing clinical cases prior to gaining proficiency seems to be an optimal way to learn (at least with current training techniques and technologies), there is a moral imperative to shorten this phase as much as possible. In order to accomplish this, the team requires "deliberate practice," or the focus of day-to-day activities on identifying and improving the specific things needed for robotic surgery to be safe.

The first step for an anesthesiologist to learn robotic heart surgery is to understand a fundamental safety concern. Robotics and minimally invasive approaches influence the safety of cardiac surgery because they handicap the surgical team's ability to protect the patient from unforeseen adverse events such as cardiac ischemia or other hemodynamic problems (Wang 2014). In an open sternotomy case, once the hemodynamics are identified as being unstable (for a variety of reasons), the patient is quickly and easily placed on cardiopulmonary bypass (CPB). Once the heart is decompressed and circulation is supported on bypass, the ongoing cardiac injury and/or systemic hypoperfusion is immediately relieved and the patient is safe from ongoing harm. A slightly longer bypass time than expected is a highly acceptable tradeoff of this approach. In contrast, a typical minimally invasive approach involves a delay before a similar chance is going to be available to protect the patient quickly with CPB or other maneuvers. When the robot is docked, it creates a barrier that reduces both the anesthesiologist's and surgeon's access to the patient. If fibrillation or hemodynamic collapse occurs, the anesthesiologist must coordinate efforts with the surgical team to be able to quickly undock the robot and move it away from the field before implementing corrective action.

Rehearsal and training are very important steps in setting up a robotic or minimally invasive program. Every member of the team must be comfortable with what needs to happen and what their role will be during the procedure. "Acting out" a routine case with the robot can help everyone see how the room is set up and what needs to be done for the case to proceed smoothly. The team should rehearse how to access the patient in a crisis scenario in "dry run" exercises prior to their first case. The anesthesiologist and surgeon should both be present during these exercises. While the surgeon is at the console, the anesthesiologist must monitor for any situations that may occur. If everyone knows his or her role in an emergency, steps can be carried out in a controlled manner to achieve the best outcome.

Preoperative Evaluation

Prior to any robotic cardiac surgery, the anesthesiologist has many factors to consider in preparing for the procedure. As with any anesthetic, the patient's comorbidities must be carefully reviewed. The patient will require one-lung ventilation for potentially 3 to 5 hours or more, so specific attention must be paid to any underlying pulmonary disease. Patients with asthma, COPD, ventilation/perfusion mismatch for any reason, or pulmonary hypertension must be further evaluated. Any patient who has contraindications to one-lung anesthesia will need further evaluation or should forgo the minimally invasive approach in favor of a median sternotomy with two-lung ventilation. We recommend room air arterial blood gas and pulmonary function tests for patients with any underlying pulmonary disease. Careful review of these studies is imperative in predicting potential success for a minimally invasive approach. Patients with severe pulmonary hypertension also need to be carefully screened. During prolonged periods of one-lung ventilation, this may be worsened, possibly forcing the team to abandon the technique in favor of a two-lung approach. Prior thoracic surgery can also affect the ability to gain the exposure afforded by the minimally invasive approach.

As these patients are known to have coronary or valvular disease, their cardiac history also needs to be evaluated. Patients with multivessel coronary disease may need more revascularization than can be done with a robotic approach. Alternatively, the location of the stenosis may affect the ability to reach the coronary vessel with a conduit and thereby prevent the approach from being used or may affect where the surgeon will place the mini thoracotomy incision. Knowing the valvular lesion will also determine where the incision will be made. During the distal anastomoses of a robotic CABG case, the hemodynamics are often stable even though these cases are done off-pump without CPB. This improved hemodynamic state in robotics is different than with off-pump CABG done via a sternotomy where the need to rotate the heart out of the chest often creates hemodynamic challenges. In robotic cases, the heart remains within the pericardium while the anastomoses are created, allowing the blood pressure to remain more stable.

As with any cardiac surgery, attention must also be paid to other comorbidities. Patients with a history of stroke, diabetes, renal or hepatic disease, to name a few, will all require some specific care. Having an adequate history will allow the anesthesiologist to achieve the best possible outcome for the patient.

Preoperative Preparation and Monitoring

There are several issues specific to robotic and minimally invasive surgery that require advanced preparation. These are all inherent to robotic cardiac surgery. The first issue is that while the robot is docked to the patient, there is limited access to the patient by either the surgeon or the anesthesiologist. Planning of the room must be well thought out in advance. It is important to know the relative positions of the operating table, the anesthesia machine, and the perfusion pump, as the robot and its arms will occupy a large amount of space. Once the procedure has begun, it is no small task to undock the robot to access the patient in an emergency situation.

Communication with the surgeon must start prior to the procedure and include the surgeon's plan and goals for the case. It is important to know ahead of time what invasive monitoring will be needed for each particular patient and any concerns the surgeon may have that might need to be addressed during the case. The discussion should include whether a coronary sinus catheter, PA vent, or endoaortic clamp might be needed. Placement of these devices takes time and planning, and their usage affects everyone in the room.

ECG, pulse oximetry, and radial arterial pressure monitoring are all standard anesthesia modalities. We have found cerebral oximetry to be extremely helpful as well. Two temperature measurements are routinely used, a core temperature and a nasopharyngeal or esophageal temperature. Central venous pressure and pulmonary artery pressure monitoring are typically used as well. All minimally invasive procedures have limited access to the patient; therefore, we use external defibrillator pads for every case. Placement of external pads needs to done to avoid the surgical field while still maintaining a vector across the heart for electricity to be delivered. Prior to incision, the pads should be hooked up to the defibrillator and the presence of an ECG trace should be confirmed. In some cases, most often minimally invasive valve surgery, a retrograde coronary sinus catheter, a pulmonary artery vent, and possibly an endoaortic balloon clamp may be employed as well. Fluoroscopy and transesophageal echocardiography (TEE) are used in the placement of these catheters. It is important to have good communication with perfusionists when using these catheters. These lines need to be checked and tested prior to their use on bypass. If a superior vena cava line is to be placed, access is usually obtained at the same time other internal jugular access is acquired.

All patients also require TEE. Information obtained from TEE is useful to evaluate the heart prior to the start of the procedure. In valve surgery, it will aid the surgeon in determining the type of surgery to be performed, whether repair or replacement might be necessary, the size of the valve, and the function of the new valve after it is placed. In all surgery it is useful in determining ventricular function and how best to treat any hemodynamic issues that may occur. Due to the limited visual field of minimally invasive surgery, information obtained by TEE can be very helpful and is often the only way to evaluate the heart. Without a good view of the surface of the heart, most decision making needs to be based on the "view" from the TEE. This information then needs to be shared with the surgeon as the case progresses.

In robotic or minimally invasive surgery, the visual field is very small and focused. While the surgeon is at the console, the picture from the console is projected in 2D so the staff in the room can have the best opportunity to anticipate what will be needed next. In our program the surgeon at the field wears a camera attached to the headlight so that after the thoracotomy incision has been made, the picture is projected onto a screen in the room for everyone to observe the progress.

Induction and Maintenance of Anesthesia

The induction of anesthesia should be performed as the anesthesiologist would perform any cardiac induction. One difference is that these patients will require lung isolation, with one-lung ventilation. The nonventilated lung will need to be allowed to decompress, as this will allow the surgeon the best view to perform the operation. We have found it best achieved with a double lumen tube, as it allows better decompression of the nonventilated lung and also allows for low-flow CPAP to the down lung if needed.

After confirmation of the endotracheal tube position, a thorough TEE exam should be performed. It is important to reevaluate any valvular disease as well as the cardiac function. The left and right sides of the heart need to be carefully examined. Comparison of these studies may need to be done at later points during the operation.

Usually 10 to 15 minutes before incision, one-lung ventilation is initiated to ensure that the patient will tolerate the extended period of lung isolation that will be required to complete the surgery. It is common to see a decrease in oxygen saturation with the onset of this severe V/Q mismatch; as hypoxic pulmonary vasoconstriction begins to occur, the shunt usually improves to allow the saturation to return to an acceptable level to comfortably proceed. If the saturation does not improve, PEEP to the ventilated lung or CPAP to the nonventilated lung may be tried. CPAP to the nonventilated lung must be used with caution as even the small amount of insufflation could affect the surgeon's ability to proceed.

Intraoperative maintenance depends on the postoperative goals of each specific case. Our goal for most robotic single-jump CABG and some double-jump CABG is extubation prior to leaving the operating room. In any robotic surgery, it is important to prevent movement while the robot is docked to the patient, as this could cause serious internal damage to the patient. We have found Rocuronium and

Remifentanyl in combination with inhalational agent and longer-acting narcotics, such as Dilaudid, to allow for quick extubation in hemodynamically stable and appropriate patients. We strive to fast-track most minimally invasive or robotic valve procedures and other robotic CABG patients with narcotics (fentanyl), muscle relaxants (Rocuronium or Vecuronium), and Propofol infusions at the end of the procedure for transport to the intensive care unit.

In robotic or minimally invasive valve surgery, some other modalities that may be used include the coronary sinus catheter for administration of retrograde cardioplegia, a PA vent for maintaining an empty heart, and an endoaortic balloon occlusive device. Retrograde cardioplegia is utilized frequently in less invasive cases. Compared to antegrade cardioplegia, this approach provides a convenient and reliable way to deliver myocardial cardioplegia with less need to interrupt the flow of the case. Problems with cardioplegia delivery should be noted by the anesthesiologist because it can predict how easy it might be to wean from CPB and maintain stable hemodynamics postoperatively. When used, these devices are all placed and positioned after induction and prior to beginning the surgical scrub. Placement of these devices requires an anesthesiologist with additional training for their use. TEE and fluoroscopy may both be required for their placement. Use of these devices also requires specific communication between the perfusionist and the anesthesiologist as well as the surgeon.

Communication

Communication among all the team members is very important throughout the case. Since an even better approach is to avoid the chance for a crisis in an actual robotic case, it is very important to discuss the patient's overall baseline state before docking the robot and starting with a less invasive approach. In ideal cases, the whole team hears the discussion and contributes to a collective judgment about whether proceeding with a less invasive approach is safe in that patient and at that time. The best time to do this is during the universal "Time Out." The circulating nurse initiates a time-out that follows the protocol as described by the World Health Organization. This checklist ensures proper access and functioning of standard equipment and supplies for a routine cardiac surgery case. For robotic surgery, there are other items needed by both the surgeon and anesthesiologist that are unique for these cases and should be discussed at this time. In our practice we have expanded the "Time Out" to include three discussions, led by the anesthesiologist, the surgeon, and the perfusionist. The purpose of anesthesiologist's report is to discuss the patient's "baseline" stability, specifically from first contact with the patient up until the time out. Verbalizing this information allows group consensus to help establish whether it is safe to proceed with the planned less invasive strategy. Specific findings related to the TEE exam, hemodynamic stability, and tolerance of one-lung ventilation can be discussed at this time. Other factors that should be discussed as they may affect patient care or surgical approach could include preoperative anticoagulation, preoperative medication usage or cessation of specific medications with rebound tendencies, and comorbidities such as renal, hepatic, pulmonary disease, or diabetes.

After the anesthesia report, the surgeon also summarizes for the team how the less invasive approach to the case is likely to increase the risk of difficulty and complications. The surgeon should have a thorough knowledge about the patient who is being treated on that day. It is the job of the cardiac surgeon to share that knowledge and make sure all staff in the room understand the unique surgical risks posed by this particular patient and/or the chance for a difficult postoperative course. Everyone should also understand the surgery being proposed by the surgeon at this time.

Finally, the perfusionist's report will discuss bypass strategies, cannula sizes for central or peripheral cannulation, and the potential need for CPB or intraaortic balloon pump support. If the plan is articulated clearly, the perfusionist can serve a valuable cross-checking role. This discussion will prevent the circulating nurse from having to scramble for this equipment later during a crisis. For instance, if the proposal was to cannulate peripherally and there is evidence of severe peripheral artery disease (i.e., can't cannulate the artery) and or a past history of vena caval filter (i.e., can't cannulate the vein), the perfusionist might suggest a plan change to an alternative approach.

Communication is also very important during the procedure. As changes are made by the anesthesiologist or the surgeon, they should be announced so everyone is aware. For example, when one-lung ventilation is initiated, everyone should be aware as there may be a change in the tone of pulse ox or a blood gas may be needed to help evaluate the patient's tolerance. The nurse and the perfusionist would then be aware that they may need to help or even change the plan based on the patient's progress. The surgeon should be aware as he or she should wait for the lung to be decompressed prior to inserting the trocars. Other situations that may require everyone being made aware include the making of the incision, chest insufflation, and anytime the bovie is used near the heart.

Intraoperative Evaluation

There are three main problems that are specific to a typical *robotic* case and, therefore, are helpful to discuss: (1) problems with diagnosing and responding to bleeding, (2) difficulties treating ventricular fibrillation, and (3) appropriately managing sudden severe hemodynamic difficulties. Each case will pose different risks for each of these problems. As discussed earlier, diagnosing bleeding can be difficult in minimally invasive procedures. The keyhole opening that exposes the heart for the attachment of the bypass graft does not allow adequate viewing of the entire field. Monitoring for bleeding is an important role for anesthesia during less invasive cases, particularly during the distal anastomosis when the robot is no longer being used. In an open cardiac case, active bleeding that causes hemodynamic abnormalities is rarely left undiagnosed for more than a few minutes. A full sternotomy affords easy visualization of all areas where bleeding might occur. In contrast, there is a far more limited field of view when performing surgery via a minithoracotomy. As a result, there is no easy way to determine if surgical sites (IMA harvest site, port sites, IMA branches, etc.) outside this limited view are actively bleeding while the case is underway. It might be necessary to put the robotic camera back in to evaluate for possible bleeding. The field of view of the camera is also limited and has no peripheral vision, so active bleeding within the chest can be missed by the camera unless it is raised as a specific concern. The anesthesiologist can help compensate for these surgical limitations by detecting hemodynamic signs of undiagnosed bleeding like the need for increased doses of vasopressors, fluids, or transfusions. The TEE can be used to assess for fluid in left chest and pericardium. If the surgeon is aware of the concern, a suction catheter can be placed into the pleural space to determine if there is a large collection. If blood is recovered, this would prompt placing the camera back into the chest to reassess surgical sites. The key step is to share concerns about anesthetic management with the surgeon so that appropriate actions can be taken. If a source of bleeding is found, then it can be treated quickly and efficiently by the surgeon.

The robotic ports are placed through the ribs at the start of robotic cases. When inserted near the heart, the ports can manipulate the heart accidentally and cause cardiac ectopy. This is usually benign and should not prompt the same diagnostic work-up and/or antiarrhythmic use when compared to unprovoked ectopy that might occur. Fibrillation during CABG can be due to cardiac ischemia, CO_2 embolism during distal anastomosis, or accidentally touching the heart with the cautery at any point. It is important to discriminate among these different etiologies because they all have a major difference in prognosis and treatment. A heart can develop fibrillation as a result of myocardial ischemia either due to native coronary disease at any point during the case or during distal anastomosis in an off-pump coronary bypass case. This cause of fibrillation often represents a dire situation that requires an aggressive response. Even if defibrillation is used, it is likely to be successful only temporarily. The underlying ischemic etiology is not treated by defibrillation, and therefore, fibrillation is likely to recur. Major changes in the operative plan may be required, possibly including initiating CPB emergently. In contrast, fibrillation can result from CO_2 embolism during a distal anastomosis off-pump and/or accidental injury from electrocautery. These events are not associated with underlying myocardial ischemia and are usually benign as long as defibrillation is quickly used and found to be effective. There are some keys to effective defibrillation during the period of one-lung ventilation:

1. The key to effective defibrillation is that it happens quickly. External pads will already have been placed while the patient was positioned preoperatively. If external pads do not work after one or two attempts, then the left lung should be inflated prior to a repeat attempt. If the lung is deflated, this can create an empty space within the thorax that does not allow an effective vector to be created between the defibrillator pads.
2. If the external pads do not work after the lung is reinflated, then internal paddles must be used. The machine needs to have the cords changed to the internal paddles and the setting changed

to 20J. A thoracotomy often needs to be rapidly made so that the paddles can be inserted into the chest. Usually pediatric paddles are used as they are easiest to place through the minithoracotomy incision. These paddles should be present on the field prior to the start of any minimally invasive procedure.

3. If the internal paddles do not work, then CPB should be initiated in order to decompress the heart so that defibrillation is able to be more effective. At this point, amiodarone and/or lidocaine may be utilized. A metabolic cause can be investigated as well, and any acidosis or electrolyte problem should be corrected.

Lung isolation and CO_2 insufflation in order to harvest the LIMA/RIMA causes a period of vulnerability that is not present in traditional open-chest CABG. Hypoxia, hypercapnia, and a low-grade tamponade effect from insufflation can lead to cardiac compromise, resulting in poor coronary perfusion and myocardial injury. Other changes that can be seen include decreased venous return, decreased cardiac output, decreased mixed venous oxygen saturation, and worsening of the V/Q mismatch, leading to a shunting situation. If this occurs, it is important to communicate this to the surgeon. Sometimes decreasing the insufflation pressure is enough to resolve the problem; other times, a rapid bailout is needed, which can range from stopping CO_2 chest insufflation all the way to the use of CPB support by peripheral (femoral artery/vein) or central (aorta/atrial) cannulation. Pulmonary hypertension may be present due to underlying cardiac disease or an inability to tolerate one-lung ventilation. Inhaled nitric oxide can be useful in situations where pulmonary hypertension is present. It can lower pulmonary pressures and reduce the work of the heart enough to complete the procedure.

It is important to monitor for signs of impending hemodynamic collapse and right heart dysfunction on TEE during the lung isolation period. In the case of off-pump coronary surgery, monitoring for ischemia during an off-pump distal anastomosis is an important role for the anesthesiologist. In median sternotomy CABG, the EKG leads are displaced and often provide an insensitive tool to detect cardiac ischemia. During sternal-sparing surgery, this is less likely to be a problem. The EKG leads remain in the correct position and provide a more sensitive measure of coronary ischemia. ST and TEE changes are very sensitive to ischemia in the off-pump situation. ST changes may show up in the first 30 seconds of occlusion. TEE provides a more specific finding of local coronary ischemia by detecting regional wall motion abnormalities in real time during coronary occlusion. In general, the LIMA to LAD anastomosis allows the heart to maintain good hemodynamics. Cardiac subluxation to expose the coronary targets is far less than during off-pump CABG via full sternotomy. A test occlusion of the coronary artery can be performed prior to a LIMA to LAD anastomosis in order to determine whether a coronary shunt will be useful. Shunting can help avoid cardiac compromise due to ischemia during the distal anastomosis on a beating heart, but makes the technical task of anastomosis more difficult. If ischemia does not resolve with the coronary shunt in place, this is a major problem that often requires a bailout maneuver – either sternotomy or peripheral-access CPB. If ischemic EKG changes do not resolve after the bypass graft is placed and it is associated with wall motion abnormality on TEE, this is another serious situation that often requires a change in the operative approach. These are the events that should be anticipated in order to facilitate rapid corrective action.

Another situation to monitor for is tamponade or right heart dysfunction. During open-chest surgery, heart surgeons are able to directly inspect the right ventricle and are easily able to detect evidence of dysfunction. In robotic cases, the minimally invasive access eliminates direct visibility of the right ventricle through the surgical wound. Echocardiography, therefore, is a key tool to monitor the right heart. There is risk of a tamponade-like effect or cardiac ischemia when CO_2 insufflation is initiated. It is important to watch for elevations in central venous pressure and pulmonary artery pressures, and decreases in systemic blood pressure (SBP) and cerebral oximetry. If any of these are present or suspected, this should be communicated to the surgeon because it could lead to a change in the operative plan. The most likely problem that would prompt a change to the operative plan is evidence of right heart dysfunction. A TEE exam should be performed continually during the case and can be used to monitor right heart function. It is possible that the surgeon could make changes in the approach that may improve the blood pressure, such as decreasing the pressure of insufflation, or make other changes in the operative plan such as using CPB assistance that will improve right heart function.

Many times, a modification in the surgical plan creates a quicker and more definitive treatment for hypotension or hypoxia.

During elective mitral valve and multivessel CABG cases, there is no access to the heart directly for cannulation, and therefore, peripheral access of the femoral artery and vein is used for bypass. The TEE exam becomes very important in determining whether there is evidence of disease in the descending thoracic aorta. This finding could complicate the safety of femoral artery cannulation and the ability to use an intraaortic balloon pump. In general, the main focus for a preop TEE is to identify intracardiac pathology and ventricular function. Femoral-access CPB is not used in every case, so the importance of reviewing the descending aorta and making this finding known to the surgeon can be forgotten at times. TEE is then used intraoperatively to ensure that the arterial wire is in place prior to the insertion of femoral arterial cannula. Using a bicaval view, the TEE is then used to guide the surgeon in placing the femoral venous cannula, ensuring its position in the superior vena cava. Prior to the initiation of CPB, the CPB machine will be primed using retrograde autologous perfusion in order to minimize hemodilution. Sometimes, volume depletion leads to difficulties in maintaining the SBP in the appropriate range. This requires two-way communication between the anesthesiologist and the perfusionist, who can adjust how quickly the volume is being removed from the patient to prevent a precipitous drop in SBP.

Weaning from CPB typically occurs within 10–20 min of removing the aortic cross-clamp. If ventricular fibrillation occurs as bypass is being weaned, it often signifies an air embolism. Such an embolism often occurs in the right coronary artery. Finding EKG evidence of right coronary artery ischemia or focal wall motion abnormality in the right coronary distribution on TEE helps confirm this as the etiology. Defibrillation is the treatment of choice at this time. Elevation of the systemic arterial pressure helps to drive the embolic air from the coronary circulation. After the patient is successfully weaned from CPB, the lungs should be gently reinflated. When there is a LIMA to LAD done robotically, the surgeon should be closely watching the position of the left upper lobe as it is inflated to confirm that it does not distort the graft. Evaluation by TEE should be done prior to weaning from CPB and removing the cannulas, looking specifically for major problems with valve function or ventricular function that should be addressed prior to attempting to remove bypass support.

Conclusion

While there are many similarities to open cases, robotic cases provide challenges that are vastly different than the corresponding conventional open approach. Anesthesiologists can contribute to success or failure of the operation by understanding how they can favorably influence the safe completion of the procedure. A great way to get through the learning curve period is to use expert coaches intimately familiar with these steps who can provide feedback to the novice. Ultimately, the culture of safety is a key aspect that allows teams to learn from mistakes made during the early initiation period. By having all personnel available for all cases while early in the learning curve, they can all gain valuable experience needed to successfully transition into an experienced program.

References

Bonaros N, Schachner T, Kofler M. Advanced hybrid closed chest revascularization: an innovative strategy for the treatment of multivessel coronary artery disease. *Eur J Cardiothorac Surg*. 2014;46(6): e94–102.

Chauhan S, Sukesan S. Anesthesia for robotic cardiac surgery: an amalgam of technology and skill. *AnnCard Anesht*. 2010;13: 169–75.

Dickey J, Damiano RJ Jr, Ungerleider R. Our surgical culture of blame: a time for change. *J Thorac Cardiovasc Surg*. 2003;126(5): 1259–60.

Edmondson A, Bohmer R, Pisano G. Speeding up team learning. *Harvard Business Review*. October 2001: 125–32.

Jeong RL. Anesthetic considerations for robotic surgery. *Korean J Anesth*. 2014;66(1): 3–11.

Mehta Y, Arora D, Jain V. Aneshtetic considerations for robotic assisted cardiac surgery. *OA Anesth*. 2014;2(1): 3.

Poston R, Tran R, Collins M, Reynolds M, Connerney I, Reicher B, et al. Comparison of economic and patient outcomes with minimally invasive versus traditional off-pump coronary artery bypass grafting techniques. *Ann Surg*. 2008;248(4): 638–46.

Sachdeva AK, Blair PG, Lupi L. Education and training to address specific needs during the career progression of surgeons. *Surg Clin North Am*. 2016;96(1): 115–28.

Suri R, Taggarse A, Burkhart HM, Daly RC, Mauermann W, Nishimura RA, et al. Robotic mitral valve repair for simple and complex degenerative disease: midterm clinical and echocardiographic quality outcomes. *Circulation*. 2015;132(21): 1961–8.

Valdis M, Chu MW, Schlachta CM, Kiaii B. Validation of a novel virtual reality training curriculum for robotic cardiac surgery: a randomized trial. *Innovations (Phila)*. 2015;10(6): 383–8.

Wang G, Gao C. Robotic cardiac surgery: an anaesthetic challenge. *Postgrad Med J*. 2014;90(1066): 467–74.

89 squamous cell carcinomas, 27 large cell tumors, and 38 bronchoalveolar tumors. There were 381 patients in pathologic stage I and 115 patients in stage II. Pathologic upstaging was seen in 22 percent of patients. There were three (0.7 percent) conversions to thoracotomy due to bleeding from the proximal pulmonary artery. Complications included atrial fibrillation (25), pneumonia (12), aspiration (3), and prolonged air leak (8). Median hospitalization was 3 days. At mean follow-up of 47.3 months, there was no local recurrence; distant metastasis was seen in 19 patients (5 percent), and 39 patients had a new lung cancer. At this follow-up period, cancer-free survival was 94 percent (372/396 patients).

Robotic technology has the potential of greatly improving the accuracy and oncologic efficacy of video-assisted lobectomy for patients with early-stage lung cancer.

Robotic Resection of Mediastinal Masses

Anterior Mediastinal Masses

In the era of VATS and robotic surgery, the approach to the diagnosis and treatment of anterior mediastinal masses (in the anterosuperior compartment) has undergone a significant change. Traditionally image-guided transthoracic needle biopsy (TTNA) and anterior mediastinotomy (chamberlain procedure), have been used for the diagnosis of lesions in this anatomic region. In this particular application, the technique of TTNA has a number of shortcomings: (1) the inability to provide adequate tissue for a meaningful diagnosis and appropriate subtyping of lymphoma, (2) the inability to differentiate lymphoma from thymoma, (3) the inability to differentiate a benign from an invasive thymic epithelial neoplasm (thymoma). In contrast, aside from the inherent risks of surgery, the anterior mediastinotomy approach suffers from (1) the inability to adequately visualize the surgical field due to a small "key hole" incision, (2) the risk of surgical complications resulting from inadequate exposure and visualization, (3) the delay in the application of radiotherapy following tissue diagnosis due to the need for wound healing prior to application of radiation, (4) occasional incisional wound breakdown following the application of radiation to the area encompassing the mediastinotomy, and (5) the need for a second definitive surgical procedure for certain types of anterior mediastinal masses.

With the advent of VATS and robotic thoracic surgery, the algorithm for the diagnosis and therapy of anterior mediastinal masses has changed. The advantages of these approaches are: (1) The incisions are placed in the lateral chest wall away from the field of radiation, which typically encompasses the entire anterior chest wall. Using the laterally placed incisions, in patients with lymphoma there is no need to delay radiation therapy while awaiting wound healing. (2) The minimally invasive videoendoscopic techniques yield adequate tissue for appropriate differentiation of thymic epithelial neoplasms from lymphoma. (3) In patients with resectable lesions, surgical resection can be accomplished in the same setting.

Lymphoma

Lymphoma is rarely solely localized to the mediastinum, and occasionally, the diagnosis of lymphoma will necessitate transthoracic open biopsy of a mediastinal mass. It is not uncommon that the diagnosis of lymphoma is suspected following a fine-needle or core biopsy, but further tissue is required to confirm the diagnosis. Given the fact that lymphoma is treated by nonsurgical means and a simple biopsy is often all that is indicated, the role for a robotic biopsy in the routine type of case is questionable. With the widespread availability of VATS, it is likely that most of the biopsies of large masses extending toward the pleural cavity can be appropriately accomplished without the robot. The exception may be a small mass extending into the left chest where dissection and preservation of the phrenic nerve will be more easily achieved utilizing the three-dimensional and magnified view of the robot together with the more precise dissection. Another use of the robot in this clinical situation is for disease in the hilar areas of the mediastinum, wherein this area is more suited to the fine dissection and visualization achieved with the robot. In the case of a suspected recurrence in a previously treated chest, the robot would also be more suitable for this type of dissection and biopsy.

Parathyroid Adenoma

In many instances, an ectopic parathyroid gland is localized to the anterosuperior mediastinum, where excision via a transcervical route is not possible. Prior techniques would have employed a median sternotomy, thoracotomy, or VATS approach for excision. Dissecting in these small and distant sites is ideally suited to fine dissection and manipulation of the robot. We have approached a number of right-sided adenomas using the robot. Others have described the successful use of the robot for excision of an adenoma in the aortopulmonary window (51).

Prior to surgery, all localization studies should be reviewed and available in order to define the optimum approach. Depending on their exact location, these lesions require dissection in difficult areas surrounded by the superior vena cava (SVC), innominate vein, phrenic nerve, aorta, and pulmonary artery. Additionally, the lesion will likely be embedded in the adipose tissue of the mediastinum or the thymus, complicating visualization. Excision of the lesion is accomplished with intraoperative monitoring of parathyroid levels to ensure complete excision of the adenoma.

Single-lung ventilation is utilized with placement of a double-lumen endotracheal tube. The patient is placed in the left lateral decubitus position. The standard approach is utilized with ports placed in a V-type configuration. The camera is placed in the seventh ICS, with the two additional ports in the fifth ICS anteriorly and posteriorly one hand breadth away. The lung is reflected away from the mediastinum using a retractor placed through an accessory incision positioned posteriorly in the sixth ICS. The robot is brought in over the head of the patient. A zero degree camera is used. We once again use a hook electrocautery and cadiere forceps. The mediastinal pleura between the SVC and the chest wall is incised in a vertical fashion. Blunt dissection creates space between the SVC and the sternum. This dissection is difficult at times given the small size of the adenoma and the surrounding fat. Patience is important as one attempts to localize the lesion. The fatty tissue is grasped and coagulated during dissection as bleeding in this small area makes further dissection hazardous and difficult. Retraction of the SVC or other neighboring structures can be performed with a simple suction catheter introduced through the auxiliary port by the assistant while simultaneously keeping the field dry. Once the lesion is identified, it is dissected free from the surrounding tissues, placed in a specimen bag, and removed. Confirmation of resection is obtained from frozen section as well as an appropriate fall in parathyroid hormone levels. We have needed to excise much of the adipose and thymic tissue in this portion of the mediastinum when we were unable to directly visualize a small adenoma. Hemostasis is ensured. Subpleural catheters are placed and the chest is drained with a chest tube positioned apically and posteriorly. The wounds are closed in the routine fashion.

Thymectomy for Myasthenia Gravis

The thymus gland is postulated to be integral in the pathogenesis of myasthenia gravis (MG). Thymectomy is currently recommended for almost all patients with MG. The younger patient and those with only ocular myasthenia are often treated nonoperatively – at least initially. Similarly, the older patient with mild disease may also be excluded from surgical management. It has, however, been demonstrated that those patients who are operated on earlier in the course of their disease tend to do better. It has also been demonstrated that the beneficial effects of thymectomy may only be realized many months after the procedure. Any surgical procedure for MG should be designed to remove all thymic tissue. Current popular surgical approaches include a transsternal approach, a transcervical combined with a transsternal approach, a transcervical approach alone, and lastly a VATS approach. A number of reports of robotic thymectomy for both MG and thymoma have been published.

While the thymus is a midline structure, we have tended to approach it from the right chest. Given the presence of the aortic arch and the heart, we learned early in our VATS experience that a left-sided approach was more difficult – as others have also found (52). No neuromuscular agents are administered. The patients are placed in a lateral decubitus position. Single-lung ventilation is achieved. Our port placement for most lesions of the anterosuperior compartment differs from our standard approach. The camera port is placed in the fifth ICS in line with the posterior axillary line. We initially use a zero-degree VATS camera to inspect the chest and to create our other ports under direct vision. Placement of our working arms is in the fourth ICS and sixth ICS in the anterior axillary line, spaced about one hand breadth from the camera port. The exact ICS will vary depending on the size of the patient. An auxiliary port is also placed in the sixth ICS in the posterior axillary line. We use a 30-degree camera. This allows a better visualization of the mediastinum and particularly when dissecting around the left phrenic nerve. A hook cautery and cadiere grasper are used. The mediastinal pleura is incised in a vertical fashion between the SVC and the sternum taking care to avoid the phrenic nerve. We then begin dissection inferiorly along the pericardium. Traction is applied to the pericardial fat and thymic tissue, which is dissected free using the electrocautery. In a stepwise fashion, all mediastinal tissues are dissected off the pericardium, SVC, and ascending aorta as the right superior pole is approached. With dissection being performed from the right chest, the likelihood of damage to the right phrenic nerve is minimal. Careful attention to the location of the phrenic nerve when mobilizing the superior pole is indicated as for any other approach to thymectomy. The arterial supply to the thymic gland is clipped during this portion of the procedure. A grasper is positioned through the auxiliary port and downward traction is applied to the gland to visualize and divide the thyrothymic ligament. Medium clips are placed and the ligament is divided using the electrocautery. We then proceed to cross the midline and to mobilize the left half of the thymic gland. The thymus is carefully dissected off the innominate vein using gentle traction and electrocautery. Any small veins are coagulated, but any larger veins draining into the innominate are clipped using clips placed with the robotic arm. Once the thymus is dissected off the innominate vein, which is skeletonized, we begin our dissection of the inferior pole of the left thymic gland. The left pleura is opened along its length, taking care to avoid the phrenic nerve, particularly proximally. With the thymic tissue being retracted by an assistant, further dissection is performed with gentle traction on the thymus together with blunt dissection and use of electrocautery to separate the gland from the pleura. The arterial supply is clipped as dissection proceeds proximally along the pleura. We then approach the left superior pole. Traction is again placed on the thymus by an assistant and the thyrothymic ligament is divided with electrocautery after placing large clips proximally with a disposable clip applier. At this point, the gland is free and placed within a specimen bag and removed from an anterior port. The mediastinum is irrigated and inspected for hemostasis. We place two soft 19-Fr drainage tubes – one into each pleural space. Subpleural catheters are placed for pain control. The lung is reinflated under direct vision and the wounds are closed in the standard fashion. If possible, all patients are extubated in the operating room.

Thymoma

The most common mediastinal mass in the anterosuperior compartment in an adult is a thymoma. These may be benign or malignant. Often a distinction between a benign and a malignant thymoma is only made during surgery by assessment of invasion into surrounding structures. Complete surgical resection remains the mainstay of management of thymomas. Spread to adjacent structures does not make a patient unresectable. Many patients with a thymoma are asymptomatic. Approximately 10–15 percent of patients with MG will have a thymoma, whereas about 30 percent of patients with a thymoma will have MG. Surgical approaches to thymoma include a median sternotomy, clamshell incision, and, more recently, a VATS approach. The VATS approach is reserved for early-stage tumors. As experience with the robot is gained, a few reports of resection of thymomas via a robotic approach have been described. We believe that a minimally invasive robotic approach to thymoma is appropriate in clinical early-stage lesions. Should the lesion appear invasive or malignant by preoperative studies, we do not attempt resection using minimally invasive techniques. For a benign-appearing centrally located thymoma, a right-sided approach is once again utilized for the reasons described above.

All preparation is identical to a thymectomy for MG as described above. The patient is not paralyzed as we have the ability to stimulate the phrenic nerve if necessary in order to better localize it. Dissection proceeds as for a standard thymectomy. As little manipulation of the mass as possible is attempted in order to prevent damage to the capsule and possible seeding of tumor cells. While resection of any involved lung is possible, we have not attempted robotic resection of any more locally advanced thymomas. Once the lesion is freed, it is placed in a specimen retrieval bag and removed through an anterior port. If necessary, a port site may be enlarged to accommodate the passage of the mass. Hemostasis is secured and drainage tubes are placed. Closure is completed in the standard fashion.

Germ Cell Tumors

These tumors may be divided into benign and malignant categories. Benign germ cell tumors include teratomas and dermoid cysts, while malignant tumors encompass seminomas and nonseminomatous tumors. The latter group includes immature teratomas, choriocarcinomas, embryonal cell carcinomas, yolk sac tumors, and mixed germ cell tumors. All anterosuperior masses in a male population in the second to fourth decade of life should have blood screened for α fetoprotein and β HCG. Malignant tumors are treated nonsurgically in the majority of cases – seminomas with radiation and nonseminomatous tumors with chemotherapy. Minimally invasive approaches are not suitable to the unusual case of a malignant tumor being managed surgically for whatever reason. Teratomas and dermoid cysts are often diagnosed preoperatively and are amenable to resection using the robot. Resection would proceed along the lines described for a thymectomy. A complete resection of all mediastinal fatty and thymic tissue in addition to the mass would not be necessary.

Lymphadenectomy

In certain clinical circumstances, mediastinal lymphadenectomy or biopsy would be indicated. This includes lymphadenopathy of unknown etiology – possible sarcoid, lymphoma or metastatic disease from lung cancer, or other malignancies are examples. The robot is ideally suited for dissection and biopsy of both mediastinal and hilar nodes – the latter may be particularly difficult to biopsy through a VATS technique. We would approach this using a standard technique. The patient is positioned in a lateral decubitus position. Single-lung ventilation is utilized. An initial skin incision in the eight ICS in the mid-axillary line is placed. An auxiliary port site in the seventh ICS medial to the camera port is placed. The lung is reflected off the nodal basin and maintained in position. Two further ports are positioned in the fifth ICS posteriorly and in the sixth ICS anteriorly. The robot is positioned over the patient's head. A hook cautery and cadiere grasper are used. The mediastinal pleura is incised and reflected off the nodal basin. Care is taken to avoid vital structures including the phrenic nerve – particularly on the left where it is more difficult to visualize. In the subcarinal space that we routinely approach from the right side, care must be taken to avoid the esophagus and vagus nerves. While dissecting in the A-P window, the dexterity and range of motion of the robot is particularly useful in avoiding damage to the recurrent laryngeal nerve. The nodes are gently elevated and dissected free using electrocautery. Retraction of structures and maintenance of a dry field is performed by the assistant using a suction catheter. All vasculature is coagulated or clipped with the latter being placed robotically. Once the node is freed, it is placed in a specimen bag and removed. Hemostatsis is ensured and the chest is closed in the standard fashion.

Posterior Mediastinal Masses

In both adults and children, the majority of posterior mediastinal masses are of neurogenic origin. Most of these masses in adults (95 percent) are benign and are usually asymptomatic. In contrast, the majority of neurogenic tumors in children are malignant. Neurogenic tumors may arise from intercostal nerves (neurofibroma, neurilemoma, and neurosarcoma), sympathetic ganglia (ganglioma, ganglioneuroblastoma, and neuroblastoma) or paraganglia cells (paraganglioma). A CT scan is usually sufficient from a diagnostic point of view, although any possibility of intraspinal extension (10 percent) should be evaluated with an MRI. Preoperative biopsy in an adult is usually not indicated unless the tumor displays unusual characteristics and a malignant tumor is likely. Although a combined VATS and neurosurgical approach has been described for dumbbell tumors, we have excluded these tumors currently from a robotic approach.

These lesions are approached in our standard fashion as described above. Single-lung ventilation utilizing a double-lumen endotracheal tube is initiated. The patient is placed in a lateral decubitus position. An initial port site is created in the eighth ICS and a standard video camera is inserted. The thorax is examined and the mass evaluated. An additional auxiliary port site of 1 cm is created under direct vision one intercostal space above and medial to the camera port, and 2–3 cm away from this port site. This is for the lung retractor. Creating any of the port sites too close to one another may lead to limitation in camera movement or robotic arms during the procedure. The retractor is placed and the lung is reflected off the mass. The retractor is then anchored to the table. The position of the two additional port sites is then determined. For posterior mediastinal masses, we use a "V"-type placement with the camera at the base of the V. Should the tumor be very low in the thorax, an inverted V-type configuration would be used with the camera being placed at a higher interspace. The additional port sites are created under direct vision prior to positioning the robot.

The robot is then brought in and positioned over the head of the patient for mid- or superiorly placed lesions. For lower lesions, the robot is brought in alongside the patient's back. The robot is positioned as close to the operating table as possible. The camera is inserted initially. We will use a 0 degree or 30 degree camera depending on the location of the lesion. The arms are then positioned through the previously established port sites. The camera is used to guide the two arms into the chest and over the retractor, positioning the instruments close to the lesion. The usual instruments that we use are a hook cautery and a cadiere grasper. Laterality for these instruments is as one would use for an open case. Lesions situated in the mid- or lower chest are easier to excise than those situated at the apex as the bony skeleton for apical lesions poses problems with access. This is particularly relevant with excision of a large apical lesion.

The pleura adjacent to the mass is incised and the mass is slowly mobilized off the ribs and vertebral bodies. The ability of EndoWrist to work in seven degrees of freedom and at 90 degrees is particularly useful when working between the mass and the ribs. When dealing with an apical mass, the apical portion should be the last area mobilized. Having mobilized all but the apex will allow more traction to be applied while freeing the apical portion and thus avoiding potential damage to the stellate ganglion and subclavian vessels. Further traction on the lesion can be applied by the surgical assistant using conventional thoracoscopic instruments via the auxiliary port. The neural origin and any vascular supply is clipped with large clips introduced through one of the port sites. The mass is thus freed and placed in a plastic specimen bag. If this is a large mass, this is in turn placed in a second specimen bag and, after lubricating the interface between the bags, the mass (within the first bag) is removed through a port site. The site is enlarged as needed in order to extract the lesion. I believe that a small utility thoracotomy – if this is needed for a large lesion – does not detract from the minimally invasive nature of the procedure and is preferable to dividing the lesion within the chest in order to remove the lesion as previously described. Hemostasis is confirmed. We use one or two subpleurally placed catheters for a constant infusion of bupivicaine 0.5 percent in the perioperative period. A single chest tube is placed posteriorly in the apex of the hemithorax through the retractor port. The lungs are reinflated under direct vision. Wounds are closed with interrupted polydiaxonone at the muscle layer. The subcutaneous tissues are approximated with absorbable sutures and the skin is closed with a subcuticular absorbable suture.

Bronchogenic Cysts

These cysts are most common in the mediastinum. They arise from the embryonic ventral foregut and are usually located in the right paratracheal or subcarinal position. They may also be located within the pulmonary parenchyma. While they are likely to be asymptomatic, the possibility of infection within the cysts or compression of the esophagus, trachea, or bronchi exists. Rarely does the cyst communicate with the tracheobronchial tree. At times, it is difficult to distinguish the cyst from subcarinal nodes. Surgical resection is indicated in all cases to confirm the diagnosis, to alleviate any symptoms, and to prevent complications. Malignant transformation has rarely been described. These cysts may be densely adherent to surrounding tissue and a complete excision is not always possible. No vital structure should be compromised and incomplete resection is adequate with de-epithelialization of the remaining wall.

The cysts are approached from the right side. Surgical technique involves placement of a double-lumen endotracheal tube. Single-lung ventilation is utilized. The patient is placed in a left lateral decubitus position. Initial camera placement is in the eighth ICS in line with the anterior axillary line. An auxiliary incision is placed in the seventh ICS about 3 cm medial to the camera port for a lung retractor. The retractor is placed and secured and the lung is reflected off the bronchogenic cyst. Two additional ports are created under direct vision in approximately the fifth ICS anteriorly and fifth ICS posteriorly about one hand breadth away from the camera site. The robot is brought into the field over the patient's head with the two arms being guided into position in the chest under direct vision. We use a cadiere grasper and a hook cautery. The cyst is grasped and an attempt is made to excise it completely. These lesions are often densely adherent to surrounding tissue, including the trachea, bronchi, and esophagus. Care must be taken to avoid damage to these structures during dissection. In the case of dense attachment to surrounding structures, we excise as much as possible of the cyst wall after aspirating its contents and gently coagulate the remaining portions of the wall. The lesion is placed in a plastic specimen bag and removed. Frozen section is obtained to ensure its benign nature. Hemostasis is confirmed. Subpleural catheters are placed for postoperative pain management. A single chest tube is placed posteriorly in the apex of the chest through the auxiliary port. All instrumentation is removed and two-lung ventilation is initiated. The wounds are closed in the standard fashion.

Pericardial Cysts

These are the second most common mediastinal cysts and are classically located in the cardiophrenic angles with 70 percent right-sided, 22 percent left-sided, and the remainder being attached to other portions of the pericardium. Communication with the pericardium is possible (5 percent). They were classically described as "spring water cysts" due to their clear fluid content. The cysts are usually asymptomatic. If diagnosed incidentally, observation or simple aspiration is the initial treatment of choice. Should these cysts recur following aspiration or should the diagnosis be questionable, then excision is indicated.

The approach to these cysts includes single-lung ventilation. The camera is placed in the eighth ICS. The lung is reflected off the pericardium and maintained in position with a retractor placed through an auxiliary incision one ICS above and 2–3 cm posterior to the camera site. Two additional port sites are placed approximately in the sixth ICS posteriorly and the sixth ICS anteriorly at least one hand breadth from the camera port. The robot is positioned at the head of the patient. Any adhesions between the cyst and the lung are divided with the electrocautery. The cyst is grasped and dissected off the pericardium using electrocautery. Should the cyst be adherent to surrounding structures, the cyst may be deroofed after aspirating the fluid. As much of the cyst wall is excised as possible. A single chest tube is placed through the retractor site at completion of the procedure. Subpleural catheters are placed and the wounds are closed in the standard fashion.

Robotic Transthoracic Sympathectomy

Although the early indications for sympathectomy range from epilepsy, toxic goiter, idiocy, exomphalos, glaucoma, angina pectoris, spastic paralysis, hypertension, and peripheral occlusive disease, presently hyperhidrosis is the only established indication for sympathectomy. Peripheral arterial occlusive disease, sympathetic reflex dystrophy, and abdominal pain syndromes represent relative indications for sympathectomy (53).

Hyperhidrosis results from excessive stimulation of the eccrine glands (54). Eccrine glands that are present throughout the body are most prevalent in the palms, axillae, and plantar regions. Consequently, hyperhidrosis most commonly presents in the hands, axilla, and the feet. The upper extremity is most commonly affected. Forty-three percent of patients have a combination of palm and axillary hyperhidrosis (55). In 37 percent of patients, hyperhidrosis is localized to the axilla, and in 20 percent only to the hand. Hyperhidrosis is seen in 1 percent of the population in the West. There is a high incidence in people of Japanese ancestry and Jews of North African, Yemeni, and Balkan descent. Although most cases of hyperhidrosis are idiopathic, secondary hyperhidrosis can be the result of hyperthyroidism, obesity, anxiety disorders, menopause, carcinoid syndrome, lymphoma, pheochromocytoma, diabetes, and tuberculosis.

A number of approaches have been advocated for the management of hyperhidrosis.

1. **Conservative management:** Aluminum chloride, glutaraldehyde, and tannic acid have been used as topical agents with disappointing results. Systemic anticholinergics have been advocated to block postganglionic acetylcholine receptors. Calcium channel blockers have also been used. The success of these techniques has been short-lived and limited. Most importantly, systemic treatments have been associated with frequent debilitating side effects (56). Also, iontophoresis that attempts to coagulate eccrine glands by the use of electrical current has had limited success (57).

2. **Alternative surgical therapies:** Surgical alternatives such as resection of the axillary sweat glands or subcutaneous curettage have been limited only to axillary hyperhidrosis. However, these techniques have had little acceptance due to the highly invasive nature of the procedures and the high complication rates.

3. **Dorsal thoracic sympathectomy:** Nonoperative methods for accomplishing dorsal thoracic sympathectomy include (a) percutaneous injection of phenol, (b) CT-guided injection of phenol, and (c) percutaneous radiofrequency thermal ablation (58–60). These techniques have been hampered by very high recurrence rates shortly after the procedure. Dorsal sympathectomy has been the only treatment for hyperhidrosis, which has resulted in long-term success.

Many surgical approaches have been described for dorsal thoracic sympathectomy. These include:

1. **Posterior thoracic approach:** The classic posterior thoracic approach was popularized by Adson and modified by White (61). This approach required

partial rib resection and resulted in prolonged painful recovery.

2. **Cervical supraclavicular approach:** Telford devised a supraclavicular approach (62). Although this approach obviated the pain associated with rib resection, it was technically demanding and associated with complications. The transcervical route requires attention to the highly complex anatomy of the cervical region, and the complications are associated with injury to these structures. The advantages of this approach include the ability to perform a bilateral sympathectomy in one sitting, minimal pain, and good cosmetic results. With this approach, due to the inability to reach the lower portion of the sympathetic chain, the T4 ganglion cannot be excised. Therefore, this approach is not as efficacious for patients experiencing axillary hyperhidrosis.

3. **Transthoracic approach:** Goetz, Marr, and Palumbo advocated an anterolateral transthoracic approach. Although this approach provided the best exposure and the most accurate sympathectomy possible, due to the significant morbidity associated with a thoracotomy, this technique did not gain popularity.

4. **Transaxillary approach:** In 1954, Atkins described a transaxillary approach, which became popular and is even used in some centers today (63). As has been noted, this technique suffers from the shortcoming of pain and lack of visualization through a very small transaxillary incision.

5. **Thoracoscopic approach:** The thoracoscopic approach to dorsal sympathectomy was used as far back as the 1940s. With the advent of advances in optics, lighting, and videoendoscopic instrumentation, VATS became the standard approach to dorsal sympathectomy. Presently, there are four video-assisted approaches to enable dorsal thoracic sympathectomy.

A. **Classic resection:** This technique involves resection of the entire sympathetic chain, including the T2, T3, and T4 sympathetic ganglia with the intervening RI.

B. **Clipping the sympathetic chain:** Proponents of this technique have emphasized the potential reversibility of the removal of the clip. However, clip removal has not been necessarily associated with the recovery of sympathetic function (64). Furthermore, some authors have postulated that clips may contribute to postoperative neuralgia (65).

C. **Thermal ablation of the dorsal sympathetic ganglion:** This approach, which can be accomplished using conventional electrocautery, diathermy with monopolar precise coagulation, or radiofrequency ablation, has become the most commonly used technique. The proponents of this technique have emphasized the ease of use, shorter operative times, ability to perform bilateral sympathectomy, and minimally invasive nature of the procedure. However, in a meta-analysis of studies of thoracoscopic sympathectomy for hyperhidrosis, Hashmonai et al. showed that resection achieved superior results (66). It is due to the complex nature of resection even with modern conventional video-assisted thoracic surgical techniques that the majority of surgeons choose thermal ablation of the sympathetic chain.

D. **Operative technique**: The room setup and preparation of the robot are covered in a separate chapter in this book.

E. **Anesthesia:** Patients undergoing robot-assisted surgery require single-lung ventilation. We prefer a left-sided double-lumen endotracheal tube over a bronchial blocker. Longer tubing is required during the robotic procedure as the anesthesiologist will occupy a more remote position away from the patient. The patient is placed in a full lateral decubitus position. We prefer to perform highly selective sympathectomy beginning with the most affected side, returning after any compensatory hyperhidrosis has subsided or plateaued in severity. This is usually within 2 weeks of the first procedure. The table is flexed to open the intercostal spaces and the position of the double-lumen tube is reconfirmed after final positioning. The patient then is prepared and draped in a routine manner. The superior portion of the drape is allowed to cover the patient's head. The table is unlocked and rotated 30 degrees from its normal position to facilitate the positioning of the robot over the patient's head.

F. Procedure started using standard **VATS instrumentation and incisions**: The surgeon stands facing the patient's back. A 2-cm incision (incision #1) is made in the sixth intercostal space in the mid-axillary line. A 10-mm metal trocar is introduced and a zero-degree Olympus

EndoEYE video endoscope is inserted into the pleural space. A second 2-cm incision (incision #2) is made in the third intercostal space in the anterior axillary line. This incision will be used by the right robotic arm. A third 2-cm incision (incision #3) is placed in the fifth intercostal space in the posterior axillary line. This incision will be used by the left robotic arm. At this point, the robot is brought in to the operating field over the patient's head. The camera arm with a 30-degree down-viewing binocular camera is introduced through incision #1 in the right pleural space. The right robotic arm with the robotic hook cautery is positioned through incision #2, and the left robotic arm with the robotic DeBakey forceps is positioned through incision #3. In the left pleural space, the right robotic arm enters the pleural space through incision #3 and the right robotic arm enters the pleural space through incision #2. The sympathetic chain is identified. The ribs are counted, and electrocute marks are placed away from the sympathetic ganglia to specify the position of ganglia #2, #, and #4. The portion of the sympathetic chain between ganglion #4 and #5 overlying rib #5 is identified, dissected with the hook cautery, and lifted with a rubber loop. Now the postganglionic fibers (RCG) can be identified easily and divided using electrocautery. Dissection is carried to the level of the second sympathetic ganglion. Following the completion of highly selective sympathectomy, flexible drain is positioned posteriorly in the pleural space and brought out through incision #1. On-Q subpleural catheters are placed traversing T2 to T8 as described elsewhere in this book for pain control. All patients are extubated and returned to the recovery room.

Robotic technology has the potential of accomplishing highly selective dorsal sympathectomy with accuracy. This technique may decrease the incidence of postsympathectomy compensatory hyperhidrosis and Horner's syndrome.

References

1. American Cancer Society. *Cancer Facts and Figures 2001*. Atlanta: American Cancer Society.
2. Jacobeus HC. Possibility of the use of the cystoscope for investigation of serous cavities. *Munch Med Wochenschr* 1910; 57: 2090.
3. Kaiser LR. Diagnostic and therapeutic uses of pleuroscopy (thoracoscopy) in lung cancer. *Surg Clin North Am* 1987; 67: 1081.
4. Kirby TJ. Invited commentary. *Ann Thorac Surg* 1997; 63: 1421–2.
5. Braimbridge MV. Thoracoscopy—a historical perspective. In Yim APC, Hazelrrig SR, Izzat MB et al. (eds). *Minimal Access Cardiothoracic Surgery*. Philadelphia: WB Saunders, 2000
6. McKenna RJ, Wolf RK, Brenner M, et al. Is lobectomy by video-assisted thoracic surgery an adequate cancer operation? *Ann Thorac Surg* 1998; 66:1903–7.
7. Mack MJ, Scruggs GR, Kelly KM et al. Video assisted thoracic surgery: has technology found its place? *Ann Thorac Surg* 1997; 64: 111.
8. Yim APC, Landreneau RJ, lzzat MB, Fung ALK. ls video-assisted thoracoscopic lobectomy a unified approach? *Ann Thorac Surg* 1998; 16: 1155.
9. Lewis RJ, Caccavale N, Boncage JP, et al. Video-assisted thoracic surgical non-rib spreading simultaneously stapled lobectomy: a more patient-friendly oncologic resection. *Chest* 1999; 116: 1119.
10. Lewis RJ. Simultaneously stapled lobectomy: a safe technique for video-assisted thoracic surgery. *J Thorac cardiovascular Surg* 1995; 109: 619–25.
11. Yim APC, Ko KM, Chau WS et al. Video-assisted thoracoscopic anatomic lung resections: the initial Hong Kong experience. *Chest* 1996; 109: 13.
12. Swanson SJ, Herndon J, D'Amico A, et al. Results of CALGB 39802: feasibility of video-assisted thoracic surgery (VATS) lobectomy for early stage lung cancer. *Am Assoc Clio Oncol* 2002; 21: 290.
13. Luketich JD, Meehan MA, Landreneau RJ, et al. Videothoracoscopic lobectomy versus open thoracotomy for early-stage non-small-cell lung cancer. *Clinical Lung Cancer* 2000; 2: 56–60.
14. Landreneau RJ, Hazelrigg SR, Mack MJ, et al. Postoperative pain-related morbidity: video-assisted thoracic surgery versus thoracotomy. *Ann Thorac Surg* 1993; 56: 1285–9.
15. McKenna RJ Jr, Fischel RJ, Wolf R, et al. Video-assisted thoracic surgery (VATS) lobectomy for bronchogenic carcinoma. *Sem Thorac Cardiovasc Surg* 1998; 10: 321–5.
16. Solaini L, Prusciano F, Bagioni P, et al. Video-assisted thoracic surgery major pulmonary resections. Present experience. *Eur J Cardiothorac Surg* 2001; 1: 437–42.

17. Daniels LJ, Balderson SS, Onaitis JT, et al. Thoracoscopic lobectomy: a safe and effective strategy for patients with stage I lung cancer. *Ann Thorac Surg* 2002; 74: 860–4.

18. McKenna RJ Jr, Houck W, Fuller CB. Video-assisted thoracic surgery lobectomy: experience with 1100 cases. *Ann Thorac Surg* 2006; 81: 421–6.

19. Kirby TJ, Mack MJ, Landreneau RJ, et al. Lobectomy video-assisted thoracic surgery versus muscle sparing thoracotomy. A randomized trial. *J Thorac Cardiovasc Surg* 1995; 109: 997.

20. Giudicelli R, Thomas P, Lonjon T, et al. Video-assisted minithoracotomy versus muscle-sparing thoracotomy for performing lobectomy. *Ann Thorac Surg* 1994; 58: 712.

21. Walker WS. VATS lobectomy: the Edinburgh experience. *Semin Thorac Cardiovasc Surg* 1998; 10: 291.

22. Craig SR, Walker WS. Potential complications of vascular stapling in thoracoscopic pulmonary resection. *Ann Thorac Surg* 1995; 59: 736.

23. Walker WS. Complications and pitfalls in video-assisted thoracic surgery. In Yim APC, Hazelrigg SR, Izzal MB, et al. (eds). *Minimal Access Cardiothoracic Surgery*. Philadelphia, WB Saunders, 2000.

24. Yim APC, Ho JKS. Malfunctioning of vascular staple cutter during thoracoscopic lobectomy. *J Thorac Cardiovasc Surg* 1995; 109: 1252.

25. Downey RJ, McCormick P, LoCicero J, et al. Dissemination of malignant tumors after video-assisted thoracic surgery. A report of twenty one cases. *J Thorac Cardiovasc Surg* 1996; 111: 954.

26. Yim APC, Wan S, Lee TW, Arifi AA. VATS lobectomy reduces cytokine response compared with conventional surgery. *Ann Thorac Surg* 2000; 70: 243.

27. Sugi K, Kaneda Y, Esato K. Video-assisted thoracoscopic lobectomy reduces cytokine production more than conventional open lobectomy. *Jpn J Thorac Cardiovasc Surg* 2000; 48: 161.

28. Leaver HA, Craig SR, Yap Pl, et al. Lymphocyte responses following open and minimally invasive thoracic surgery. *Eur J Clin Invest* 2000; 30: 230.

29. Walker WS, Leaver HA, Craig SR, Yap PL. The immune response to surgery: conventional and VATS lobectomy. In Yim APC, Hazelrigg SR, Izzat MB, et al. (eds). *Minimal Access Cardiothoracic Surgery*. Philadelphia: WB Saunders, 2000.

30. Yim APC, Ko KM, Chau WS, et al. Video-assisted thoracoscopic anatomic lung resections: the initial Hong Kong experience. *Chest* 1996; 109: 13.

31. Demmy TL, Curris JJ. Minimally invasive lobectomy directed toward frail and high-risk patients: a case control study. *Ann Thorac Surg* 1999; 68: 194.

32. Landreneau RJ, Mack MJ, Hazelrigg SR, et al. Prevalence of chronic pain after pulmonary resection by thoracotomy or video-assisted thoracic surgery. *J Thorac Cardiovasc Surg* 1994; 107: 1079.

33. Nakata M, Saeki H, Yokoyama N, et al. Pulmonary function after lobectomy: video-assisted thoracic surgery versus a thoracotomy. *Ann Thorac Surg* 2000; 70: 938.

34. Kaseda S, Aoki T, Hangai N, et al. Better pulmonary function and prognosis with video-assisted thoracic surgery than with thoracotomy. *Ann Thorac Surg* 2000; 70: 1644.

35. Sugiura H, Morikawa T, Kaji M, et al. Long-term benefits for the quality of life after video-assisted thoracic lobectomy in patients with lung cancer. *Surg Laparosc Endosc* 1999; 9: 403.

36. Yim APC, liu HP. Complications and failures from video-assisted thoracic surgery: experience from two centers in Asia. *Ann Thorac Surg* 1996; 61: 538.

37. Yim APC, Liu H, Izzat MB, et al. Thoracoscopic major lung resection: an Asian perspective. *Semin Thorac Cardiovasc Surg* 1998; 10: 326.

38. Kaseda S, Aoki T, Hangai N. Video-assisted thoracic surgery (VATS) lobectomy: the Japanese experience. *Sem Thorac Cardiovasc Surg* 1998; 10: 300.

39. Roviaro G, Varoli I, Vergani C, et al. VATS major pulmonary resections: the Italian experience. *Semin Thorac Cardiovasc Surg* 1998; 10: 313.

40. McKenna RJ Jr, Wolf RK, Brenner M, et al. Is VATS lobectomy an adequate cancer operation? *Ann Thorac Surg* 1998; 66: 1903.

41. Yim APC. Thoracoscopic surgery in the elderly population. *Surg Endosc* 1996; 10: 880.

42. Demmy TL. VATS lobectomy for frail or complex patients. *Chest* 2003; 124: 234.

43. Mack MJ, Hazelrigg SR, Landreneau RJ, et al. (eds.). The first international symposium on thoracoscopic surgery. *Ann Thorac Surg* 1993; 56: 605.

44. Yim APC, Landreneau RJ, Izzat MB, et al. Is video-assisted thoracoscopic lobectomy a unified approach? *Ann Thorac Surg* 1998; 66: 1155.

45. Heitmiller RF, Mathison DJ. French incision. In Grillo HC, Austen WG, Wilkins EW, et al. (eds). *Current Therapy in Cardiothoracic Surgery*. Toronto, BC: Decker, 1989.

46. Brunelli A, Monteverde M, Borri A, et al. Predictors of prolonged air leak after pulmonary lobectomy. *Ann. Thorac Surg* 2004; 77: 1205–10.

47. Okereke I, Murthy SC, Alster JM, et al. Characterization and importance of air leak after lobectomy. *Ann Thorac Surg* 2005; 79: 1167–73.

48. Larry R, Kaiser LR, David W, et al. Trial of a novel synthetic sealant in preventing air leaks after lung resection. *Ann Thorac Surg* 2001; 71: 1623–9.

49. Belboul A, Dernevik L, Aljassim O, et al. The effect of autologous fibrin sealant (Vivostat®) on morbidity after pulmonary lobectomy: a prospective randomised, blinded study. *Eur J Cardiothorac Surg* 2004; 26: 1187–91.

50. Gharagozloo F, Tempesta B, Margolis M, et al. Video-assisted thoracic surgery lobectomy for stage I lung cancer. *Ann Thorac Surg* 2003; 76: 1009–15.

51. Bodner J, Wykypiel H, Greiner A. Early experience with robot-assisted surgery for mediastinal masses. *Ann Thorac Surg* 2004; 78: 259–65.

52. Yim AP, Lee TW, Izzat MM, et al. Place of video-thoracoscopy in thoracic surgical practice. *World J Surg* 2001; 25: 157–61.

53. Royle JP. History of sympathectomy. *Aust N Z J Surg* 1999; 69: 107–12.

54. Gaskell WH. *The Involuntary Nervous System*. London: Longman, Green and Co, 1916.

55. Bernard C. Sur les effets de la section de la portion cephalous du grand sympathique. *Comptes rend Soc Biol* 1852; 4: 168–70.

56. Brown-Sequard CE. Experimental researches applied to physiology and pathology. *M Exam* 1852; 8: 481,548,617,698.

57. Alexander W. *The Treatment of Epilepsy*. Edinburgh: Y J Pentland, p. 228, 1889.

58. Adler OB, Engel A, Sageno D. Palmar hyperhydrosis treated by percutaneous transthoracic chemical sympaticolysis. *Eur J Radiol* 4: 57–62.

59. Wilkinson HA. Radiofrequency percutaneous upper thoracic sympathectomy. Technique and review of indications. *N Engl J Med* 1984; 311: 34–38.

60. Telford ED. The technique of sympathectomy. *Br J Surg* 1935; 23: 448–450.

61. Adson AW, Brown GE. Treatment of Raynaud's disease by lumbar ram section and ganglionectomy's and per vascular sympathetique neurectomy of the common iliacs. *JAMA* 1925; 84: 1908–10.

62. Telford ED. The technique of sympathectomy. *Br J Surg* 1935; 23: 448–50.

63. Atkins H. Sympathectomy by axillary approach. *Lancet* 1954; 1: 538.

64. Wittmoser R. Toracoscopic sympathectomy and agronomy. In Cuschieri A, et al. (eds). *Operative Manual of Endoscopic Surgery*. Berlin: Sringer Verlag, 1992.

65. Teleranta T. Secondary sympathetic chain reconstruction after endoscopes thoracic sympathectomy. *Eur J Surg* 1998; suppl. 1: 1–8.

66. Hashmonai M, Assalia A, Kopelman D. Thoracoscopic sympathectomy for palmar hyperhydrosis. Ablate or resect? *Surg Endosc* 2001; 15: 435–41.

Chapter

12

Robotics in Thoracic Surgery 2

Benign and Malignant Esophageal Disease

Farid Gharagozloo

ENDOSCOPIC ROBOTIC ESOPHAGECTOMY

Historical Background

"The history of esophageal surgery is a tale of men repeatedly losing to a stronger adversary yet persisting in this unequal struggle until the nature of the problems became apparent and the war was won."

A discussion on robotic esophagectomy is appropriately prefaced by this quote by Emslie, which provides the most accurate perspective for the struggle of surgeons with this elusive organ (1).

The anatomic remoteness of the esophagus, along with the many challenges of intraoperative management, have dictated the approach to esophagectomy through the ages. Galen described the patient with esophageal cancer in the second century AD. In the tenth century, Avicenna described esophageal tumors as the most common cause of dysphagia (2). Although surgery of the esophagus was first recorded by the Egyptians in 2500 BC with "repair of the gullet," the first successful resection of cervical esophageal cancer was performed by Czerny in 1877 (3). This work was predicated on Billroth's work in 1871 who demonstrated the feasibility of resection and re-anastomosis of the cervical esophagus in an animal model (4). However, it was six decades later that a successful esophageal resection with intrathoracic anastomosis was performed (5).

In 1913, Torek performed the resection of a squamous cell carcinoma (SCCA) of the thoracic esophagus through the left chest (6). Esophageal gastric continuity was established using a rubber tube that connected the cervical esophagus to the stomach. The patient survived 13 years. For the first decades of the twentieth century, many techniques for the establishment of continuity of the alimentary tract were investigated. In 1911, Kelling described the use of colon for esophageal replacement (7). The use of stomach, based on the right gastroepiploic artery and the right gastric artery, was first demonstrated in the laboratory by Kirschner in 1920 (8). In 1933, Ohsava of Japan performed the first successful esophagectomy with an intrathoracic esophagogastric anastomosis through the left chest (9). This pioneering work was followed by similar reports from Marshall, Adams, Phemister, Churchill, and Sweet in the United States who advocated a left transthoracic approach (10–12). In 1946, Ivor Lewis reported esophageal resection through separate laparotomy and right chest incisions with an intrathoracic anastomosis at the apex of the right chest (5). In order to avoid the consequences associated with an intrathoracic anastomotic leak in 1972, McKeown advocated the placement of the esophagogastric anastomosis in the neck through a separate cervical incision after the Ivor Lewis procedure (13). It is of interest that presently the issue of intrathoracic anastomotic leaks continues to dictate the approach to esophageal resections. Furthermore, it should be noted that the present controversy between the advantages of transthoracic esophagectomy (TTE) versus transhiatal esophagectomy (THE) is not new. Indeed, this controversy has its roots in two different approaches that were advocated throughout the twentieth century.

The transhiatal approach (THA) began in 1913 when Denk demonstrated in cadavers the feasibility of blunt dissection of the esophagus by working from the neck down and up through the esophageal hiatus (14). This approach was performed by a laparotomy and a cervical incision and obviated the need for a thoracotomy. In 1933, Turner reported the first "blunt" esophagectomy followed by an antethoracic skin tube reconstitution of the esophagogastric continuity (15). Ong and Lee in 1916 and LeQuesne and Ranger in 1966 reported a small series of patients with "blunt" esophagectomy with transhiatal gastric pull up and a cervical esophagogastrostomy (16,17). In 1978, Oringer resected the technique of transhiatal transcervical esophagectomy without a thoracotomy (18).

Epidemiology

Cancer of the esophagus is one of the most common malignancies worldwide. Approximately 13,000 new cases of esophageal cancer were diagnosed in the United States in 1998. Almost 12,000 patients died within the first year (19). Presently the rate of esophageal cancers has increased dramatically. Esophageal cancer is unusual compared to other solid tumors due to the geographic variations in incidence and the cell type. Although SCCA is the most common histologic subtype of esophageal cancer globally, the primary esophageal adenocarcinoma (ACA) is the predominant histologic subtype in North America (20).

In 1991, Blot and colleagues examined more than 9,000 esophageal cases registered in nine National Cancer Institute surveillance, epidemiology, and end results program areas (21). They found that:

1. Adenocarcinoma of the lower esophagus accounted for 17 percent of primary esophageal cancers overall.
2. From 1976 to 1987, the average rate of increase for primary esophageal adenocarcinoma exceeded that of any other cancer.
3. During the last 3 years of this study, 1984–1987, adenocarcinoma accounted for 34 percent of all esophageal tumors in white males.

By 1993, adenocarcinoma accounted for 48.1 percent of all cancers of the lower esophagus in the United States (22). In the 1998 update of the original study by Blot, Devasa et al. reported a 350 percent increase in the rate of adenocarcinoma of the esophagus in white North American males from 1976 to 1994 (23).

With the observation that many adenocarcinomas of the esophagus occur in association with Barrett's epithelium, the metaplasia–dysplasia–carcinoma sequence has been clearly demonstrated (24). Prospective studies estimate that patients with Barrett's epithelium have at least a 30- to 40-fold higher risk for development of invasive adenocarcinoma (25). Presently Barrett's epithelium, which exhibits mutation of the P53 tumor suppressor gene, is considered premalignant (26). This marked change in the biology and epidemiology of esophageal cancer has impacted the therapeutic strategy for this disease significantly. As noted, there has been a shift from predominance of SCCA associated with tobacco and alcohol exposure to adenocarcinoma arising in a Barrett's esophagus as a consequence of reflux disease. In contrast to SCCA, the clearly delineated metaplasia–dysplasia–carcinoma sequence with adenocarcinoma provides an opportunity for early detection and better outcomes after resection.

Historically the role of surgery in SCCA of the esophagus has been one of palliation. The risk of surgical procedures associated with the locally advanced nature of SCCA of the mid-esophagus has prevented oncologically efficacious procedures. The shift from SCCA of the mid-esophagus to adenocarcinoma of distal esophagus and gastroesophageal junction makes these tumors more amenable to complete resection. Furthermore, recent refinements in operative technique and perioperative management have enabled greater safety in accomplishing the more efficacious en bloc tumor resection and nodal exoneration. Not only has there been a shift in the cell type and location of esophageal carcinoma, there has also been a shift in the surgical approach from palliation to one with curative intent.

Therapeutic Strategies

Although surgery has been the mainstay of treatment of esophageal carcinoma, the high morbidity and mortality rates associated with surgery have necessitated more palliative procedures as well as the search for nonsurgical therapies. Results of surgical resection have improved. In the 1960s and 1970s, the operability rate of esophageal carcinoma was 58 percent, resectability rate was 39 percent, mortality associated with resection was 29 percent, with an overall 5-year survival of 4 percent (27). In the 1980s, the resectability rate was 56 percent, mortality rate with resection was 13 percent, and 5-year survival was 10 percent (28). Presently in specialized centers that perform greater than 50 procedures per year, the mortality rate is reported at 4.5 percent with a 5-year survival of 50.4 percent overall (29). Clearly, this dramatic change in the overall survival and operative risk is due to the earlier diagnosis of esophageal carcinoma, refinement of surgical technique and perioperative care, and greater use of multimodality therapy.

Preoperative Neoadjuvant Chemotherapy Alone

The use of preoperative chemotherapy in locally advanced esophageal carcinoma has been the subject of numerous trials. Most trials have evaluated preoperative chemotherapy, given for one to six cycles followed by a definitive surgical procedure (30–33). Later trials have given chemotherapy both preoperatively and postoperatively. Overall preoperative chemotherapy with cisplatin-based combination therapy has achieved a major response in 17–66 percent of patients with pathologically confirmed complete response of 3–10 percent. Operability has ranged from 50 to 100 percent with resectability of tumors ranging from 40 to 90 percent. Operative mortality after preoperative chemotherapy has been comparable to surgery alone. However, the overall survival of patients treated with preoperative chemotherapy has been disappointing. The median 5-year survival has ranged from 10 to 26 percent. In support of smaller studies, the landmark American Intergroup Trial reported by Kelsen and colleagues showed no benefit for neoadjuvant chemotherapy over surgery alone (34).

Preoperative Neoadjuvant Radiotherapy Alone

Trials of neoadjuvant radiotherapy have failed to show increased resection rate or improved survival compared to surgery alone (35).

Preoperative Neoadjuvant Combined Chemoradiation Therapy

The Radiation Therapy Oncology Group (RTOG 85-01) randomized trial showed superiority of neoadjuvant chemoradiation therapy over radiation alone (36,37). The combination of chemoradiation with surgery has resulted in significant disease downstaging and has increased the proportion of R0 resections. However, a consistent survival advantage for neoadjuvant chemoradiation followed by surgery has not been demonstrated. All these studies have been hampered by the inclusion of both SCCA and adenocarcinoma and inconsistent surgical procedures. A survival advantage with neoadjuvant chemoradiation followed by surgery over surgery alone was shown in two trials of patients with adenocarcinoma. Three-year survival rates were 32 percent for combined modality therapy versus 6 percent for surgery alone. From the limited data available, it seems that chemoradiation may help local disease control, when combined with surgical resection (38). No randomized trials have directly compared chemoradiation with surgery when the surgical procedure has been performed with curative intent rather than palliation. Urschell et al. performed a meta-analysis of randomized trials comparing neoadjavent chemoradiation and surgery versus surgery alone. There were nine studies with 1,116 patients. Combined modality therapy was superior to surgery alone with respect to (1) 3-year survival, (2) complete resection, (3) locoregional tumor recurrence, and (4) distant recurrence. Twenty-one percent of patients obtained complete pathologic response. Results were best when chemo and radiation therapy were given concurrently. Operative mortality was higher after multimodality therapy.

Furthermore, although it has been suggested that chemoradiation alone can be adequate without surgical resection, a number of considerations argue against the omission of surgery:

1. False complete response rates based on imaging modalities are commonly seen, and true complete response can only be determined after resection.
2. With chemoradiation alone, persistent local or locally recurrent disease is seen in approximately 50 percent of patients. The addition of surgery reduces local disease recurrence (39). Furthermore, even with sterilization of the primary tumor, persistent nodal disease is observed. Surgery cleans any persistent nodal disease and provides posttherapy pathologic staging of the disease.
3. Surgical treatment following chemoradiation provides far more superior relief of dysphagia and resumption of oral intake compared to chemoradiation alone. In one report, solid food intake was 100 percent with surgery as compared to 45 percent without surgery (40). In a perspective study, O'Rourke et al. reported incidence of stricture as 16 percent with surgery and 50 percent after chemoradiation alone (41). Furthermore, postoperative anastomotic strictures respond to dilation very easily as compared to postchemoradiation malignant strictures, which do not respond to dilation and require stenting or other endoscopic procedures.

Even though further clinical studies are needed to identify the best multimodality regimens, their dose levels, and methods and schedules of administration, an increasing number of patients are receiving neoadjuvant therapy. As shown by Rice et al., patients with advanced disease (T_3N_1) who respond to neoadjuvant therapy have better outcomes than with surgery alone (42). These authors have shown that neoadjuvant therapy has not been beneficial in patients with clinical early-stage disease. Consequently, at the present time, surgery remains the standard treatment for resectable early-stage cancer of the esophagus. Patients with advanced local regional disease should be offered preoperative chemoradiation therapy prior to surgery in order to achieve cytoreduction and improved resectability. As a majority of patients with carcinoma of the esophagus are diagnosed at a late stage, the majority of patients are candidates for preoperative neoadjuvant chemoradiation therapy followed by surgery.

Surgical Therapy

Currently, most esophagectomies are carried out either through the transhiatal approach (THE) or through the Ivor Lewis transthoracic approach (TTE). Other procedures such as left thoracoabdominal approach (43), left thoracoabdominal cervical approach (44), left transthoracic approach (45), synchronous combined abdominothoracic cervical approach (46), and transabdominal approach (47) are either of historic interest or reserved for unusual circumstances.

Transhiatal Esophagectomy

Transhiatal esophagectomy without a thoracotomy was resurrected and popularized by Orringer in 1978. This procedure, which uses a laparotomy and cervical incision, removes the esophagus "bluntly" and, after passing the stomach tube through the hiatus and the bed of the esophagus, a cervical esophagogastrostomy is accomplished. The advantage of THE is that it avoids the morbidity associated with a thoracotomy. Furthermore, the proponents of THE note that cervical anastomotic leaks are not associated with the mediastinitis and high mortality associated with leaks of the intrathoracic anastomosis.

Although a number of small series has been reported, the largest reported series by Oringer and colleagues presents data on 1,085 patients with THE (48). In this series, THE was possible in 98.6 percent of patients and a stomach was used in 96 percent of patients. A total of nine patients (0.8 percent) had excessive intraoperative hemorrhage with three intraoperative deaths. Other complications included entry into the pleural spaces (77 percent), splenectomy (3 percent), recurrent laryngeal nerve injury (7 percent), chylothorax (<1 percent), pneumonia (2 percent), wound dehiscence (3 percent), anastomotic leaks (13 percent), and hospital mortality (4 percent).

Even though mortality from an anastomotic leak is very low, it is important to note that the leak rate after THE is quite high. In fact, a leak rate has been reported to be as high as 25 percent in less experienced centers (49). The cervical esophagogastrostomy is positioned on the highest point in the stomach, which has worse perfusion and relies on blood flow through transmural vessels connecting with the gastroepiploic artery. A cervical anastomotic leak usually results from using the portion of stomach conduit with porous blood flow. Furthermore, although mortality is low with a cervical anastomotic leak, the morbidity of a draining esophagogastric fistula in the neck and future stricture formation is quite daunting.

An additional shortcoming of THE is the high rate of phrenic nerve injury with its associated sequela. Aside from the technical concerns relating to cervical esophagogastrostomy, the critics of THE have asserted that it gained popularity in an era when esophageal surgery was associated with high mortality and morbidity. A significant part of morbidity and mortality of esophagectomy was associated with a thoracotomy, which is obviated by THE technique. Furthermore, the critics have noted that THE violates the basic surgical principles of adequate hemostasis and exposure and falls short as a "cancer operation" by avoiding an en bloc dissection of mediastinal lymph nodes. These authors have observed that recent studies showing better survival with en bloc resection and mediastinal nodal exoneration as well as advances in surgical and anesthetic techniques relegate THE to the era of palliation versus era of surgery with curative intent. These observations suggest that with better staging, earlier diagnosis, and combined modality therapy, the traditional focus of surgery, which has been palliation for dysphagia typically in patients with end-stage esophageal cancers, should be abandoned. In contrast, many investigators have asserted that surgical treatment of esophageal adenocarcinoma should have cure as the driving force.

Ivor–Lewis Procedure, Right Thoracic Abdominal Approach

If the primary goal of treatment of esophageal cancers is cure of the neoplasm, with the relief of dysphagia as an important secondary concern, surgical resection should encompass the entire tumor, draining lymph nodes, and adequate proximal and distal margin. The combined laparotomy and right thoracotomy approach with an intrathoracic esophagogastrostomy, which was originally described by Ivor Lewis in two stages, has evolved into a single-stage procedure (50). The potential advantage of this procedure is a complete resection of the tumor with surrounding nodes under direct vision.

The greatest concerns with the Ivor–Lewis procedures are the requirement for thoracotomy and morbidity and mortality associated with intrathoracic anastomosis. Matheson and other proponents of the Ivor–Lewis approach have emphasized that the leak rate can be very low in the chest and have stressed the importance of how anastomosis is performed rather than where it is performed (51). In centers with high volumes of esophagectomy, leak rates of intrathoracic anastomoses have ranged from 0 to 2 percent (52). In a study from the Lahey Clinic comparing THE and TTE with the same surgeons performing the procedures, respiratory insufficiency and atelectasis occurred more commonly after TTE versus THE (27±19 versus 13±8) (53). With TTE recurrent nerve palsy, chylothorax and posterior tracheal tears were very uncommon. Historically, despite the theoretical advantages of en bloc dissection and full lymphadenectomy, studies comparing TTE and THE have shown no difference in overall survival.

In a single-institution nonrandomized study, Matheson has shown improved survival with TTE (51). In a recent study of 263 patients with resectable esophageal adenocarcinoma from the single institution, Portale et al. showed better survival after TTE versus THE (70 percent versus 35 percent in all stages). Furthermore, the survival trends persisted for each stage of the disease. In a European study of 425 patients undergoing TTE versus THE, Gockel et al. showed a survival advantage with TTE as compared to THE (54). Based on this data, these authors have advocated complete en bloc resection. Altorki and Skinner have reported a 40 percent 5-year survival after en bloc resection of tumors of the lower esophagus (55). Sihvo and colleagues showed the 5-year survival of 50 percent after esophagectomy with extensive lymphadenectomy compared to 23.2 percent with less extensive procedures (56).

In a randomized trial, Hulscher and co-workers showed a trend toward better survival after TTE versus THE (57). The survival benefit of TTE is not limited only to patients with early-stage disease. Collard et al. and Swanson et al. showed that TTE esophagectomy for adenocarcinoma is superior to THE in patients with transmural esophageal adenocarcinoma with as many as eight involved lymph nodes (58,59). In these studies, there was a virtual absence of local recurrence within the operative field, an observation which may explain the superior results with TTE. In addition, this observation would make TTE more appropriate when resection is performed as a "clean-up" and staging maneuver following neoadjuvant chemoradiation therapy.

The McKeown variation on the Ivor–Lewis procedure is carried out in three stages.

1. Right thoracotomy
2. Abdominal exploration
3. Cervical incision.

In this procedure, esophagogastrostomy is placed in the neck. Therefore, the McKeown procedure suffers from problems associated with cervical esophagogastrostomy as were outlined for THE. In our view, the McKeown procedure is hampered by the shortcomings of both TTE and THE approaches and is best suited for tumors, usually SCCAs in the upper esophagus where an adequate proximal resection may not be possible through the chest.

Video-Assisted Minimally Invasive Techniques for Esophagectomy

With the advent of video-assisted techniques and their application to procedures in the abdomen and chest, there has been an attempt to apply these techniques to resection of the esophagus. The investigators have reasoned that minimally invasive techniques can decrease morbidity associated with an esophagectomy.

Thoracoscopic esophageal mobilization combined with conventional THE: The first attempt was to use video-assisted thoracoscopy to mobilize the esophagus followed by a laparotomy and a cervical esophagogastrostomy (60). Akaishi et al. showed less postoperative pain and more complete recovery of vital capacity as compared to a conventional esophagectomy (61). Other authors, however, were not able to demonstrate a clear advantage for thoracoscopic esophageal mobilization (62).

Total laparoscopic THE: DePaula et al. reported a laparoscopic THE with a cervical esophagogastrostomy (63). Others have reported a similar approach.

Although operative mortality has been very low, this procedure has been hampered by a number of problems: (1) unsatisfactory completion of intrathoracic esophageal mobilization, (2) unsatisfactory lymph node dissection, and (3) complications associated with conventional THE.

Combined laparoscopic and thoracoscopic THE with cervical esophagogastrostomy: This procedure was championed by Luketich et al. (63). The esophagus is mobilized by thoracoscopy followed by laparoscopic mobilization of the stomach and a cervical esophagogastrostomy. The early results of this technique for minimally invasive esophagectomy were reviewed by Luketich (64). Twenty-five of 77 patients (32 percent) were operated on for Barrett's esophagus with high-grade dysplasia. Ninety percent of patients had adenocarcinoma. The majority of patients underwent combined thoracoscopic and laparoscopic THE. Twelve of 77 patients (16 percent) required conversion to a laparotomy or thoracotomy. The mean operative time was 7.5 hours, mean ICU stay of 1 day, and mean hospital stay of 7 days. Thirty-day operative mortality was 0. 27 percent for patients who suffered from major complications. There were seven (10 percent) anastomotic leaks. Mean lymph node yield was 16, with 60 percent of the nodes removed from the abdomen. At 20 months, overall survival was 81 percent. However, with the same 20-month follow-up, 18 of 77 patients (23 percent) had cancer recurrence (10 percent distant recurrence and 13 percent local recurrence).

Our experience with combined laparoscopic and thoracoscopic esophagectomy has been similar. Based on this experience, a number of conclusions can be made:

1. A laparoscopic approach to gastric mobilization and intraabdominal lymphadenectomy is not comparable to the degree of gastric mobilization and nodal dissection that is obtained by a laparotomy. Although the laparoscopic approach may be ideal for patients with Barrett's esophagus with high-grade dysplasia, in patients with more advanced locoregional disease, the present laparoscopic techniques do not enable en bloc lymphadenectomy and violate the principals of oncologic efficacy. In practice, firing a stapling device across the left gastric axis leaves a significant amount of tissue behind. This tissue would be easily dissected with an open procedure.
2. The combined laparoscopic and thoracoscopic approach suffers from the shortcomings of THE, which were outlined earlier. Consequently, in its present form, this approach may represent a return to the palliative error of esophageal surgery at a time when curative intent should be emphasized.
3. Although thoracoscopic mobilization of the esophageus is feasible, complete mediastinal exoneration with the removal of paraesophageal tissue requires deeper dissection into the mediastinum. In our experience, by virtue of the shortcomings of thoracoscopic instrumentation, a degree of dissection is not comparable by thoracoscopy to that which can be obtained by a thoracotomy during conventional Ivor–Lewis esophagogastrostomy. These concerns are highlighted by the very high rate of local recurrence, which is seen shortly after conventional minimally invasive procedures. Based on this experience, we have concluded that a more sophisticated minimally invasive approach to en bloc esophageal resection and nodal exoneration with an intrathoracic esophagogastrostomy is required.

Robotic Esophagectomy

Over the past decade, our program for esophageal carcinoma has followed the concept of en bloc resection of the tumor with extensive periesophageal lymphadenectomy. The en bloc resection of esophageal cancer has been accomplished using the Ivor–Lewis approach. In 2011, based on the Society of Thoracic Surgeons database, for patients undergoing esophageal resection using this technique at our institution, the mortality rate was 2 percent, pneumonia was seen in 11 percent of patients, and there were no anastomotic leaks.

This experience has formed the basis for robotic esophagectomy program at our institution. At the outset of the robotic esophagectomy program, a number of parameters were identified:

1. Our experience with VATS and laparoscopy had clearly demonstrated the feasibility of esophagectomy using minimally invasive techniques. However, in our experience the thoracoscopic approach impaired the ability to perform mediastinal nodal exoneration, which has been a requirement of our conventional

The EndoWrist

The EndoWrist is a cable-driven wrist at the end of the robotic arm. The placement of the robotic arm through the VATS hole is comparable to the chopstick maneuvers of conventional VATS instruments. The EndoWrist at the distal end of the robotic arm is then positioned in the confined space and brings four more degrees of freedom and six more directions of movement to the maneuverability already possible by the movement of the robotic arm pivoting at the entry site. The movement of EndoWrist allows for movement of distal instruments much like the movements of the surgeon's wrist during conventional surgery.

Downscaling

The da Vinci robotic system is designed to provide downscaling from the motion of the surgeon's hands to that of the robotic arm. This is invaluable in dissecting the fine and fragile tissues of distal esophagus. Furthermore, a fixed Hz motion filter is used to filter out the tremor in the surgeon's hand and enhance the accuracy of surgical dissection.

Binocular Vision

The binocular robotic camera provides superb three-dimensional visualization and, by nature of being mounted on the central robotic arm, it is manipulated by the surgeon. The result of this is an immobile field of vision with high resolution and magnification and total control of movements by the surgeon. The ability to manipulate the camera and the robotic arms recreates the surgeon's own natural head, eye, and wrist motions as used during open procedures and enhances hand–eye coordination.

Operative Technique

Anesthesia

Patients undergoing video-assisted thoracic surgical Heller myotomy require single-lung ventilation. We prefer a left-sided double-lumen endotracheal tube over a bronchial blocker. With a double-lumen tube, lung collapse is superior and hilar manipulation does not result in movement of the blocker and inadvertent expansion of the lung. As is addressed in a separate chapter in this book, the facility of the anesthesiologist with robotic techniques is crucial to the conduct of the surgery. Following the induction of anesthesia, with the patient in the supine position, upper GI endoscopy is performed. The gastroesophageal junction is identified and a nasogastric tube is positioned under direct vision into the stomach. Decompression of the stomach facilitates retraction of the diaphragm and enhances visualization of the gastroesophageal junction. While the patient is in the supine position, the gastroscope is pulled back to the distal esophagus and secured for patient positioning. As described by Pellegrini et al., the gastroscope plays a significant role during the myotomy procedure. First, it allows for identification of the left lateral wall of the esophagus without the need for extensive mobilization of a circumferential dissection of the esophagus. Second, it transilluminates the esophageal mucosa and helps in identification of the area of incomplete myotomy. Third, by application of intraluminal suction to the mucosa during the myotomy procedure, the mucosa is pulled toward the lumen of the esophagus, thereby exposing the anterior plane between the esophageal mucosa and the muscle of esophagus.

Patient Positioning

The patient is placed in an extended right lateral decubitus position. The table is fully flexed to enlarge the space between the ribs. The surgeon stands behind the patient. A monitor is positioned at the patient's feet and a second monitor is positioned in front of the patient facing the surgeon. The robot is positioned in front of the patient. During the robotic portion of the procedure, the robot is brought into the operative field from an anterior to posterior direction facing cephalad at 30 degrees to the axis of the patient.

Myotomy

After the patient is prepped and draped, a 2-cm incision (#1) is made in the seventh intercostal space in the mid-axillary line. This incision will serve as a camera port during the VATS and robotic portions of the operation. A second 2-cm incision (#2) is made in the sixth intercostal space anteriorly at the anterior axillary line. A third 2-cm incision (#3) is made in the sixth intercostal space posteriorly at the mid-scapular line. A fourth 1-cm incision is made one interspace below the anterior incision and as far inferiorly as possible. This incision will be used for the placement of diaphragmatic retractor, and at the conclusion of the procedure, it will be used for the placement of drainage chest tubes. It is paramount that this incision be positioned as far anteriorly from incision #2 in order to decrease interference with the robotic arm. As has been described in Chapter 19 in this book, we prefer the Olympus EndoEYE video endoscopic system. A 10-mm 0-degree end-viewing scope is positioned initially viewing cephalad over the diaphragm. The inferior pulmonary ligament is divided and the lung is retracted superiorly. The table is positioned in Trendelenburg to allow the lung to fall into the apex of the chest. The camera is then rotated 180 degrees to view the distal esophagus at the diaphragm. The surgeon and the surgical team then rotate their field of vision and use the video monitor at the patient's feet for the next phase of the procedure. In order to retain intuitive spatial relationships, it is imperative that the surgical team view the surgical site in the same direction and axis as the video endoscope. The gastroscope is rotated to the patient's left and its tip is flexed, thus allowing the surgeon to visualize the distal esophagus without the need for further dissection. Using conventional Endosheers (Ethicon Endosurgery, Cincinnati, OH) with cautery attachment, the pleura overlying the esophagus is divided. An Endostitch instrument (Auto Suture, US Surgical, Norwalk, CT) with a 2-0 Ethibond suture is used to place retraction sutures on the two edges of the pleura. The sutures are then brought out through the anterior and posterior incisions (incisions #2 and #4) and fixed to the drapes. This maneuver creates a pleural sling and elevates the esophagus from its normal mediastinal location into the left pleural space. A fan retractor (Ethicon Endosurgery, Cincinnati, OH) is introduced through the anterior (#4) incision and positioned on the posteromedial aspect of the diaphragm and used to retract the diaphragm inferiorly. This retractor is fixed to the table by the use of a mechanical holder (Mediflex; Velmed, Inc., Wexford, PA). The esophageal hiatus is identified and the left lateral limb of the right crus of the diaphragm is divided using the Endosheers with cautery. The dissection is discontinued with the visualization of the phrenoesophageal ligament on the underside of the diaphragm. Using the Endostitch instrument with a 0 Ethibond suture, full-thickness retraction sutures are placed on the cut edges of the diaphragm and brought out through the anterior and posterior incisions, respectively (#2 and #4). The sutures are fixed to the drapes. This maneuver allows for a full visualization of the esophagogastric junction. At the end of the procedure, the cut edges of the right limb (RL) of the right crus of the diaphragm are reapproximated using an Endostitch instrument with 0 Ethibond suture. Usually, three such sutures are necessary. By avoiding disruption of the anterior crural arch and by restoring the integrity of the RL of the right crus of the diaphragm, the crural sling is preserved and the antireflux barrier remains intact. At this point, the VATS camera is removed and the robot is positioned. The robot is brought in from the anterior aspect of the patient. It is positioned caudad to cephalad with 30-degree rotation in the cephalad direction on the patient's axis. The camera port is positioned in the camera incision (#1) and a 30-degree down-viewing scope is positioned viewing caudally onto the distal esophagus. The right robotic arm with a hook end-effector instrument connected to a cautery is placed through the anterior incision (#2) and its EndoWrist is positioned directly over the distal esophagus. A left robotic arm with a DeBakey forceps as its distal end-effector instrument is positioned through the posterior incision (#3) and its EndoWrist is positioned directly over the distal esophagus. A metal suction with a blunt tip is positioned through the anterior incision below the entry point of the right robotic arm. The suction is used by the assistant to evacuate cautery smoke, control bleeding, and provide downward force on the esophageal mucosa during the myotomy, should this become necessary. With binocular view and depth perception and the facility of EndoWrist movements, the performance of esophageal myotomy is quite accurate and uncomplicated. The muscular wall of the esophagus is exposed and the muscle is divided with a hook cautery at the midpoint of exposed esophagus. The anatomic plane between the mucosa and the muscle is identified. The blunt metal suction is positioned on the mucosa, endoluminal suction is also applied using the video gastroscope. The robotic forceps are used to elevate the muscle layers. The culmination of these maneuvers allows for the hook cautery (blended coagulation current set at 30 W) to be used to divide the muscle of the esophagus. As the distal aspect of the esophagus and the intussuscepted portion of the esophagus into the proximal stomach is approached, the robotic forceps are used to reduce the intussusception by pulling the esophagus in a cephalad direction. The hook cautery then completes the myotomy approximately 1 cm onto the cardia of the stomach. Myotomy is discontinued when the submucosal vascular plexus of the stomach wall is visualized. At this point, the gastroscope is advanced past the gastroesophageal junction into the stomach. The ease of movement of the gastroscope into the stomach and the lack of resistance confirms a complete division of the esophageal muscles at the gastroesophageal junction. Furthermore, the gastroscope is retroflexed to view the gastroesophageal junction from a caudad to cephalad direction. The observation of the transilluminated mucosa of the proximal portion of stomach cardia from the light of the robotic camera serves as the final confirmation for a completion of esophageal myotomy. Following the completion of myotomy, the chest is filled with saline and the gastroscope is used to insufflate air into the stomach and esophagus to rule out any mucosal perforation. Any mucosal perforations are easily repaired by the endoscopic techniques and use of 4-0 Prolene sutures. The robotic arms are retracted and the robot is moved away from the table. At this juncture, the conventional VATS EndoEYE camera is inserted through the camera port, and the left limb (LL) of the right crus of the diaphragm is reapproximated as described earlier. At this point, a 2-cm square piece of Vicryl mesh (Ethicon, Inc., Somerville, NJ) is positioned at the distal aspect of the mediastinum. This absorbable mesh is attached to the edges of the mediastinal pleura using the Endostitch with 2-0 Ethibond sutures. We have found that the Vicryl mesh, which is absorbed and replaced by scar tissue approximately 8 weeks following implantation, reestablished the integrity of the pleura on the left lateral aspect of the esophagus and repositions the distal esophagus into the mediastinum. Furthermore, this maneuver with the resultant scarring of the pleura prevents the formation of a mucosal diverticulum at the distal portion of the esophagus. It has been hypothesized that the mucosal diverticulum may be one of the causes of chronic dysphagia even with an adequate myotomy when a fundoplasty is not performed. In fact, some authors have proposed that one of the benefits of fundoplasty is the prevention of a mucosal diverticulum by placing external pressure on the mucosa. Prior to the employment of this technique, we had observed mucosal outpouching at the distal esophagus and the level of gastroesophageal junction in a number of patients. This technique seems to have addressed that issue without any negative sequelae. Following pleural closure, the diaphragmatic retractor is removed. The lung is reinflated under direct vision. A 28-Fr straight chest tube is inserted through incision #4 and positioned posteriorly in the pleural space. ON-Q Pain Buster catheters are positioned in a subpleural tunnel extending from the second to the eighth intercostal spaces and the incisions are closed as described in Chapter 19 for video-assisted surgery. The gastroscope is used to confirm the appropriate position of the nasogastric tube. The patient is extubated in the operating room. Postoperatively, we routinely obtain an upper GI contrast study with water-soluble contrast to rule out mucosal perforation and to confirm completeness of distal esophageal myotomy. With a satisfactory study, a soft diet is started, the chest tube is removed, and most patients are discharged on the second postoperative day.

ROBOTIC LAPAROSCOPIC BELSEY MARK IV FUNDOPLASTY

Gastroesophageal reflux disease is the most common disease of human, affecting approximately 20 percent of Americans (70). Normal individuals experience some GERD on a regular basis (71,72). Pathologic reflux results in injury to the esophagus and the upper aerodigestive tract. GERD has been shown to be a strong risk factor for esophageal carcinoma (73). Curiously, esophageal adenocarcinoma has nearly quadrupled in frequency in the United States since the 1980s, when oral and acid medications have had their greatest use (74,75). GERD classically presents as heartburn and regurgitation. In addition to the classic presentation, GERD can present with a number of atypical symptoms that stem from exposure of the upper aerodigestive tract to gastric contents (76).

This procedure combines the excellent visualization and maneuverability of the da Vinci robot for the dissection and identification of hiatal structures, with the speed and ease of laparoscopic suturing techniques.

The procedure has two parts: (1) robotic dissection and exposure, (2) conventional laparoscopic crural closure and fundoplasty.

Robotic Dissection and Exposure

The patient is placed in the lithotomy position. The surgeon stands between the legs. Two laparoscopic insufflators are used. We prefer to use the Visiport instrument (US Surgical Corp.) for initial port entry into the peritoneum. Port #1 (camera port) is placed inferior to the umbilicus. A small curvilinear incision is made under the umbilicus. A Kocker clamp is used to grasp the frenulum of the umbilicus and to elevate the anterior abdominal wall. Upward traction on the clamp provides a countertraction, which is necessary for safe peritoneal entry under video endoscopic guidance using the Visiport instrument. Pneumoperitoneum is created using CO_2 gas to a maximum pressure of 15 mmHg. The table is placed in a steep reverse Trendelenburg position. Under direct video endoscopic guidance, four other ports are placed. We prefer to use the 10–12 Visiport trocar (US Surgical Corp.) for all ports. These ports do not require reducer caps. The capless design of these ports enables rapid instrument change without loss of pneumoperitoneum. A 0-degree Olympus EndoEYE video endoscope is introduced through port #1. Port #2 is placed in the right paraumbilical region at the right mammary line. Port #3 is placed in the left paraumbilical region in the left mammary line. An endoscopic paddle retractor is introduced through port #2 and used to place downward traction on the gastroesophageal junction and to expose the phrenoesophageal ligament. Using the video endoscope, the left and right limbs of the right crus are identified. Port #4 is placed in the subcostal region halfway between the umbilicus and the xiphoid just to the left of the midline. This port is aligned with the RL of the right crus of the diaphragm. Port #5 is placed in the subcostal region two finger breaths to the left and caudad to port #4. Port #5 is aligned with the LL of the right crus of the diaphragm. A Diamond-Flex retractor (Snowden Pencer, Tucker, GA) is placed through port #5 and fixed to the table using a self-retaining system (Mediflex). The laparoscopic insufflator is disconnected from port #1 and attached to port #4. A second insufflator is attached to port #5. The use of two high-flow insufflators facilitates rapid extracorporeal knot placement while preserving pneumoperitoneum and exposure of the esophageal hiatus.

At this point the da Vinci robot is brought in over the patient's head. The head of the table is rotated 30 degrees away from the anesthesia machine on its longitudinal axis to facilitate docking of the robot. A 30-degree down-viewing robotic binocular camera is introduced through port #1. The right robotic arm with a hook cautery instrument is introduced through incision #5. The left robotic arm with a Debakey grasper instrument is introduced through port #3. The entire dissection uses electrocautery and meticulous hemostasis. Port #5 is used to vent smoke out of the peritoneal cavity. Blood and fluid accumulate in the hiatus, are difficult to evacuate, and tend to discolor the structures. We avoid using a suction irrigator system. The right crural arch is identified. The phrenoesophageal ligament is divided. The hepatogastric omentum is divided and the caudate lobe of the liver is identified. This maneuver necessitates division of the hepatic branch of the anterior vagal nerve and a small arterial branch of the left gastric artery. This vessel is to be distinguished from a large aberrant left hepatic artery, which arises from the left gastric artery in 25 percent of patients. In these patients the hepatic artery should be avoided and dissection should be confined to the superior aspect of the artery. At this point the RL of the right crus is visualized. The lateral and medial borders of the RL are identified. This maneuver facilitates the identification of the esophagus. Lateral traction is placed on the esophagus. The fatty tissue overlying the RL is excised and the RL is followed inferiorly to its junction with the LL of the right crus. Next the dissection of the RL is carried superiorly onto the crural arch and around to the LL of the right crus. The LL is dissected inferiorly by taking down the angle of His and gastric fundal attachments. Medial traction moves the esophagus medially and facilitates the exposure of the entire crural sling. *Importantly, encirclement of the esophagus or division of the short gastric vessels is not required.*

After complete dissection of the esophageal hiatus, the robot is undocked. The remainder of the procedure is accomplished by conventional laparoscopy.

Conventional Laparoscopic Crural Closure and Fundoplasty

Posterior Crural Closure

A 30-degree Olympus EndoEYE video endoscope is introduced through port #1. Posterior crural closure is accomplished by reapproximating the RL and LL with three sutures. We prefer the Endostitch instrument (Auto Suture) with 0 Ethibond suture. The Endostitch instrument is an ideal suturing device for laparoscopy as it facilitates one-handed suturing thereby allowing the surgeon's left hand to provide appropriate exposure. Furthermore, when approximating the RL and LL of the right crus posterior, the straight needle of the Endostitch instrument passes in a tangential plain to the anterior aspect of the aorta and carries a lower risk of inadvertent aortic injury, which results from deep suture placement. Conversely, the curved needle used with a laparoscopic needle driver can pass deeper than intended and can engage the anterior wall of the aorta.

The grasper in the surgeon's left hand is placed on the medial aspect of the esophagus and used to retract the esophagus lateral and to the left. The maneuver exposes the "V"-shaped posterior junction of the RL and LL of the right crus. A 1 cm^2 absorbable pledget cut from Vicryl mesh (Ethicon, Inc.) is passed through port #4. The end stitch with 0 Ethibond is passed through port #5. Intracorporeally the pledget is loaded onto the needle. The needle is passed through LL and RL. Next intracorporeally the needle is passed through a second Vicryl pledget, which is introduced with the grasper in the surgeon's left hand. The Endostitch carrying the suture is withdrawn out of the entry port #5 and extracorporeal knots are placed using a knot pusher. The suture is cut above the knot. This technique is repeated for all the posterior crural sutures.

Anterior Crural Closure

In a similar manner to the posterior crural closure, 0 Etibond sutures on the Endostitch instrument with intracorporeally loaded pledgets of Vicryl mesh are used to reap proximate the anterior portion of the crural arch. This step represents a modification of the original Belsey Mark IV technique. However, in our experience, the anterior crural closure allows for the formation of an acute angle at the gastroesophageal junction and recreates one of the important features of the normal antireflux barrier. The sutures are passed through port #5, a Vicryl pledget is loaded on the suture intracorporeally, and the suture is passed through the RL and LL of the crural arch. A second Vicryl pledget is loaded intracorporeally onto the suture and the suture is tied using extracorporeal technique as outlined previously. Usually two or three interiorly placed sutures are required. The crural closure is sized properly based on the passage of a 60-Fr bougie. After an extensive number of cases, we have determined that the ability to pass a grasper freely between the esophagus and the anterior crural closure reapproximates the sizing of the crural closure, which is achieved with the bougie. Presently we prefer this technique for crural sizing. Following crural closure, the Belsey fundoplasty is performed.

Belsey Fundoplasty

The anterior intussesption of the esophagus into the stomach is accomplished for the anterior 270 degrees (from RL to LL of the right crus) of the 360-degree circumference of the esophagogastrectomy junction. The esophagogastrectomy fat pad is removed. The esophagus is marked 2 cm above the esophagogastric junction at the medial border of the left vagus nerve (E1), the lateral border of the right vagus nerve (E3), and half way in-between (E2). The stomach is marked 2 cm below the gastroesophageal junction at the greater curvature (G1), the lesser curvature (G3), and at a point half way between G1 and G3 (G2). The Endostitch instrument with 00 Ethibond is introduced through port #5. The first Belsey suture (E1-G1, greater curve) passes in mattress fashion from G1 to E1 back to G1. A Vicryl pledget is introduced with a grasper through port #4. The pledget is loaded onto the Endostitch intracorporeally before and after it is passed through E1. Placement of absorbable pledget on the two sides of the esophageal "bite" decreases the risk of tears of the esophageal muscle. Consequently the order of suture placement is (G1-pledget-E1-pledget-G1). The suture is withdrawn through port #5. Metal clips are placed on the free ends of the suture to facilitate identification and recovery of the suture at a later point. The untied suture is reintroduced through port #5 and deposited in the left upper quadrant away from the gastroesophageal junction. This suture is tied a later time. Placing a tie on the "G1-E1" suture at this time will obscure the precise placement of "E2-G2" and "E3-G3" sutures. A second Belsey suture ("E3-G3," lesser curve) is passed in a similar manner from G3 to E3 back to G3, withdrawn through port #5, tagged with metal clips, and deposited in the right upper quadrant away from the gastroesophageal junction. This suture will be tied a later time. The third Belsey suture ("E2-G2," midpoint) is introduced in the same manner from G2 to E2 back to G2. This suture is withdrawn from port #5 and tied using a knot-pusher and extracorporeal knots. Next the "E1-G1" suture is withdrawn out of port #5 and tied. Finally the "E3-G3" suture is withdrawn out of port #5 and tied.

Placement of the first row of mattressed Belsey sutures results in the intussusception of the esophagus into the stomach by 2 cm for 270 degrees.

Next three mattressed sutures of 00 Ethibond are placed from the stomach at G1, G2, and G3 onto the anterior crural closure at LL, midpoint of the crural arch, and RL of the right crus, respectively. This second row of sutures places the entire fundoplast under the diaphragm. An Endostitch instrument with 00 Ethibond is introduced through port #5. The suture is passed into the stomach just below G1 and through the RL of the right crus. The suture is withdrawn from port #5 and tied by extracorporeal technique. A second 00 Ethibond suture is placed on the stomach just below G2, passed through the midpoint of the anterior crural closure and tied. A third 00 Ethibond suture is passed just below G3, passed through the LL of the right crus of the diaphragm and tied. The trocar sites are closed using an EXIT instrument and 0 Vicryl (Ethicon Endo-Surgery). Subcutaneous tissues are closed with 00 Vicryl and the skin is closed with staples.

References

1. Emslie RG: Perspectives in the Development of Esophageal Surgery. In Jamieson GG (Ed): *Surgery of the Esophagus*. Melbourne: Churchill Livingstone, 1988, pp. 3–8.
2. Law SYK, Wong J: Management of Squamous Cell Carcinoma of the Esophagus. In Pearson FG, et al. (Ed): *Esophageal Surgery*. Melbourne: Churchill Livingston, 2002, pp. 705–724.
3. Czerny V: Neue Operationen. *Zentralbl Chir* 4: 433, 1877.
4. Billroth T: Uber die Resektion des Oesophagus. *Arch Klin Chir* 13: 65, 1871.
5. Lewis I: The Surgical Treatment of Carcinoma of the Esophagus: With Special Reference to a New Operation for Growths of the Middle Third. *Br J Surg* 34: 18, 1946.
6. Torek F: The First Successful Case of Resection of the Thoracic Portion of the Esophagus for Carcinoma. *Surg Gynecol Obstet* 16: 614, 1913.
7. Kelling G: Osophagoplastik mit Hilfe des Querkolon. *Zentralbl Chir* 38: 1209, 1911.
8. Kirschner MB: Eines neues verfahren der Osophagoplastik. *Arch Klin Chir* 114: 606, 1920.
9. Ohsava T: The Surgery of the Esophagus (in Japanese). *J Jpn Surg Soc* 34: 1518, 1933.
10. Marshall SF: Carcinoma of the Esophagus: Successful Resection of Lower End of Esophagus with Reestablishment of the Esophageal Gastric Continuity. *Surg Clin North Am* 18: 643, 1938.
11. Adams W, Phemister DB: Carcinoma of the Lower Thoracic Esophagus: Report of a Successful Resection and Esophagogastrostomy. *J Thorac Surg* 7: 621, 1938.
12. Churchill ED, Sweet RH: Transthoracic Resection of Tumors of the Stomach and Esophagus. *Ann Surg* 115: 897, 1942.
13. McKeown KC: Trends in Esophageal Resection for Carcinoma, with Special Reference to Total Esophagectomy. *Ann R Coll Surg Engl* 51: 213, 1972.
14. Denk W: Zur Radikaloperation des Osophaguskarzinomen. *Zentralbl Chir* 40: 1065, 1913.
15. Turner GG: Excision of Thoracic Esophagus for Carcinoma with Construction of Extrathoracic Gullet. *Lancet* 2: 1315, 1933.
16. Ong GB, Lee TC: Pharyngogastric Anastomosis after Esophagopharyngectomy for Carcinoma of the Hypopharynx and Cervical Esophagus. *Br J Surg* 48: 193, 1960.
17. LeQuesne LP, Ranger D: Pharyngolaryngectomy with Immediate Pharyngogastric Anastomosis. *Br J Surg* 53: 105, 1966.
18. Orringer MB, Sloan H: Esophagectomy without Thoracotomy. *J Thorac Cardiovasc Surg* 76: 643, 1978.
19. Kirby TJ, Rice TW: The Epidemiology of Esophageal Carcinoma: The Changing Face of the Disease. *Chest* 4: 217–225, 1994.
20. Henteleff H, Casson AG: Epidemiology of Malignant Neoplasms. In Pearson FG (Ed): *Esophageal Surgery*. Philadelphia: Churchill Livingston, 2002, pp. 668–676.
21. Blot WJ, Fraumeni JF: Trends in Esophageal Cancer Mortality among US Blacks and Whites. *Am J Public Health* 77: 296, 1987.
22. Daly JM, Karnell LH, Menck HR: National Cancer Database Report on Esophageal Carcinoma. *Cancer* 78: 1820, 1996.
23. Devesa SS, Blot WJ, Fraumeni JF: Changing Patterns in the Incidence of Esophageal and Gastric Carcinoma in the United States. *Cancer* 83: 2049, 1998.
24. Portale G, Hagen JA, Peters JH, et al: Modern Five-Year Survival of Resectable Esophageal Adenocarcinoma: Single Institution Experience with 263 Patients. *J Am Coll Surg* 2006; 202: 588–596.
25. Cameron AJ, Ott BJ, Payne WS: The Incidence of Adenocarcinoma in Columnar-Lined (Barrett's) Esophagus. *N Engl J Med* 313: 856, 1985.
26. Casson AG, Mukhopadhyay T, Cleary KR, et al: P53 Gene Mutations in Barrett's Epithelium and Esophageal Cancer. *Cancer Res* 51: 4495, 1991.
27. Earlam R, Cunha-Melo JR: Esophageal Squamous Cell Carcinoma: I – A Critical Review of Surgery. *Br J Surg* 67: 381, 1980.
28. Muller JM, Erasmi H, Stelzner M, et al: Surgical Therapy of Esophageal Carcinoma. *Br J Surg* 77: 845, 1990.
29. Patti MG, Costantini M, Godwin DH, et al: A Hospital's Annual Rate of Esophagectomy Influences the Operative Mortality Rates. *J Gastrointest Surg* 2: 186, 1998.
30. Kelsen D, Hilaris B, Coonley C, et al: Cisplatin, Vindesine, and Bleomycin Chemotherapy of Local,

Regional, and Advanced Esophageal Carcinoma. *Am J Med* 75: 645–652, 1983.

31. Kelsen DP, Minsky B, Smith M, et al: Preoperative Therapy for Esophageal Cancer: A Randomized Comparison of Chemotherapy Versus Radiation Therapy. *J Clin Oncol* 8: 1352–1361, 1990.
32. Roth JA, Pass HI, Flanagan MM, et al: Randomized Clinical Trial of Preoperative and Postoperative Adjuvant Chemotherapy with Cisplatin, Vindesine, and Bleomycin for Carcinoma of the Esophagus. *J Thorac Cardiovasc Surg* 96: 242–248, 1988.
33. Schlag P, Herrmann R, Raeth V, et al: Preoperative Chemotherapy in Esophageal Cancer: A Phase II Study. *Acta Oncologica* 27: 811–814, 1988.
34. Kelsen DP, Ginsberg R, Pajak TF, et al: Chemotherapy Followed by Surgery Compared to Surgery Alone for Localized Esophageal Cancer. *New Engl J Med* 339: 1979–1984, 1998.
35. Al-Sarraf M, Martz K, Herskovic A, et al: Superiority of Chemoradiotherapy (CT-RT) Versus Radiotherapy (RT) in Patients with Esophageal Cancer. Final Report of an Intergroup Randomized and Confirmed Study. *Proceedings of the American Society of Clinical Oncology*, Vol. 15, 1996, p. 206.
36. Herskovic A, Martz K, Al-Sarraf M, et al: Combined Chemotherapy and Radiotherapy Compared with Radiotherapy Alone in Patients with Cancer of the Esophagus. *N Engl J Med* 326: 1593–1598, 1992.
37. Al-Sarraf M, Martz K, Herskovic A, et al: Progress Report of Combined Chemoradiotherapy Versus Radiotherapy Alone in Patients with Esophageal Cancer: An Intergroup Study. *J Clin Oncol* 15: 277–284, 1997.
38. Yau P, Jamieson GG: Adjuvant and Neoadjuvant Therapy for Cancer of the Esophagus. In Pearson FG, et al. (Ed): *Esophageal Surgery*. Philadelphia: Churchill Livingston, 2002, pp. 748–750.
39. Rice TW, Blackstone EH, Adelstein DJ, et al: N_1 Esophageal Carcinoma: The Importance of Staging and Downstaging. *J Thorac Cardiovasc Surg*: 454–464, 2001.
40. Halvorsen RA, Jr, Thompson WM: CT of Esophageal Neoplasms. *Radiatr Clin North Am* 136: 1051–1056, 1989.
41. Inculet RI, Keller SM, Swyer A: Evaluation of Noninvasive Tests for the Preoperative Staging of Carcinoma of the Esophagus. *Ann Thorac Surg* 40: 561–565, 1985.
42. Tio TL, Cohen P, den Hartog Jager FC, et al: Preoperative TNM Classification of Esophageal Carcinoma by Endosonography. *Hepatogastroenterology* 37: 376–381, 1990.
43. Wilkins EW, Jr: Classic Left Thoracoabdominal Approach. In Pearson FG (Ed): *Esophageal Surgery*. Philadelphia: Churchill Livingston, 2002, pp. 802–809.
44. Ginsberg RJ: Left Thoracoabdominal Cervical Approach. In Pearson FG (Ed): *Esophageal Surgery*. Philadelphia: Churchill Livingston, 2002, pp. 809–813.
45. Park BJ, Ginsberg RJ: Left Transthoracic Esophagectomy. In Pearson FG (Ed): *Esophageal Surgery*. Philadelphia: Churchill Livingston, 2002, pp. 813–818.
46. Pearson FG: Synchronous Combined Abdomino-Thoraco-Cervical Esophagectomy. In Pearson FG (Ed): *Esophageal Surgery*. Philadelphia: Churchill Livingston, 2002, pp. 828–834.
47. Bains MS: Transabdominal Esophagogastrectomy. In Pearson FG (Ed): *Esophageal Surgery*. Philadelphia: Churchill Livingston, 2002, pp. 854–859.
48. Orringer MB, Marshall BM, Iannettoni MB: Transhiatal Esophagectomy: Clinical Experience in Refinements. *Ann Surg* 230: 392, 1999.
49. Katariya K, Harvei JC, Pina E, et al: Complications of Transhiatal Esophagectomy. *J Surg Oncol* 57: 157, 1994.
50. Mathisen DJ: Right Thoracoabdominal Approaches. In Pearson FG (Ed): *Esophageal Surgery*. Philadelphia: Churchill Livingston, 2002, pp. 818–828.
51. Mathisen DJ, Grillo HC, Wilkins EW, et al: Transthoracic Esophagectomy: A Safe Approach to Carcinoma of the Esophagus. *Ann Thorac Surg* 45: 137, 1988.
52. Ellis FH, Gibb SP, Watkins E, Jr: Esophagogastrectomy: A Safe, Widely Applicable and Expeditious Form of Palliation for Patients with Carcinoma of the Esophagus and Cardia. *Ann Surg* 198: 531, 1983.
53. Shahian, DM, Neptune WB, Ellis FH, et al: Transthoracic Versus Extrathoracic Esophagectomy: Mortality, Morbidity, and Long-Term Survival. *Ann Thorac Surg* 41: 237, 1986.
54. Gockel I: Surgical Therapy of Esophageal Cancer. *W J Surg Onc*, 2005.
55. Altorki N, Skinner D: Should En Bloc Esophagectomy be the Standard of Care for Esophageal Carcinoma. *Ann Surg* 234: 581–587, 2001.
56. Fihvo EI, Luostarinen ME, Salo JA: Fate of Patients with Adenocarcinoma of the Esophagus and the Esophagogastric Junction: A Population-Based Analysis. *Am J Gastroenterol* 99: 419–424, 2004.
57. Hulscher JB, Van Sandik JW, DeBoer AG: Extended Transthoracic Resection Compared with Limited Transhiatal Resection for Adenocarcinoma of the Esophagus. *N Engl J Med* 21: 1663–1669, 2001.

58. Collard JM, Otte JB, Fiasse R, et al: Skeletonizing En Bloc Esophagectomy for Cancer. *Ann Surg* 234: 25–32, 2001.

59. Swanson SJ, Batirel HF, Bueno R, et al: Transthoracic Esophagectomy with Radical Mediastinal and Abdominal Lymph Node Dissection and Cervical Esophagogastrostomy for Esophageal Carcinoma. *Ann Thorac Surg* 72: 1918–1924, 2001.

60. Dexter SPL, Martin IG, McMahon MJ: Radical Thoracoscopic Esophagectomy for Cancer. *Surg Endosc* 10: 147–151, 1996.

61. Akaishi T, Kaneda I, Higuchi N, et al: Thoracoscopic En Bloc Total Esophagectomy with Vertical Mediastinal Lymphadenectomy. *J Thorac Cardiovasc Surg* 112: 1533–1541, 1996.

62. Luketich JD, Nguyen NT, Schauer PR: Laparoscopic Transhiatal Esophagectomy for Barrett's Esophagus with High-Grade Dysplasia. *J Soc Laparoendosc Surg* 2: 75–77, 1998.

63. DePaula AL, Hashiba K, Ferreira EAB, et al: Transhiatal Approach for Esophagectomy. In Toouli J, et al. (Ed): *Endosurgery*. New York: Churchill Livingston, 1996, pp. 293–299.

64. Luketich JD, Schauer PR, Urso K, et al: Future Directions in Esophageal Cancer. *Chest* 113(1 suppl): 1205–1225, 1998.

65. Shimi S, Nathanson LK, Cushieri A: Laparoscopic Cardiomyotomy for Achalasia. *J R Coll Surg Edinb* 36: 152, 1991.

66. Pelligrini CA, Leichter R, Patti M: Thoracoscopic Esophageal Myotomy in the Treatment of Achlasia. *Ann Thorac Surg* 56: 680–682, 1993.

67. Patti MG, Pelligrini CA, Arcerito M: Caomparison of Medical and Minimally Invasive Surgical Therapy for Primary Esophageal Motility Disorders. *Arch Surg* 130: 609–616, 1995.

68. Patti MG, Pelligrini CA, Horgan S: Minimally Invasive Surgery for Achalasia. *Ann Surg* 230: 587, 1999.

69. Finley RJ, Clifton JC, Stewart KC, et al.: Laparoscopic Heller Myotomy for Achalasia: A Clinical and Scintigraphic Swallowing Followup. *Can J Surg* 42(suppl): 25, 1999.

69. Stewart KC, Finley RJ, Clifton JC, et al.: Thoracoscopic Versus Laparoscopic Modified Heller Myotomy for Achalasia: Efficacy and Safety in 87 Patients. *J Am Coll Surg* 189: 164–170, 1999.

70. Locke GR, Talley NJ, Felts SL, et al.: Prevalence and Clinical Spectrum of Gastroesophageal Reflux Disease: A Population-Based Study in Olmsted County, Minnesota. *Gastroenterology* 112: 1448–1450, 1997.

71. Hiebert CA: Surgical Management of Esophageal Reflux and Hiatal Hernia. *Ann Thorac Surg* 52: 159–60, 1991.

72. DeMeester TR, Wang CI, Weraly JA, et al.: Technique, Indications and Clinical Use of 24-Hour pH Monitoring. *J Thorac Cardiovasc Surg* 79: 656, 1980.

73. Souba WW: Links in the Chain: Gastroesophageal Reflux Disease, Barrett's Esophagus, Dysphasia, and Carcinoma. *Contemporary Surg* 56: 57–58, 2000.

74. Richter JE: Chest Pain and Gastroesophageal Reflux Disease. *J Clin Gastroenterol* 30: S39–S41, 2000.

75. Devesa SS, Blot WJ, Fraumeni JF Jr: Changing Patterns in the Incidence of Esophageal and Gastric Carcinoma in the United states. *Cancer* 15: 2049-2053, 1998.

76. Ormseth EJ, Wong RKH: Reflux Laryngitis: Path Physiology, Diagnosis and Management. *Am J Gastroenterology* 94: 2812–2817, 1999.

Chapter 13

Transoral Robotic Surgery

Applications in the Management of Benign and Malignant Diseases of the Pharynx

Jan Akervall and Paul Hoff

Introduction

Transoral minimal invasive surgery for benign or malignant conditions has dramatically changed the plan field for head and neck surgery. What used to be lengthy, complicated procedures, often requiring two teams (resecting and reconstructing), with often poor functional outcome, has over the last 5 years changed into well-tolerated, fast, and functionally superior treatments with improved outcomes. In this chapter, we will describe the paradigm shift that transoral minimal surgery, especially using robotic techniques, has had on how we look at treatment options. In the case of benign conditions, e.g., obstructive sleep apnea (OSA), robotic base-of-tongue (BOT) resections challenge the standard of care – continuous positive airway pressure (CPAP); and in case of malignant conditions, robotic and other transoral procedures are challenging concomitant chemoradiation, which has been the dominant therapy for locoregionally advanced head and neck cancers (HNCs) over the last decade. We will also discuss anesthesia-related concerns, such as laser vs. standard endotracheal (ET) tubes, nasal vs. oral intubation, and extubation vs. tracheostomy.

Transoral Robotic Surgery for OSA

Obstructive sleep apnea is characterized by intermittent episodes of complete (apnea) or partial (hypopnea) airway obstruction. The American Academy of Sleep Medicine defines OSA based on the apnea–hypopnea index (AHI), which is a combination of the number of apneic and hypopneic episodes that occur in 1 hour as determined during polysomnography. Patients are categorized as mild (5–15), moderate (16–30), and severe (>30). Morbidity and mortality increase as the degree of OSA increases above 15 events per hour (1). Quality-of-life measures are also affected by OSA as demonstrated by the Functional Outcomes of Sleepiness Questionnaire (FOSQ) (2).

OSA affects patients of all age groups, but reaches its peak in middle age and beyond. This condition has been linked to cardiovascular disease, hypertension, cognitive decline, sexual dysfunction, diabetes, obesity, and many other morbid conditions. The prevalence of adult patients demonstrating daytime symptoms and known OSA is 2 percent of women and 4 percent of men (3). The prevalence of OSA increases to 24 percent of men and 9 percent of women in those who demonstrate obstructive breathing without daytime symptoms. Unfortunately, it is generally estimated that 80–90 percent of adults remain undiagnosed in the population.

The gold standard treatment for OSA is CPAP, first introduced in the 1980s. Intolerance of CPAP is high and compliance is variable with an overall compliance rate of less than 50 percent (4). Even those patients who do use CPAP successfully may not use it long enough to gain maximal effect.

Success in the surgical literature is defined as a reduction in AHI of 50 percent and an AHI less than 20. Stuck and Maurer describe the adjusted AHI, which accounts for both the time patients wear CPAP during the night compared to ideal (6 hours) (5). The adjusted AHI success rate with CPAP is similar to published surgical reports. With the advent of multilevel surgery as well as the new Inspire hypoglossal nerve stimulator (Inspire Medical Systems, Maple Grove, MN), surgical treatment of properly selected patients is reaching equivalence with the "gold standard" CPAP.

The surgical treatment of OSA dates back to Fujita's introduction of the uvulopalatopharyngoplasty (UPPP). At the time of his publication, Fujita recognized the importance of multilevel obstruction including the BOT (6). Over the past 30 years, a number of techniques have been introduced to address BOT obstruction, including CO_2 laser resection, radiofrequency ablation, suture suspension

(7), skeletal framework surgery, and Coblation (ArthroCare, Austin, TX). Success has been modest and the gold standard surgical technique remains bimaxillary advancement with a success rate greater than 80 percent in experienced hands (8). For the morbidly obese patient, weight loss and bariatric surgery are recommended and are highly effective (9).

In 1991, Croft and Pringle introduced drug-induced sedated endoscopy (DISE). This technique has gained wide acceptance in Europe and is rapidly gaining popularity in North America as surgeons have recognized its utility in identifying both sites of obstruction and planning of site-specific surgery (10,11). DISE is performed with the patient supine, awake, and sedated in the operating room with both the transoral robotic surgery (TORS) surgeon and an anesthesiologist.

The application of TORS for the treatment of OSA was introduced by Vicini et al. in 2010 (12). TORS was recognized as a unique tool offering the capability to safely and effectively access the BOT in patients with retrolingual obstruction. TORS for BOT evolved from the very effective but morbid transcervical BOT reduction with hyoepiglottoplasty (TBRHE) procedure (13). TBRHE provides excellent exposure as well as the ability to remove a large volume of obstructing tissue (up to 50 ml) as well as a success rate of 80 percent. The morbidity associated with this procedure – including tracheostomy, feeding tube, tongue weakness, and fistula – has limited acceptance by both patients and surgeons. Vicini recognized the capability of TORS to replicate the best features of TBRHE including wide exposure as well as the ability to safely resect large volumes of tissue through a transoral approach, thereby significantly limiting morbidity. TORS for OSA has rapidly gained acceptance among sleep surgeons as a part of a multilevel approach in highly selected patients.

Since the first publication of TORS for OSA in 2009, numerous publications representing over 800 patients have been studied. In 2014, the FDA gave its approval for removal of benign tissue from the BOT, but stopped short of approving TORS for the clinical indication of OSA. A detailed description of patient selection as well as outcomes will be discussed in the section on benign TORS outcomes.

Minimally Invasive HNC Surgery

Since the VA trial (14), the EORTC (15), and RTOG 91-11 (16) studies, primary concomitant chemoradiation has been the main treatment for HNC, especially in the anatomic subsites of oropharynx, pharynx, and larynx. Prior to that era, open surgery using a transcervical approach to the pharynx or via a mandibular swing was the predominant preliminary therapy followed by adjuvant radiation, but that changed with these three randomized trials that all compared chemotherapeutic and radiation protocols with traditional open surgery followed by radiation. The studies showed similar outcome with regard to overall survival but better results with regard to organ preservation. However, in none of these studies, minimal invasive surgery was offered to patients, which is the surgical equivalent to organ preservation.

However, open approaches to HNCs, followed by reconstructive surgery using regional flaps, e.g., pectoralis major and more lately free tissue transfer, predominantly radial forearm flaps, carry significant downsides. Some include extended operating room time, necessity for large multidisciplinary teams, slow postoperative recovery, high risk for tracheostomy and chronic PEG tube dependency, long rehabilitation, and often poor functional outcome. Due to these shortcomings, minimal invasive head and neck surgery has developed, which is faster and easier for the patient and the surgeon, with improved rehabilitation of swallowing and speech functions. Traditional head and neck surgeons have argued that margins are compromised with minimal invasive surgery and that it is harder to locally control the disease. However, outcomes data now clearly show that that is not the case. Rich et al. showed that transoral laser microsurgery (TLM) with or without adjuvant therapy offers 94 and 88 percent 2- and 5-year survival, respectively, for stage III and IV tumors of the oropharynx (17).

TLM or TORS has now developed into what looks like a paradigm shift in head and neck surgery. Every progressive head and neck program in the country is now adding TLM or TORS to their repertoire. The transition has taken decades though; when Professor Wolfgang Steiner, Göttingen, Germany, first presented his outcomes data from a large series of patients treated with TLM, he was heavily criticized for compromising basic surgical principles, e.g., cutting through the tumor to get it out through the endoscope. However, his long-term survival results were the same or better than results from traditional open surgical resections (18), and for everyone who watched him operate and saw his patients start eating the first postoperative day, the future choice of surgical technique was obvious. TLM was slow to gain ground due to the steep learning curve. To orient yourself through a long and narrow endoscope is hard, and to remove a large tumor from a tight space can certainly be a challenge, so the more intuitive robotic approach is what has sparked the interest significantly.

The CO_2 laser was introduced for larynx in the 1970s, and Steiner, as mentioned above, took the technique to the next level in the 1980s and 1990s with regard to oropharynx and pharynx. The minimal thermal trauma, resulting in less swelling and faster post-operative recovery and more precise dissections, has taken head and neck surgery in a new direction. TORS uses mainly bovie, which has more thermal impact, but the transoral approach still results in fewer free flaps, shorter hospital stay, less need for feeding tubes, fewer tracheostomies, and better functional outcomes. Weinstein and O'Malley introduced TORS, and the technique has given surgeons who never jumped on the endoscopic train an option to get a shortcut to minimally invasive surgery. TORS uses a wide-angle HD camera, and the improved overview of the surgical field facilitates the orientation.

For both TORS and TLM, airway management is a major concern. Since TORS utilizes monopolar cautery (bovie) for resection, a regular ET tube (oral or nasal) is used, but for TLM an oral laser tube (normally a size 6 metal laser tube) is preferred. A regular usage of ET tube is convenient since these patients often are left intubated overnight in the surgical intensive care unit (SICU), but in the case of using a laser tube for TLM, the situation is different. The laser tube is not appreciated for overnight intubation and should be switched out for a regular ET tube when the resection is completed. This can be done using the GlideScope (Verathon, Seattle, WA) or a Cook airway exchange catheter.

The discussion has intensified now that we see more and more HPV-related squamous cell HNC in younger patients without smoking and drinking history. These patients have much improved prognosis (85–90 percent 5-year survival vs. 65 percent as was the case in RTOG 91-11) and do better during treatment since their performance status is much higher than traditional HNC patients. With better prognosis comes the interesting dilemma of possibly scaling back on the aggressiveness of treatment. Surgery followed by radiation alone is back in the discussion and is in many institutions challenging concomitant chemoradiation.

Robotic Setup

Whether transoral surgical techniques are applied to benign or malignant conditions, the setup and general surgical principles are the same. In this section, we will discuss these principles and compare the results to those from traditional surgical techniques.

Trans-oral Robotic Surgery requires organization and efficiency from a multispecialty team. The team includes the surgeon, anesthesiologist, a surgical technician who has dedicated time to train and scrub robotic cases, and a consistent bedside assistant familiar with TORS. There is a basic instrument setup that is standard for TORS, and familiarity of the team with this set is essential. The retractor typically used for OSA cases is the Davis Meyer mouth gag with suction ports (Figure 13.1), although the McGyver, Crow-Davis, Dingman, and Feyh-Kastenbauer (F-K) retractor can also be used.

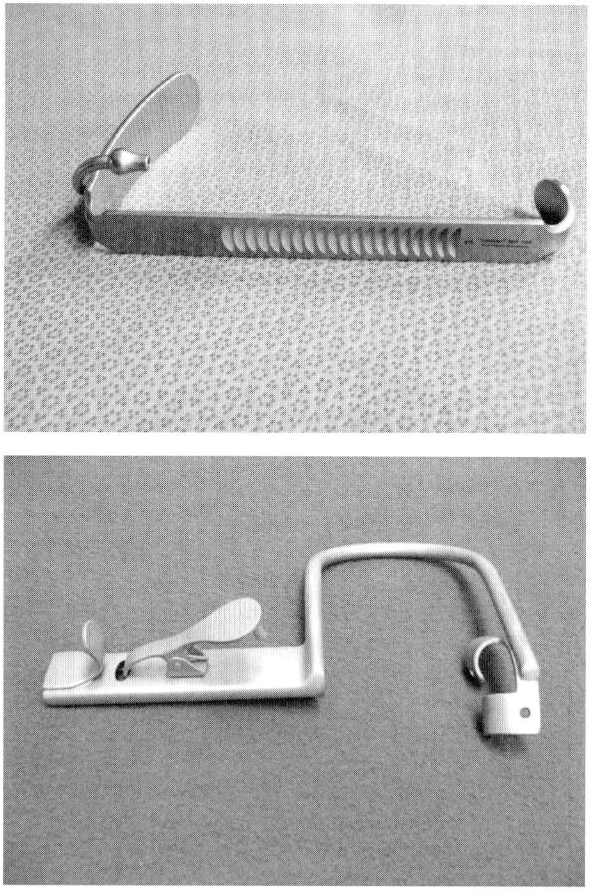

Figure 13.1 Davis Meyer mouth gag with tongue blade that includes a suction channel.

The basic operating room configuration is shown in Figure 13.2a and b. Note that the bed is rotated 180 degrees away from the anesthesiologist. The Maryland dissector is the primary instrument used for grasping tissue. The paired robotic arm is used for cutting tissue and can be equipment with either a monopolar cautery or two different laser options: the Revolex LISA laser (Thulium) or the Omniguide CO_2 laser. The configuration of the mouth gag and the arrangement of instruments in the mouth are shown in Figure 13.3a and b.

Perioperative Concerns for the Anesthesiologist for Patients Undergoing Treatment of OSA and HNC with TORS and TLM

TORS for OSA

Candidates for TORS who suffer from OSA are patients who have been diagnosed with moderate to severe OSA and have failed conservative therapy (weight loss and CPAP). A typical patient will be middle-aged with an American Society Anesthesiology (ASA) classification of 2 and a BMI under 30. As part of the clinical exam, the ENT surgeon will have assessed the airway and selected patients with a Malampati score of 3 or less without significant retrognathia.

The preoperative surgical evaluation to determine candidacy for TORS multilevel surgery for OSA includes a DISE. DISE is performed with the patient under supervised sedation in the operating theater with the use of Propofol administered by either target-controlled infusion (19) or manual infusion (20). In most centers, bispectral analysis (BIS; Covidien, Boulder, CO) at a level between 50 and 60 is used to assist the surgeon attain a proper level of sedation. Airway observations are performed using a flexible video nasopharyngoscope with the patient both awake and sedated in supine position (Figure 13.4). Supplemental oxygen may be administered as needed during the procedure, and resuscitative equipment should always be available.

If a patient is found to be a suitable candidate for multilevel surgery for OSA, the patient may undergo TORS immediately or at a later date depending on the surgeon's preference. In most cases, patients undergoing TORS for OSA undergo nasal intubation; if nasal procedures such as septolasty and turbinate reduction are to performed, this should be done at the time of DISE in which case the patient can immediately either undergo laryngeal mask airway (LMA) or ET intubation to safely complete the nasal surgery.

The anesthesia concerns unique to TORS for OSA include nasal intubation, airway fire, and a 180-degree turn of the patient away from anesthesia. To perform TORS efficiently, the surgeon will often request transnasal intubation. The nasal RAE tube is anchored over the forehead with tape. Protective eye shield is mandatory. With the airway secure, the bed is then rotated 180 degrees away from the anesthesiologist to allow for docking of the robot. During the preinduction and preincision time out, it is important to affirm that the risk of fire is real and that FiO_2 should be kept below 30 percent throughout the case; if the patient requires additional oxygen, this should be communicated to the surgeon who will discontinue the use of electrocautery until oxygen requirements allow for resumption of the procedure. Patients routinely receive perioperative steroids (Decadron 8–10 mg) and antibiotics (Unasyn or Clindamycin).

At the completion of the procedure, the bed is rotated back to the anesthesiologist for planned extubation in the operating room. If there is concern for airway swelling due to prolonged surgery time or if there has been excessive bleeding, the patients may remain intubated overnight and observed in the intensive care unit. Reintubation is very uncommon (<1 percent). Rarely is unplanned tracheostomy necessary in these patients and is usually due to individual patient concerns (cardiac disease, obesity, severe OSA).

Postoperative care is focused primarily on analgesia and airway maintenance. Patients have considerable pain for up to 2 weeks following surgery. Patients who are able to tolerate CPAP are encouraged to use their device for the first 2 weeks after surgery to counter the effects of edema and narcotics. Because the average length of stay is typically less than 2 days, patients must quickly transition from IV analgesics (Dilaudid) to oral medication (Oxycodone, Acetaminophen, and nonsteroidal antiinflammatory medications). The readmission rate following TORS for OSA can be as high as 15 percent due primarily to dehydration and poor pain control.

TORS and TLM for HNC

The airway concerns for HNC patients are different than for OSA, since these patients may have an

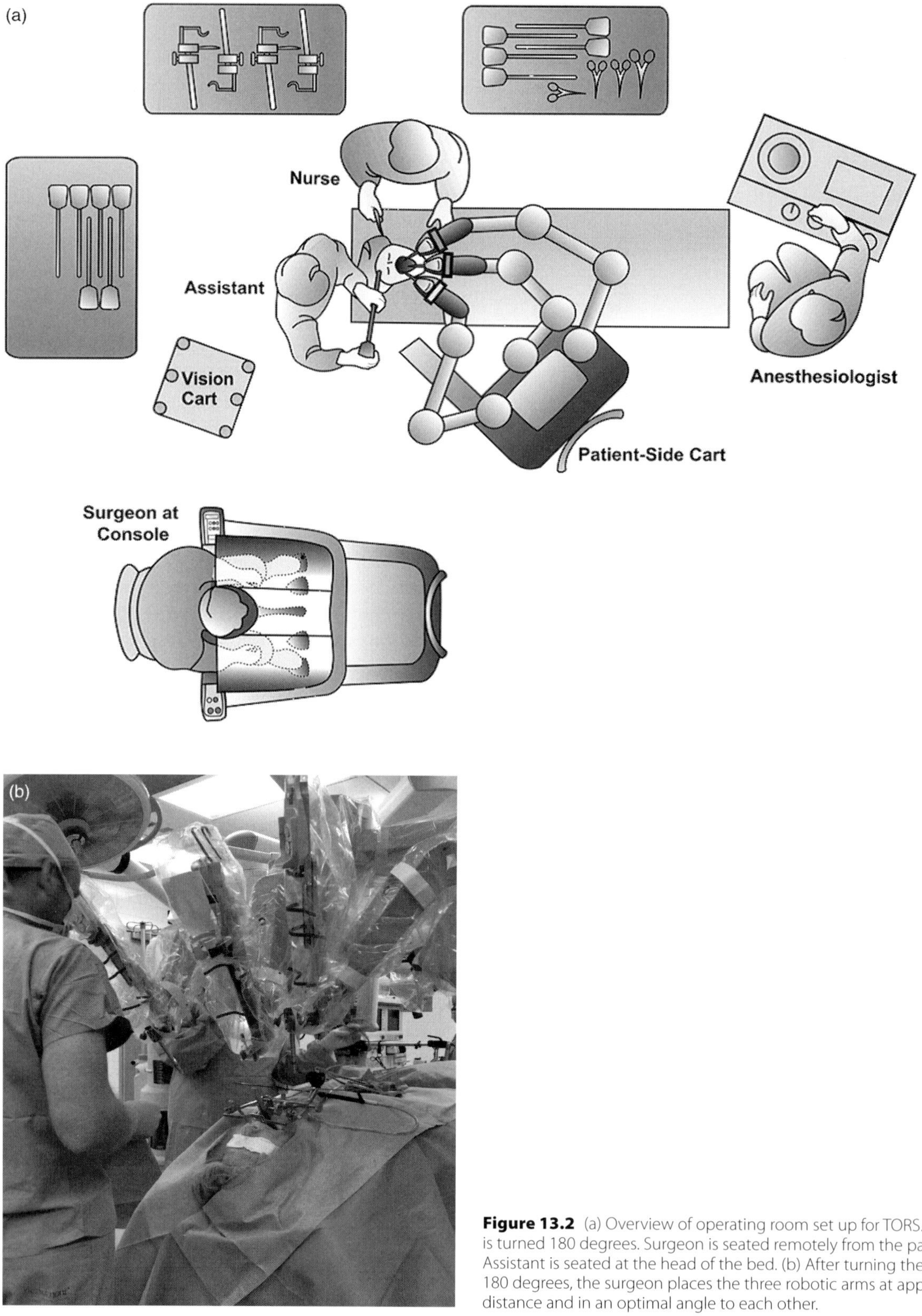

Figure 13.2 (a) Overview of operating room set up for TORS. Table is turned 180 degrees. Surgeon is seated remotely from the patient. Assistant is seated at the head of the bed. (b) After turning the bed 180 degrees, the surgeon places the three robotic arms at appropriate distance and in an optimal angle to each other.

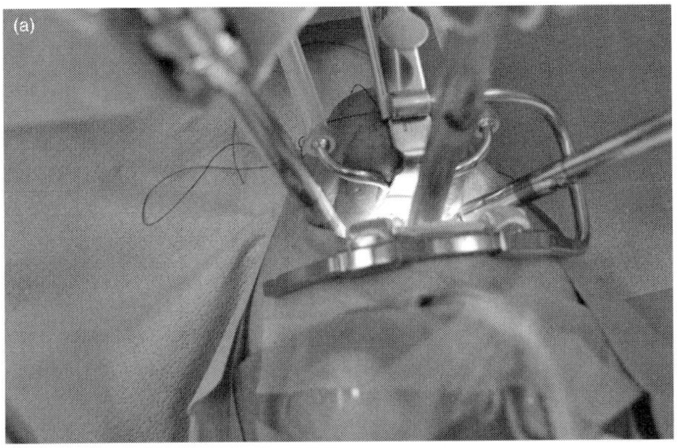

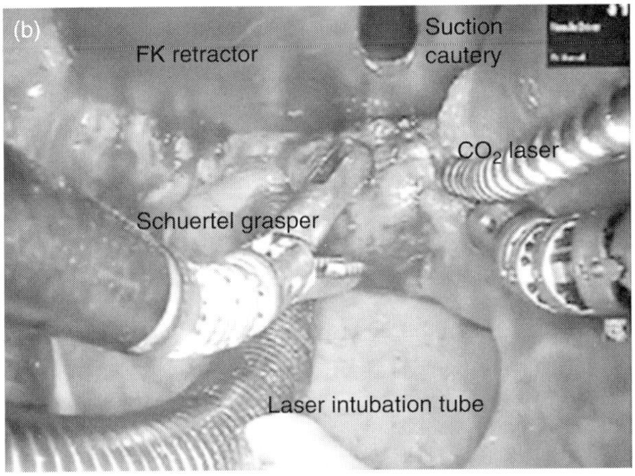

Figure 13.3 (a) Intraoperative view of the TORS instrument configuration for OSA. Nasal intubation is commonly used. Eye shields are mandatory. Instrument cannulas are used to retract the oral commissures. Custom-made mouth guards are used to protect upper and lower incisors. (b) Intraoperative view of the TORS instrument configuration for a BOT resection. An oral size 6 metal laser tube is used, and the CO_2 laser is clipped on to the needle driver.

obstructing mass in their pharynx/larynx, or the exposure may be affected by previous treatment, e.g., radiation. Indication for a wake tracheostomy will be the same whether open or transoral surgical approach is considered. However, if a transoral approach is the method of choice, oral or nasal intubation will be done. For TORS, some surgeons use oral and some nasal RAE tubes, and for TLM, a size 6 metal laser tube. Postoperatively, immediate extubation in the operating room can be considered but – due to the risk for postoperative bleedings, and this is especially the case after deep or lateral resections where the bigger vessels are located, or if there is significant swelling – a conversation between the surgeon and the anesthesiologist should take place to decide if keeping the patient intubated overnight in the SICU is a better option. In the case of TORS, this is straight-forward since the patient already has an appropriately sized ET tube in place, but in the case of TLM, the laser tube needs to be replaced with a regular ET tube. The safest way to do this is by using a GlideScope, and if visualization is good, just pull the laser tube and place a regular properly sized ET tube. If there is swelling or if visualization is limited, a Cook airway exchange catheter can be used. Since it does not fit through a size 6 metal laser tube, it can be introduced into the trachea next to the laser tube, after which the laser tube is removed. Postoperatively, the patient is kept on IV Decadron 6 mg BID, and the following morning a simple cuff leak test should be done to confirm that it is safe to extubate the patient.

Outcome of TORS for OSA

Since its inception in 2006, the application of TORS for benign disease has been dominated by sleep surgeons who recognized the advantage of this technology to address the BOT; this interest is reflected by the breadth of peer-reviewed articles that have appeared in the literature over the past 6 years. The focus of this section will be on outcomes following TORS for the treatment of OSA.

The surgical treatment of OSA can be divided into three groups: skeletal framework surgery, soft tissue surgery, and nerve stimulation. The surgical gold standard remains bimaxillary advancement (MMA) with an overall success rate of 87 percent (8). Unfortunately, MMA is not widely available and many patients are fearful of surgery involving alteration of the mandible and/or maxilla, as well as concerns about cosmesis, malocclusion, and facial numbness.

Patients with OSA who have failed conservative therapy (CPAP) are typically searching for a solution that will both eliminate the need for mechanical assistance and have minimal morbidity. Multilevel surgery addresses these concerns, but does come with significant short-term morbidity including dysphagia, pain, and dysguesia. Fortunately, these symptoms resolve within 1–3 months in most patients.

Since the recognition that OSA is often caused by collapse of the airway at different levels, surgeons have turned to DISE to help determine the appropriate surgery for each patient. DISE should be considered a standard part of the evaluation of patients with OSA, including patients are being considered for multilevel sleep surgery, or TORS, as well as patients with stridor

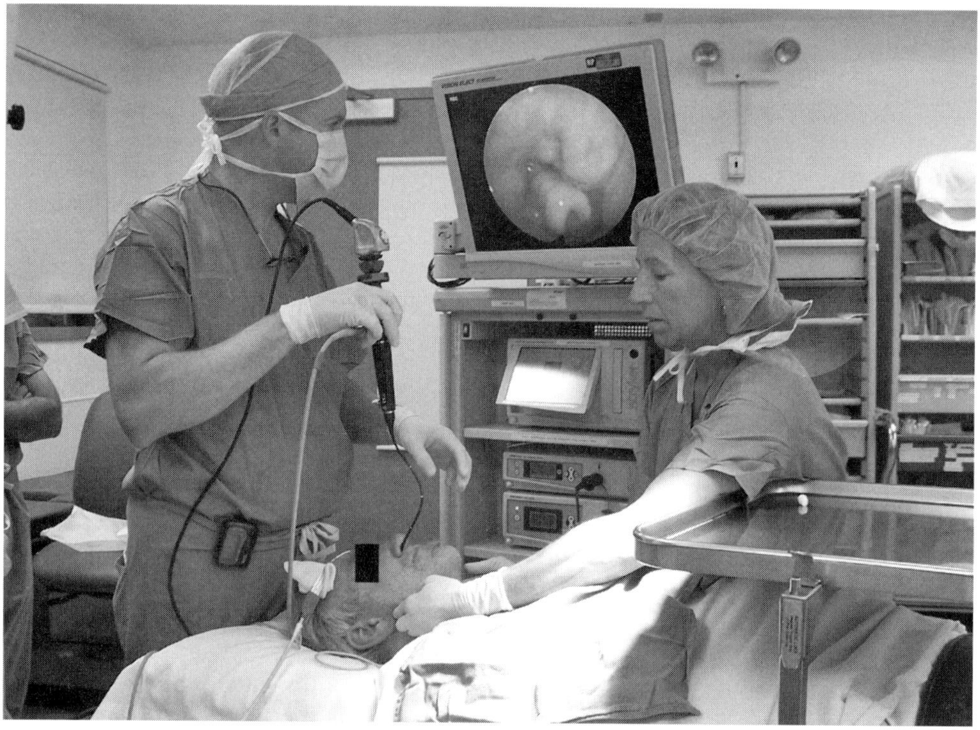

Figure 13.4 Intraoperative setup of DISE. Surgeon stands at the head of the bed, sharing the airway with the anesthesiologist.

and discordant examination (OSA despite small tonsils in a pediatric population).

Several DISE grading systems are available, but the most widely accepted are the VOTE and NOHL (11,12). In 2014, the European Position Paper was published and consensus was reached in all areas except (1) a standardized scoring system and (2) which system should be used by all – systems were found to be too simple or too complex (21). At this time, DISE is a useful tool for establishing a patient's candidacy for surgery and to develop individualized surgical plans; however, in its current state, DISE is it not a predictor of *success*. However, DISE has been found to be helpful in predicting treatment failure, specifically in patients being evaluated for hypoglossal nerve stimulation (22).

The introduction of TORS for OSA occurred in 2010 (12). The first studies were performed as part of a multilevel approach including UPPP, TORS BOT reduction, and tracheostomy. Tracheostomy was performed for patient safety in these early patients. In order to better define the role of BOT reduction in the improvement of both AHI and excess daytime somnolence, Lin et al. (23) studied 12 patients with moderate to severe OSA who underwent isolated BOT reduction. This group of 12 included patients who had failed previous UPPP as well as patients who had no prior surgery. Patients had an average postoperative follow-up of 4 months and both pre- and postoperative AHI (43.9±41 vs. 17.6±16.2) and ESS (13.7±5 vs. 6.4±4.5) improved. The efficacy of TORS BOT resection for OSA had been clearly demonstrated.

In 2014, the combined work of leading TORS sleep surgeons from seven nations was published. In this retrospective cohort of 243 patients, improvements were demonstrated in AHI (43.3 vs. 17.5, $p < 0.001$), lowest O_2 (79.5 vs. 83.9, $p < 0.001$), and ESS (12.5 vs. 5.8, $p < 0.001$). The overall success rate was 67 percent, and 55 percent of patients were able to discontinue CPAP as determined by an AHI <15 without excess daytime somnolence (24).

In 2014, the FDA gave its approval for TORS removal of benign tissue from the BOT using the da Vinci robot (Intuitive Surgical). The procedure and device were found to safe. Postoperative complications were described as major (6.6 percent) and minor (19.3 percent): major complications included bleeding (4.2 percent), dysphagia, and aspiration pneumonia.

Minor complications included dehydration, pain, globus, and dysguesia. Factors correlating with complication included the number of pharyngeal procedures performed and a higher ASA classification (>2). In the United States, FDA approval of TORS for the clinical indication of OSA is pending prospective data; the International Sleep Surgery Society has developed a multicenter collaborative study (ISCORE) with this goal in mind (25).

Surgeons embarking on a comprehensive sleep surgery program are as interested in predictors of success as they are in outcome. Several studies have attempted to improve patient selection. In general, the ideal patient would have a BMI under 30, age under 65, large volume of lingual tonsil tissue, DISE showing no concentric collapse in the velum or oropharynx, hyoid to mandibular plane distance <35 mm, and no prior upper airway surgery (26–28).

One of the main concerns following TORS multilevel surgery is long-term morbidity due to dysphagia that may arise from reshaping of the BOT and, in some cases, epiglottis. Easa et al. (29) performed a retrospective study assessing both short-term and long-term dysphagia. In this study, all 72 patients underwent TORS BOT resection and epiglottoplasty. The average follow-up period was 20±7.1 months and swallowing function was determined by both MDADI and FVSS and NG tube dependence. There was minimal impact on pre- and postoperative MDADI and VFSS although 6 percent demonstrated short term (1 week). NG tube feeds were not required in any patients. There were no long-term swallowing complaints registered in this study. In addition, there was no correlation between the volume of BOT tissue and epiglottis removed and aspiration as demonstrated by VFSS. Easa et al. (29) reported a retrospective study from a single institution where tracheostomy performed with TORS multilevel surgery was standard practice at the time. The role of epiglottis in airway protection cannot be overemphasized. In this patient population with benign disease, the surgeon should be extremely circumspect when considering supraglottoplasty. Improving OSA at the expense of airway protection and a lifetime of dysphagia is not a good trade-off. If supraglottoplasty is being considered, a modification of the supraglottoplasty (V-epiglottoplasty) as described by Magnuson should be considered (unpublished). Alternatively, a staged supraglottoplasty or thryohyoidopexy can be offered to the patient if, after postoperative PSG and DISE, there is demonstrated persistent supraglottic collapse and OSA.

Comparison of the Two Major Minimally Invasive Head and Neck Surgical Techniques – TLM and TORS

There are two major minimally invasive transoral head and neck surgeries that both have transformed the way we look at HNC treatment – TLM and TORS. TLM uses CO_2 laser, which was introduced, in 1967, by Jako and Polanyii on cadaveric larynges (30) and then, in 1968, in a canine model, the first in vivo laryngeal laser experiment (31). Bredemeier's invention of the micromanipulator to deliver CO_2 energy through a microscope was the beginning of the current laryngeal laser surgery era (32). In the 1980s and 1990s, Steiner developed the technique further and larger tumors of larynx, pharynx, and oropharynx became the target for TLM (33), after developing a wide variety of endoscopes to get access to any subsite of the pharynx and larynx (Figure 13.5). As of today, there are no stages of HNC that is a limitation for TLM. The limitations are rather defined by the tumor growth pattern (e.g., tumor growing through the pharynx into the carotid space) or by anatomic restrictions of the pharynx, limiting the access of the endoscopes to certain subsites.

TORS operates under the same principles as TLM; by resecting tumors transorally, the functionality of the pharynx is preserved. However, there are some fundamental differences as outlined in

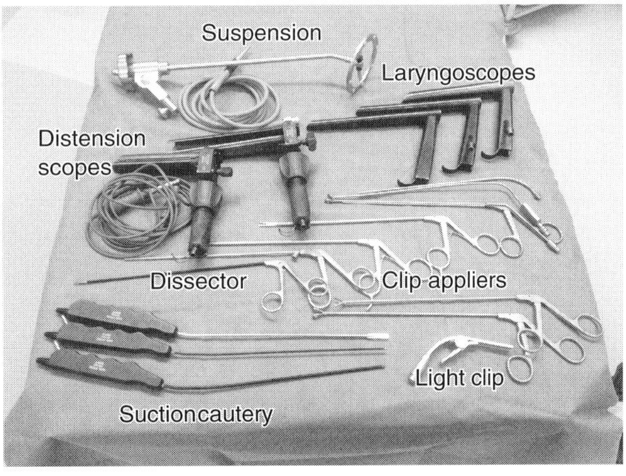

Figure 13.5 There are a number of endoscopes and instruments available for TLM, designed for tumor resections of the pharynx and larynx, that share the airway with the metal laser tube.

Table 13.1 Minimal invasive head and neck surgery performed by TLM and TORS

	TLM	TORS
Tactile feedback	Yes	No
Access	Good	Great
Optimal anatomic subunit	Larynx	Oropharynx
Setup	Fast	Complex
No. of surgeons needed	1	2
Visualization		
Overview	Limited	Superior
Detailed	Superior	Good
Control of bleeding		
Cautery, clips	Yes	Yes
Need for assistant	No	Yes
Instruments (bovie vs. laser)		
Bovie	No	Yes
Suction cautery	Yes (surgeon)	Yes (assistant)
Laser	Yes (CO_2)	Yes (CO_2, Thulium)
Retractors	Yes (wide variety)	Yes (limited options)
Mouth gag	No need	Yes (couple of options)
Control of margins	Good	Good
Skilled assistant needed	No	Yes (suction, retraction)
Ergonometric qualities	Poor	Superior
Teaching	Difficult	Easy

Table 13.1. The main advantages of TORS over TLM are the wide-angle camera, which improves overview, and the robotic arm flexibility. With TLM, the CO_2 laser needs a "straight shot" to the target through the endoscopes, but with TORS, the rotating arms can access tumors in difficult locations. The main advantages of TLM over TORS are that it is a one-person operation and microscopic precision (Figure 13.6). Despite its relatively short history (34–36), TORS has had a fundamental impact in HNC surgery. The main reason for its growth is the rapid adaptation the head and neck surgeons experience. TLM takes years to master, but with TORS, surgeons are operational in months.

Both techniques are superior to open procedures, especially with regard to functional outcome. PEG tube and tracheostomy frequencies are significantly lower; there is no need for mandibular swings for access reasons; and, in addition, the patients are quickly discharged to home (36). Furthermore, inset of free flaps for the reconstruction of oropharynx can be performed with TORS without a mandibulotomy (37,38). This is again a result of the versatile, rotating, and flexible robotic arms and the wide-angle camera. An additional advantage of not performing mandibulotomies for inset of free flaps is a more accurate assessment of the size and design of the flap. It is easy to misjudge the defect and, therefore, harvest and inset too large flaps after a mandibultomy. This is in addition to more obvious downsides to mandibulotomies, such as scaring, decreased oral function, and frequent trismus due to the dislocation of temporomandibular joint.

According to Weinstein et al., about 93 percent of patients who are screened for TORS can actually have the surgery. The remaining 7 percent have to have open procedures due to poor access (39). Limitations of this technique are mainly related to poor access due to the patients' anatomic characteristics, e.g., small oropharynx or mouth, large teeth, and/or stiff neck. Cancers of the oropharynx are the low-hanging fruit. The F-K retractor (Olympus, Tokyo, Japan) gives good exposure down to the vallecula, but due to restrictions in angling the retractor and thus the inability to follow the natural tract into the larynx, false cords and endolarynx are better handled with TLM.

For the oropharynx, a 30-degree forward, wide-angle 3D HD camera (Panasonic, Osaka, Japan) offers great visualization of anatomic subunits, including inferior BOT, vallecula, and lateral pharyngeal walls. With the 540-degree movement of the robotic arms and by using the clutch, the surgeon can intuitively reposition the instruments as needed and get access to any anatomic subunit of the pharynx.

The only spot that offers some serious challenges is the glossotonsillar sulcus. This area, if deep and if the oropharynx is small, can be hard to expose due to the abovementioned limitations of the F-K retractor. If facing such cases, the surgeon should have the Karl Storz (Tuttlingen, Germany) TLM set handy and switch over since the narrow endoscopes used by that technique can penetrate that space more efficiently. A novel, thin, impact-resistant dental guard, which rapidly can be custom-fitted for protection during intubations and transoral procedures such as TORS and TLM, can provide benefit (Figure 13.7a and b).

The da Vinci system offers a standard monopolar cautery device for cutting, with different blades. There are also a few options for lasers that can be added to the system (Omniguide [CO_2] and Lisa [thulium] lasers). The Omniguide CO_2 laser can be clipped on to the needle driver and works relatively well. The cutting is precise though, and with energy levels at 10–15 W, the BOT can be easily resected. Another advantage of CO_2 laser over bovie is less thermal trauma, which results in less swelling and subsequently an easier extubation phase.

With both TLM and TORS, postoperative overnight intubation is the safest way to avoid tracheostomies. The laser tube should be switched to a regular ET tube in the operating room when the resection

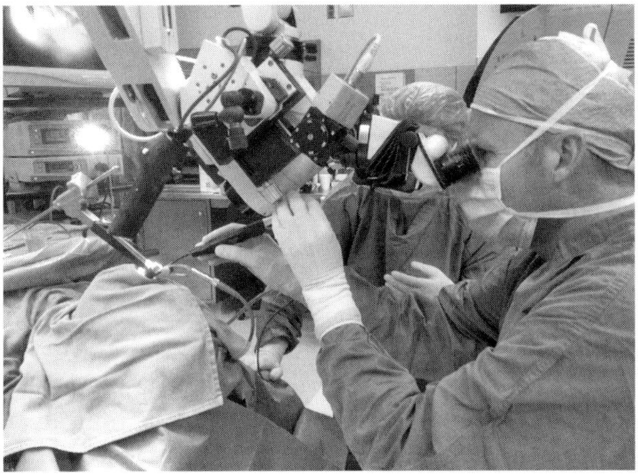

Figure 13.6 TLM is performed by a single surgeon, visualizing the tumor through a microscope, directing the CO_2 laser beam with a micromanipulator through endoscopes. A size 6 metal laser tube is used for intubation.

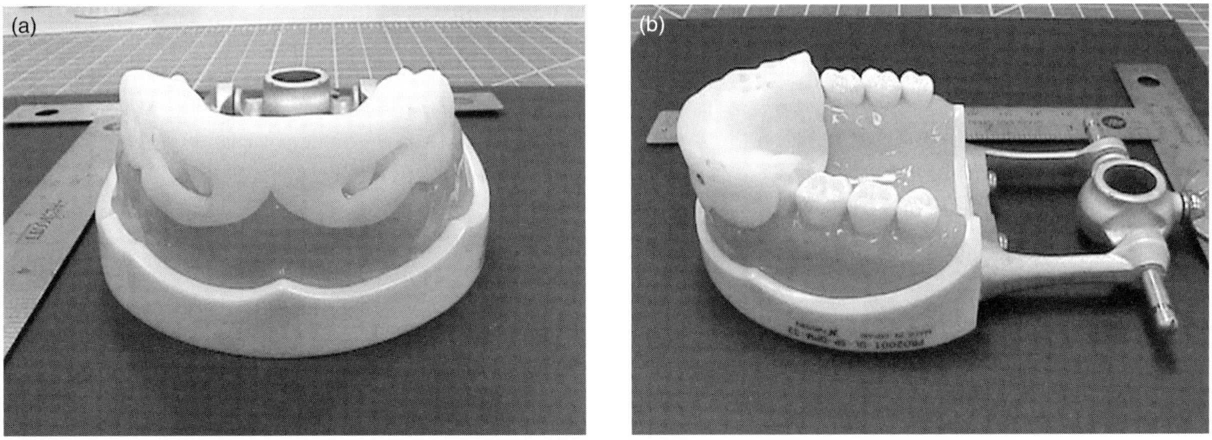

Figure 13.7 A novel, thin, impact-resistant dental guard that rapidly can be custom-fitted on site by hospital staff or at home preoperatively by the patient for protection during intubations and transoral procedures such as TORS and TLM (Akervall technologies Inc., Saline, MI). (a) Front view showing force-absorbing lateral slits. (b) Side view exposing the palatal extension that provides stabilization of the dental guard during transoral instrumentation.

is completed, and after 12- to 24-hour postoperative ventilator care with the patient on IV steroids and a simple cuff leak test in the ICU, patients can routinely be extubated without assistance of anesthesia and without any major risk for airway obstruction.

Survival Outcome of TORS and TLM for Patients with HNC

As mentioned earlier, transoral minimally invasive surgical techniques are challenging the mainstay of modern organ preservation therapies for HNC – concomitant chemoradiation. We have discussed the functional advantages transoral approaches have as compared with open, transcervical procedures. However, none of those advantages would be important if it was not for comparable or even improved survival outcomes. Although there are no randomized trials comparing oncologic outcomes between primary chemoradiation protocols and primary transoral minimally invasive surgical resections, retrospective comparisons support an advantage of primary surgery. In addition, functional outcomes may be superior following transoral surgical treatment. Management of oropharyngeal SCC will most likely continue to be multidisciplinary with an ongoing effort to deescalate treatment to reduce morbidity (40). Ford et al. also concluded that the oncologic outcome is the same for TORS as it is for open surgical approaches (41).

Steiner evaluated 48 previously untreated patients with stage III and IV BOT squamous cell carcinoma, treated with TLM. The Kaplan-Meier 5-year local control rate was 85 percent (42). Haughey et al. presented 3-year overall survival, disease-specific survival, and disease-free survival of 86, 88, and 82 percent, respectively, in a multicenter study of 204 patients with stage III and IV oropharynx cancer. Local control was 97 percent, and 87 percent of patients had normal swallowing or episodic dysphagia (42). In another study of 171 p16-positive HNC cases, Haughey reported the 3- and 5-year Kaplan-Meier estimates for DFS were 91 and 88 percent, respectively, whereas for DSS they were 95.5 and 94.4 percent, respectively (43). Rich reported similar findings in 84 stage III and IV p16-positive oropharynx cancer. Overall survival at 2 and 5 years was 94 and 88 percent, respectively, and disease-specific survival at 2 and 5 years was 96 and 92 percent, respectively. Adjuvant radiation was given in roughly 50 percent of these studies, and the survival rates are comparable or better than for chemoradiation (44).

Paradigm Shift in Treatment of HNCs – Is the Era of Chemoradiation Coming to an End?

Prior to the last two decades of HNC treatment, dominated by organ preservation protocols using mainly chemoradiation for oropharynx and larynx HNSCC, radical but also disruptive surgery and sometimes adjuvant radiation was dominating. These major surgical procedures could involve subtotal BOT resections, mandibulectomy, and neck lymphatics on bloc, which would leave large defects that need to be reconstructed. Bigger was determined to be better for many decades. For reconstructions, regional flaps, predominantly pectoralis major and, to some extent, latissimus dorsi and trapezuis flaps, were the work horses, but over time more sophisticated and versatile free flaps got introduced. The radial forearm flap dominated for many years, and recently anterolateral thigh flaps have gained popularity since the size can easily be personalized and the donor site morbidity is less of an issue. However, even with the introduction of these improved reconstructive alternatives, patients still had and still have suboptimal functional outcome in many surgical scenarios. Free fibula grafts are still the main alternative for mandibular reconstructions. Reconstructing the pharynx with free flaps improved cosmetic and also functional outcome, but basic dilemma remained; any external approach to the pharynx involves disruption of normal structures, including but not limited to constrictor and other deep musculatures of the neck. In addition, external surgical approach to the neck disrupts normal sensory nerve functions of the pharynx. Subsequently, the procedure carries a 35 percent risk for chronic dysphagia.

With the VA trial and the RTOG 91-11 studies, the pendulum shifted to a more conservative approach. Chemoradiation was introduced and gave patients hope for preserving the larynx and swallowing function. However, as time has passed and with improved survival rates, thanks to the current increased incidence of HPV rather than smoking- and drinking-related tumors, the significant side effects – e.g., dysphagia and xerostomia, and the extended treatment time with often lengthy leave of absence for patients – have prompted a discussion of whether the degree of aggressiveness in treatment can be scaled back. Maybe bigger is not better after all, not for surgery and not even for radiation-based treatment protocols. The introduction of intense modulated radiation therapy, often in conjunction with concomitant chemotherapy, has certainly reduced side effects and improved outcome, but we are still looking for ways to speed up treatment times and shorten rehabilitation. A full treatment course of chemoradiation takes at least 7 weeks, with an additional 2–6 months of healing. Minimally invasive transoral head and neck surgery takes a few hours, and patients eat and drink the next day and heal up from postoperative soreness within 1–2 weeks.

Subsequently, when the minimal invasive techniques described briefly above got introduced and accepted, they certainly have made an impact on HNC treatment. Just like radiation can be scaled back, surgery can too. At first, small tumors of the larynx and oropharynx were the target, or palliative procedures, but as time has passed, larger and larger cancers have been proven to be successfully removed, with much improved functional outcomes. The paradigm shift from a surgical perspective lies in the concept of (a) just remove the tumor and a margin, (b) do not disrupt normal tissue on your way to the tumor, and (c) leave the resected area open for healing by secondary intention.

TML for the larynx seemed to be easier to accept, but Steiner's transoral approach to larger oropharyngeal, supraglottic, and hypopharyngeal cancers was a much harder concept to accept for many institutions during the 1990s. There are many reasons for this; we have already mentioned difficulties to accept the concept of piecemealing the tumor during resection, and another issue has been how to control the margins with somewhat limited visibility through an endoscope. Overall, there seems to have been a mental block for many surgeons to accept that there was an alternative way to do head and neck surgery, other than what they were trained for. However, piecemealing is absolutely not necessary. When minimal invasive head and neck surgeons get more skilled and experienced, they understand that transoral en bloc resections are possible even for large tumors. However, as mentioned above, TLM takes time to learn, mainly due to limited visualization through long and narrow endoscopes.

With the introduction of TORS for HNC and its FDA approval in 2010, there was all of a sudden a minimally invasive alternative for all head and neck surgeons that never added TML to their therapeutic arsenal. TORS offers a leap in technology that has had and still has an instant and profound impact on the acceptance for transoral resections in institutions all over the world. TORS, using the da Vinci/Intuitive equipment and techniques, is so intuitive that a well-trained head and neck surgeon can pick up and implement the technique after a few training sessions.

Summary

TORS has become increasingly popular for the treatment of OSA and HNC. For HNC, TLM is an alternative technique to TORS. The advantages offered by TORS have also found application in the resection of benign parapharyngeal space tumors (45), lingual thyroid (46), tumors of the clivus (47), and others. Both TORS and TLM offer significant advantages as compared to traditional open approaches for HNC surgery, especially with regard to functional outcome and reduced need for both tracheostomy and long-term feeding tube. Patients undergoing evaluation for TORS undergo DISE; DISE requires IV sedation of patients with moderate to severe OSA. Protocols for safe and efficient administration of sedation have been developed. TORS for OSA does have some differences in perioperative management when compared to traditional surgical techniques. From an anesthesia standpoint, these consist of nasal instead of oral intubation and the rotation of the operating table 180 degrees away from the anesthesiologist to accommodate proper docking of the robot platform; TLM, in contrast, does not require rotation of the bed beyond 90 degrees and requires an oral metal laser ET tube. In both TORS and TLM, special attention must be exercised to protect dentition with custom-molded mouth guards (48).

In this chapter, we discussed both surgical and outcome-related advantages of these techniques that are now challenging the standard of care in both sleep surgery and HNC surgery.

For the management of HNC, TORS and TLM may challenge the dominant treatment modality of concomitant chemoradiation in favor of surgery followed by adjuvant radiation alone, without chemotherapy; studies have demonstrated similar or improved 3- and 5-year survival outcomes with minimally invasive surgery. With regard to functional outcome, there is no doubt that TORS and TLM offer superior results with regard to rapid recovery and minimal need for either tracheostomy or long-term feeding tube. In case of OSA, transoral surgical techniques have been used in the past, but TORS has gained popularity due to its superior exposure of the BOT and more accurate resection of obstructing tissue located at the BOT.

Postoperative management is now dominated by a policy of either extubation in the operating room (TORS for OSA) or extubation the following day after overnight observation in the SICU for HNC patients undergoing TORS or TLM. Most patients can easily be extubated the following morning, and very few require a tracheostomy. This is especially true after TLM since thermal trauma from CO_2 laser is less than the trauma and subsequent swelling from monopolar cautery (TORS). Intravenous steroids and antibiotics are standard practice in the perioperative period and are discontinued after extubation. Patients undergoing TORS for OSA are maintained on postoperative antibiotics for 1 week.

In conclusion, transoral surgical techniques for OSA and HNC, such as TORS and TLM, are rapidly gaining popularity due to both lower morbidity and similar survival compared to open approaches. For anesthesiologists these techniques present specific challenges, particularly in the OSA patient undergoing TORS. However, compared to traditional open HNC surgery, the advent of transoral surgery should be seen as positive development. Coordination of airway management between surgeon and anesthesiologist remains the guiding principle in transoral surgery.

References

1. Marin JM, et al. Long-term cardiovascular outcomes in men with obstructive sleep apnoea-hypopnoea with or without treatment with continuous positive airway pressure: an observational study. *Lancet* 2005;365:1046–53.
2. Weaver TE, et al. An instrument to measure functional status outcomes for disorders of excessive sleepiness. *Sleep* 1997;20:835–44.
3. Young T, et al. Epidemiology of obstructive sleep apnea. *American Journal of Respiratory and Critical Care Medicine* 2002;165:1217–39.
4. Weaver TE, et al. Adherence to continuous positive airway pressure therapy: the challenge to effective treatment. *Proc Am Thorac Soc.* 2008;5:173–8.
5. Stuck BA, et al. Effects of continuous positive airway pressure on apnea-hypopnea index in obstructive sleep apnea based on long-term compliance. *Sleep Breath* 2012;16:467–71.
6. Fujita S, et al. Obstructive sleep apnea: pathophysiology, upper airway evaluation and surgical treatment. *ENT J* 1993;72:67–72.
7. Omur M, et al. Tongue base suspension combined with UPPP in severe OSA patients. *ACTA Oto Ital* 2004.
8. Holty JE, et al. Maxillomandibular advancement for the treatment of OSA: a systematic review and meta-analysis. *Sleep Medicine Reviews* 2010;14:287–97.
9. Buchwald H, et al. Bariatric surgery: a systematic review and meta-analysis. *JAMA* 2004;292:1724–37.
10. Vicini C, et al. The nose oropharynx hypopharynx and larynx (NOHL) classification: a new system of diagnostic standardized examination for OSAHS patients. *Eur Arch Otorhinolaryngol* 2012;269:1297–300.
11. Kezirian EJ, et al. Drug-induced sleep endoscopy: the VOTE classification. *Eur Arch Otorhinolaryngol* 2011;268:1233–6.
12. Vicini C, et al. Transoral robotic tongue base resection in obstructive sleep apnoea-hypopnoea syndrome: a preliminary report. *ORL J Otorhinolaryngol Relat Spec* 2010;72:22–7.
13. Chabolle F, et al. Tongue base reduction with hyoepiglottoplasty: a treatment for severe obstructive sleep apnea. *Laryngoscope* 1999;109:1273–80.
14. Wolf G, et al. Induction chemotherapy plus radiation compared with surgery plus radiation in patients with advanced laryngeal cancer. *N Engl J Med* 1991;324:1685–90.
15. Lefebvre JL, et al. Larynx preservation in pyriform sinus cancer: preliminary results of a European Organization for Research and Treatment of Cancer phase III trial. EORTC Head and Neck Cancer Cooperative Group. *J Natl Cancer Inst* 1996;88:890–9.
16. Forastiere AA, et al. Concurrent chemotherapy and radiotherapy for organ preservation in advanced laryngeal cancer. *N Engl J Med* 2003;27:2091–8.
17. Rich JT, et al. Transoral laser microsurgery (TLM) with or without adjuvant therapy for advanced stage oropharyngeal cancer: outcomes and prognostic factors. *Laryngoscope* 2009;119:1709–19.
18. Steiner W, et al. Transoral laser microsurgery for squamous cell carcinoma of the base of the tongue. *Arch Otolaryngol Head Neck Surg* 2003;129:36–43.
19. Berry S, et al. Validity of sleep nasendoscopy in the investigation of sleep related breathing disorders. *Laryngoscope* 2005;115:538–40.
20. Borek RC, et al. Quantitative airway analysis during drug-induced sleep endoscopy for evaluation of sleep apnea. *Laryngoscope* 2012;122:2592–9.

21. De Vito A, et al. European position paper on drug-induced sedation endoscopy (DISE). *Sleep Breath* 2014;18:453–65.
22. Woodson BT, et al. Three-year outcomes of cranial nerve stimulation for obstructive sleep apnea: the STAR trial. *Otolaryngol Head Neck Surg* 2015.
23. Lin HS, et al. Transoral robotic surgery for treatment of obstructive sleep apnea-hypopnea syndrome. *Laryngoscope* 2013;123:1811–6.
24. Vicini C, et al. Clinical outcomes and complications associated with TORS for OSAHS: a benchmark for evaluating an emerging surgical technology in a targeted application for benign disease. *ORL J Otorhinolaryngol Relat Spec* 2014;76:63–9.
25. Hoff P, et al. Transoral robotic surgery in benign diseases including obstructive sleep apnea: safety and feasibility. *Laryngoscope* 2015;125:1249–53.
26. Hoff PT, et al. Body mass index predicts success in patients undergoing transoral robotic surgery for obstructive sleep apnea. *ORL J Otorhinolaryngol Relat Spec* 2014;76:266–72.
27. Spector ME, et al. Addressing the retrolingual space in obstructive sleep apnea: outcomes stratified by Friedman stage in patients undergoing transoral robotic surgery. *ORL J Otorhinolaryngol Relat Spec* 2015;78:1–8.
28. Thaler ER, et al. Outcomes for multilevel surgery for sleep apnea: obstructive sleep apnea, transoral robotic surgery, and uvulopalatopharyngoplasty. *Laryngoscope* 2015.
29. Easa M, et al. Swallowing outcome after TORS for sleep apnea: short- and long-term evaluation. *Eur Arch Otorhinolaryngol* 2015;272:1537–41.
30. Jako GJ. Laser surgery of the vocal cords. An experimental study with carbon dioxide lasers on dogs. *Laryngoscope* 1972;82:2204–16.
31. Shapshay SM. Laser surgery of the vocal cords: an experimental study with carbon dioxide lasers on dogs. *Laryngoscope* 1996;106:935–8.
32. Polanyi TG, et al. A CO_2 laser for surgical research. *Med Biol Eng* 1970;8:541–8.
33. Steiner W, et al. Endoscopic laser surgery of the upper aerodigestive tract, with special emphasis on cancer surgery. *Thieme* 2000.
34. Dean NR, et al. Robotic-assisted surgery for primary or recurrent oropharyngeal carcinoma. *Arch Otolaryngol Head Neck Surg* 2010;136:380–4.
35. White HN, et al. Transoral robotic-assisted surgery for head and neck squamous cell carcinoma: one- and 2-year survival analysis. *Arch Otolaryngol Head Neck Surg* 2010;136:1248–52.
36. Weinstein GS, et al. Selective neck dissection and deintensified postoperative radiation and chemotherapy for oropharyngeal cancer: a subset analysis of the University of Pennsylvania transoral robotic surgery trial. *Laryngoscope* 2010;120:1749–55.
37. Song HG, et al. Robot-assisted free flap in head and neck reconstruction. *Arch Plast Surg* 2013;40:353–8.
38. Selber JC, et al. Transoral robotic reconstructive surgery. *Semin Plast Surg* 2014;28:35–8.
39. Weinstein GS, et al. Transoral robotic surgery: a multicenter study to assess feasibility, safety, and surgical margins. *Laryngoscope* 2012;122:1701–7.
40. Hinni ML, et al. Oropharyngeal cancer treatment: the role of transoral surgery. *Curr Opin Otolaryngol Head Neck Surg* 2015;23:132–8.
41. Ford SE, et al. Transoral robotic versus open surgical approaches to oropharyngeal squamous cell carcinoma by human papillomavirus status. *Head Neck Surg* 2014;151:606–11.
42. Haughey BH, et al. Transoral laser microsurgery as primary treatment for advanced-stage oropharyngeal cancer: a United States multicenter study. *Head Neck* 2011;33:1683–94.
43. Haughey BH, et al. Prognostic factors and survival unique to surgically treated p16+ oropharyngeal cancer. *Laryngosopce* 2012;122:S13–33.
44. Rich JT, et al., Transoral laser microsurgery (TLM) +/- adjuvant therapy for advanced stage oropharyngeal cancer: outcomes and prognostic factors. *Laryngoscope* 2009;119:1709–19.
45. Arshad H et al. Transoral robotic resection of selected parapharyngeal space tumors. *Eur Arch Otorhinolaryngol* 2013;270:1737–40.
46. Prisman E, et al. Transoral robotic excision of ectopic lingual thyroid: case series and literature review. *Head Neck* 2015;37:88–91.
47. Dallan I, et al. The natural evolution of endoscopic approaches in skull base surgery: robotic-assisted surgery? *Acta Otorhinolaryngol Ital* 2011;31:390–4.
48. Akervall et al. Dental protection during intubations and rigid laryngoscopy (unpublished).

Chapter 14

Robotic Technology in Neurosurgery

Past, Present, and Future Perspectives

Alisson R. Teles and Tobias A. Mattei

Introduction

The word "robot" was originally coined in 1923 by Karel Capek (1890–1938) to describe a mechanical man performing *robota*, a Czech term meaning forced labor. Nowadays, robots are defined as manipulators that, through variable programmed motions, are designed to move materials or tools to perform a variety of tasks. In minimally invasive surgery, robotics (i.e., the science and technology of robots, and their design, manufacture, and application) can improve the dexterity of conventional instruments, helping the surgeon with augmented visual and haptic inputs.

Advanced surgical robotic concepts are now beginning to emerge with the use of voice control, real-time holography, robotics for both positioning and micromanipulation, and, the more recently acquired concept of telerobotics for the performance of remote surgeries, with the surgeon operating with an adjuvant surgeon working in a virtual reality environment and the secondary robotic transfer taking place within the actual patient care area (1).

As during any technological revolution, robotics is finding increased usage in the medical field. Between the years 1980 and 1990, the first robots were introduced into neurosurgery (2,3) to guide the needle in stereotactic biopsies. Later, the use of robotic holders was extended to many procedures, including the localization and treatment of brain tumors, vascular malformations, epilepsy, and functional neurosurgery (localizing the temporal horn to place depth electrodes, movement disorder surgery), and endoscopic surgery. The same has occurred in the field of spine surgery, in which promising applications have been demonstrated with robot-assisted screw placement and puncture-based procedures such as vertebral augmentation and biopsies.

Over the past 30 years since first robotic-assisted neurosurgical procedure (4), an increasing number of research articles has been published on robotics in neurosurgery (5). The growth in neurosurgical robots, as well as the evolvement of general surgical robotics (6,7), has been closely linked to specific improvements in visualization systems, lesion localization techniques, microsurgery technologies, and positive trends in minimally invasive surgeries (1,5,8–20).

While the main factors that motivated the adoption of robotic technology in the industrial setting were related to automation, mass production, and manpower safety, the increased interest in the application of robotics as an adjuvant surgical tool has been mainly related to the possibility of increasing surgical precision, stability, and dexterity in order to overcome human limitations related to spatial accuracy, precise quantitative analysis of movements, and fatigue (6). The concept of integration between biomechanical tools with navigation systems theoretically allows access to target areas in the brain in a safe and minimally invasive way (1). It is clear that surgical tools that can aid improve surgical outcomes through higher accuracies, shorter procedure duration, and/or lower costs would be beneficial (21). Despite such potential advantages, the actual incorporation of robotic technology to the surgical routine is counterbalanced by several challenges involving sterilization, hardware maintenance, and precision reliability. Moreover, the ideal protocol for maintaining patient safety by assuring precise control over robotic maneuvers as well as the exact timeframe and mode of the human–machine interaction has not yet been established (22).

Neurosurgical Robotic Systems

The design paradigm for the first and many current neurosurgical robots is based on stereotactic frames (5,23). Not less important than mechanical framing aspect, progressive developments in the imaging field were also crucial for the evolvement of robotic-assisted neurosurgery. In fact, advances in imaging of the central nervous system have been the basis of the majority of breakthroughs in the history of neurosurgery (22,24).

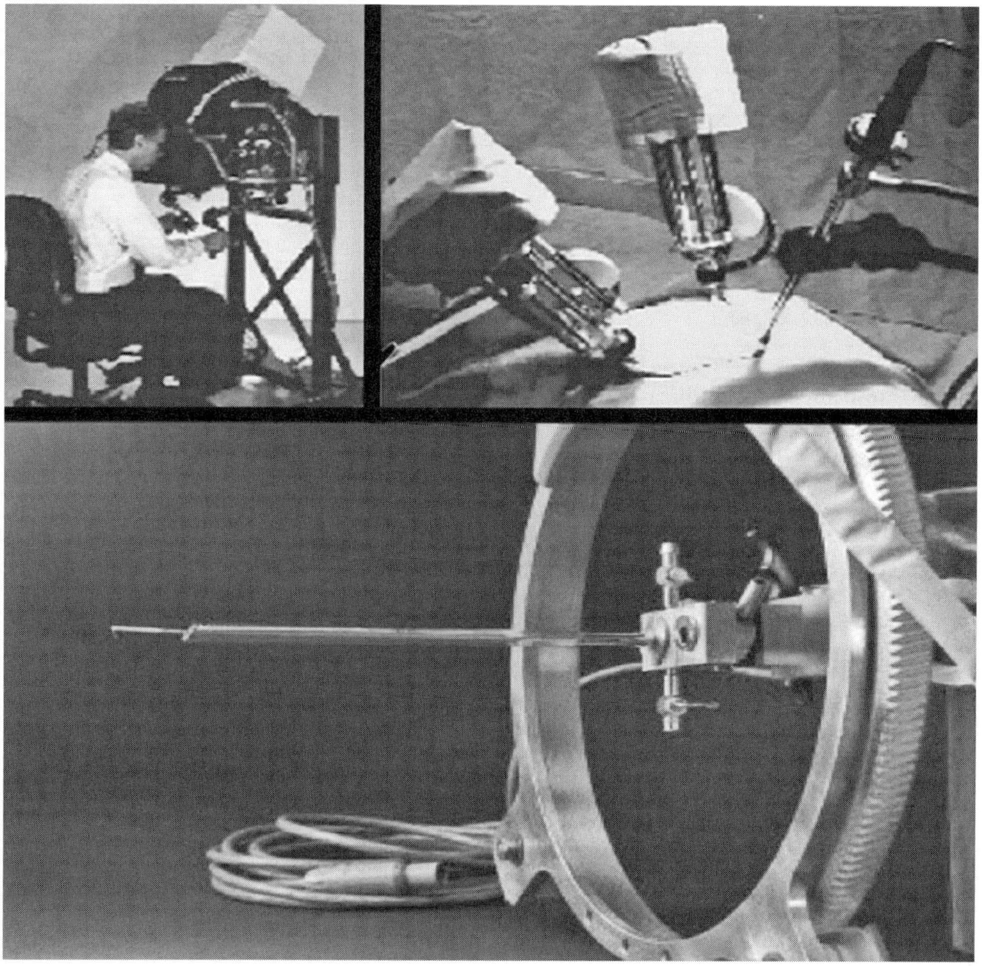

Figure 14.1 The programmable universal machine for assembly (PUMA 200), a system for CT-guided intracranial stereotactic biopsy, was the first robotic platform employed in neurosurgery in 1985.

Shortly after a proof-of-concept percutaneous nephrostomy robot in late 1984 (25), the first clinical trials for a surgical robot began in Vancouver, Canada, in 1985, with the Arthrobot, a voice-activated orthopedic surgical assist system for positioning of a patient's knee (5). A few months later, Kwoh et al. (4) conducted a stereotactic biopsy on a brain lesion using an off-the-shelf PUMA 200 (Figure 14.1). Drake et al. (26), in 1991, reported the use of PUMA 200 as adjuvant in the surgery for thalamic astrocytomas in six children. In 1995, the MINERVA system was the first robotic system to use real-time CT guidance during a stereotactic brain biopsy (5). The integration of imaging with stereotactic frame robots was key to the development of high-precision adaptable neurosurgical robots such as the NeuroArm (Figure 14.2), NeuroBlate, and NeuroMate. Table 14.1 presents an overview of the current active neurosurgical robots and groups.

Clinical Applications in Neurosurgery

During the last decades, robotic technologies have emerged as powerful adjuvant tools in the field of interventional medical procedures. Currently, robotic technologies have already been successfully employed to assist in several surgical tasks in neurosurgery, such as instrument positioning, trajectory planning, needle biopsy insertion, placement of deep brain stimulators (DBS) and epilepsy monitoring electrodes, pedicle screw placement, vertebroplasty, as well as soft tissue cutting using the x–y coordinates.

Table 14.1 Summary of active neurosurgical robots and groups

Project	Reg approval	Group	Task	Subjects	Note
CyberKnife	US FDA, CE	Accuracy Inc. (USA)	Image-guided radiotherapy	100 k patients (2010)	Mature technology
iSYS	CE, ISO, US FDA	ARC Seiberdorf Research (Austria)	CT- and US-guided biopsies	Gel phantoms	Validating for neurosurgery
NeuroBlate/ AutoLITT	US FDA, Health Canada	Montesis Medical Inc. (USA/Canada)	MRI-guided neuro. tumor ablation	275+ clinical procedures (US)	Real-time MR-compatible
NeuroMate	US FDA, CE & Saudi FDA	Renishaw PLC (UK)	Stereotactic neurosurgery	"Thousands" of procedures (2012)	Introduced in 1989, commercialized in 1997
Novalis	US FDA, CE	Varian (US) and Brainlab (Germany)	Image-guided radiotherapy	1M "patient treatments" (2014)	Mature technology
Renaissance/ SpineAssist	CE, US FDA, Korean FDA, Chinese FDA	Mazor Robotics (Israel)	Spinal and brain neurosurgery	"Approx. 10,000 procedures" (2015)	1st transcerebellar brainstem biopsy (2015)
ROSA Brain/ Spine	US FDA, CE, Health Canada	Medtech S.A. (France)	Stereotactic neurosurgery	1,200 procedures (2014)	Haptic feedback
SYMBIS & NeuroArm	Health Canada	IMRIS & University of Calgary (Canada)	Microsurgery and stereotactic neurosurgery	58 patient cases (2015)	MR-compatible
TMS-Robot	CE, Health Canada	Axilum Robotics (France)	Transcranial magnetic stimulation	4 human subjects (2014)	Brain-to-brain interface
Active System	No	FP7 ACTIVE (EU)	General neurosurgery	No	Includes Kuka and Renishaw
Arata-Fujimoto	No	Nagoya Inst. Tech (Japan)	Stereotactic neurosurgery, phantom tumor	Rapid prototypes	Custom robot and controller
CAS-BH5	No	Navy General Hospital (China)	Frameless stereotactic neurosurgery	17 patients (2007, 2014)	1,300 km telesurgery
EXPERT & Neurobot	No	Shinshu Uni. (Japan)	Simulated neurosurgical suturing	13 surgeries (2013)	Armrest for surgeon
MARS	No	Uni. Luebeck (Germany)	Stereotactic neurosurgery	Human trial biopsy (2012) 72)	Hybrid manual/ auto positioning
MINIR I & II	No	University of Maryland (USA)	Intracranial surgery	No49	Shape memory alloy acutation
MiroSurge	No	DLR (Germany)	Cranial surgery, pedicle screw placement	Phantoms, ex vivo bones	"Soft" robot, on-arm optical, haptics
Morita Microsurgical	No	Uni. Tokyo (Japan)	Deep-field microneurosurgery	Cadavers, phantoms (2005, 2013)	Micromanipulation focus
Neuroglide	No	EPFL/KB Medical (Switzerland)	Spinal (cervical interbody fusion)	6 cadavers (2013)	Co-manipulated
Neurostar	No	Neurostar GmbH (Germany)	Monitorized stereotaxy	Mouse and rat trials	Deep brain stimulation
RAVEN I & II	No	Applied Dexterity & Uni. Washington (USA)	Neurosurgery and laparoscopy	3 cadavers (2013)	"Open source" design
SemiAuto Trepanation	No	RWTH Aachen Uni. (Germany)	Trepanation and craniotomy	Phantom skulls	Handheld unit
Uni. Bern Robot	No	Uni. Bern (Switzerland)	Stereotactic cochlear implants	Cadavers and phantoms	Semiauto marker search

Source: Smith et al. (5).

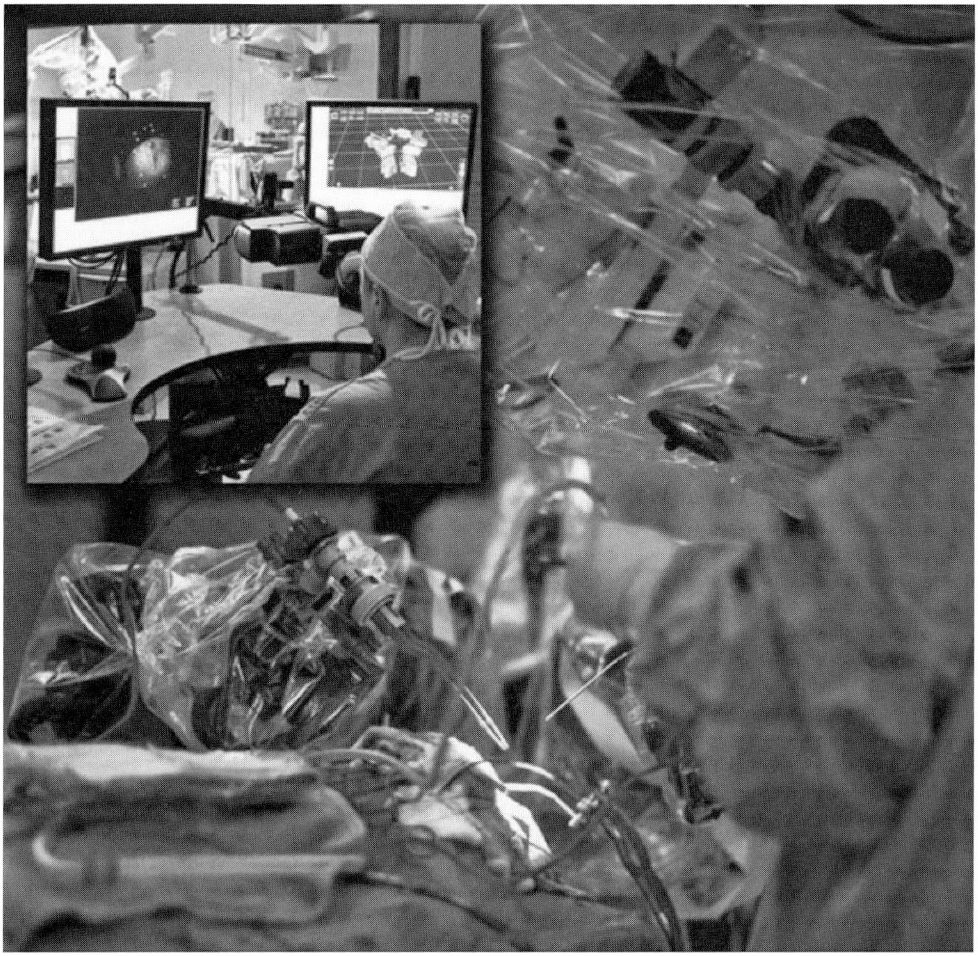

Figure 14.2 NeuroArm platform positioned for removal of an olfactory groove meningioma. The right arm holds a bipolar forceps and the left a bayonet-shaped sucker. Stereoscopic images from two high-definition cameras attached to the operating microscope are projected to the surgeon at the workstation (insert). Also shown in the insert are the 3D MRI display (left) and virtual manipulators registered to the radiofrequency coil (right). (Reproduced with permission from Lang MJ, Greer AD, Sutherland GR. Intra-operative robotics: NeuroArm. *Acta Neurochir Suppl*. 2011;109:231–6. doi:10.1007/978-3-211-99651-5_36.)

In the sequence, we present some of the outcomes reported in the literature regarding the incorporation of robotic technology to specific fields in neurosurgery (Box 14.1).

Stereotactic Neurosurgery

The possibility of flexibility and automation of target coordinates through the use of new software applications has significantly attracted the attention of experts in stereotactic neurosurgery for robotic technology (3). In recent years, many groups have demonstrated the feasibility, safety, and accuracy of frameless biopsy employing robotic techniques (2,27–30).

Haegelen et al. (30) reported good results with NeuroMate robot in a series of 15 patients submitted to robotic-guided stereotactic biopsy of brain stem lesions. From a total of 17 biopsies, transcerebellar approach was used in 12 cases and a double-oblique anterior frontal approach in 5 cases.

Bekelis et al. (28) reported the use the SurgiScope system (ISIS Intelligent Surgical Instruments & Systems, Grenoble) for stereotactic image-guided robotic biopsy in 41 patients. A biopsy arm was affixed to the SurgiScope microscope, enabling the robotic instrument to function primarily as an instrument holder, positioned in alignment to the chosen

Box 14.1 Examples of Current Applications of Robot-Assisted Neurosurgery

- Stereotactic and functional neurosurgery
  - Stereotactic biopsies of brain lesions
  - Deep-brain stimulator implantation
  - Insertion of depth electrodes for intraoperative localization of epileptic foci
  - Implantation of brain catheters for chemotherapy
- Neuroendoscopy
  - Third ventriculostomy
  - Approaches to skull base
- Brain tumor surgery
- Spine surgery
  - Pedicle screw fixation
  - Vertebroplasty
  - Biopsies
  - Anterior lumbar interbody fusion
- Peripheral nerve surgery
  - Nerve transfer
  - Nerve tumors

trajectory. The mean operative time was reported to be 54.7 min in the first half of cases and 34.5 min in the latter half, demonstrating a progressive learning curve with the use of robot-assisted technology. The authors reported a diagnostic yield per procedure of 97.8 percent. Complications included transient worsening of a preexisting deficit (2 percent) and permanent deficit (2 percent) (28).

Lefranc et al. reviewed their experience with the robotic ROSA device in 100 frameless stereotactic biopsies (27). In their series, the robotic arm of ROSA device was used as an instrument holder (as arcs with frames); surgeons performed the biopsy manually through the reducers after the robotic arm was automatically positioned along the planned trajectory. They reported that, after matching between preoperative planning and postoperative CT scans, all biopsy sites were inside the tumor target. Histological diagnosis was established in 97 patients, and no deaths or permanent morbidity related to surgery. Postoperative bleeding was observed in 10 patients, 2 of them presented transient neurological deficit. Twenty-eight lesions were deep brain lesions and 20 were less than 15 mm in diameter. The operative time, as reported by the authors, was less than 1 hour for the last 50 frameless robotic biopsies, including positioning of the head, installation of the robot and draping, and less than 2 hours when the robot was coupled with the O-arm and bone fiducial registration.

Functional and Epilepsy Surgery

Following the progressive evolvement of robotic-assisted stereotactic neurosurgical biopsies, promising results have been demonstrated in the field of functional neurosurgery such as DBS implantation, image-guided insertion of depth electrodes for epilepsy foci localization, as well as robot-assisted stereotactic laser ablation of epilepsy foci.

In an in vitro study using the NeuroMate neurosurgical robot (Renishaw-Mayfield), Varma and Eldridge (31) demonstrated an accuracy of 1.29 mm in a large series of 113 DBS implantations. Recently, von Iasngsdorff et al. (32) quantified application accuracy of NeuroMate robot during frame-based DBS procedures for movement disorders in 30 basal ganglia targets (13 globus pallidus internus, 10 subthalamic nucleus, 7 ventralis intermedius nucleus) in 17 consecutive patients. The authors demonstrated that the in vivo application accuracy of the NeuroMate neurosurgical robot was better than 1 mm, at least similar to the accuracy of stereotactic frame arms (32).

Heuer et al., using the StimPilot system (StimPilot-Medtronic Inc., Minneapolis, MN), which consists of a neuronavigation station, a microdrive control, and a microelectrode recording display and control, have reported successful implantation of 262 DBS leads in 147 patients, targeting the intermediate nucleus, globus pallidus internus, and anterior thalamic nucleus, with only 1 patient in this series requiring lead repositioning (33).

Another successful application of robotic technology to functional neurosurgery is the image-guided insertion of depth electrodes for intraoperative localization of epileptic foci in patients with drug-resistant epilepsy. A pioneering study of robot-assisted surgery has demonstrated successful implantation of recording electrodes in three patients, with significant reduction in the operating time in comparison to procedures performed before the use of robotic technology (34). Spire et al. (35) also reported the use of SurgiScope robot for placement of intracranial depth electrodes for epilepsy surgery with good results.

Later on, in 2013, Cardinale et al. (36) published a large study of 500 stereoelectroencephalography (SEEG) procedures, including a study of localization error (LE) in a series of 1,050 frame-based electrode implantations assisted by the NeuroMate robotic system. The authors assessed the LE on both cortical entry point and deep target point. Because the SEEG electrodes are semirigid and are implanted without any guide tubes, the target point LE, even if excellent (median error = 1.77 mm, interquartile range = 1.25–2.51 mm), can be certainly affected by slight intracranial deviations. In order to verify the intrinsic accuracy of the stereotactic system, it is therefore advisable to consider the entry point LE as the most important measure. The authors obtained a median LE of 0.78 mm, with an interquartile range of 0.49–1.08 mm.

Similarly, Lefranc et al. (37) reported the accuracy in 52 frame-based implantations performed in vivo (mean 0.81 mm, SD 0.39 mm) using the ROSA robotic-assistance device (Medtech, Montpellier, France). In 2015, Gozález-Martínez et al. (38) also reported their experience with ROSA robotic system in 101 SEEG procedures. The time of implantation planning was 30 min on average (range, 15–60 min). The average operative time was 130 min (range, 45–160 min). In vivo accuracy (calculated in 500 trajectories) demonstrated a median entry point error of 1.2 mm (interquartile range, 0.78–1.83 mm) and a median target point error of 1.7 mm (interquartile range, 1.20–2.30 mm). Of the group of patients who underwent resective surgery (68 patients), 45 (66.2 percent) gained seizure freedom status. Mean follow-up was 18 months. The total complication rate was 4 percent. The authors highlighted the safety, accuracy, and efficiency in anatomically defining the epileptogenic zone and subsequently promoting sustained seizure freedom status in patients with difficult-to-localize seizures.

Recently, Gonzalez-Martinez et al. (39) reported their first experience with robot-assisted stereotactic laser ablation in a 19-year old woman with a 10-year refractory focal seizure history using ROSA robot in 2014. The authors highlighted that the procedure was minimally invasive, quick and safe, with only minimal discomfort to the patient who was discharged from the hospital the day after the treatment.

Endoscopic Brain Surgery

Neuroendoscopy is a well-established treatment modality for hydrocephalus, intracranial cystic lesions, tumor resection or biopsy, and any kind of microsurgical procedures that can be assisted by an endoscope, in order to achieve sufficient additional control of the operative field without retraction of neurovascular structures. One potential disadvantage and possible source of complication of neuroendoscopy is the guidance of the endoscope within the cranium by the surgeon. Endoscopes are either moved freehand or are temporarily fixed using mechanical or pneumatic fixation devices. In this sense, using a robot for positioning and holding the endoscope enables the surgeon to carry out very smooth and slow motions inside very critical anatomical regions (40–42).

In 2002 and 2003, Goto et al. (43,44) presented their first results of endoscopic brain surgery using the NeuRobot system (Shinshu University School of Medicine and Hitachi Ltd.), a master–slave micromanipulator system for neurosurgery, which consists of a 3D endoscope and three robotic arms. Takasuna et al. (45) described the feasibility of applying NeuRobot to intraventricular procedures commonly treated with the neuroendoscope (third ventriculostomy, fenestration of the septum pellucidum, biopsy of the thalamus, and biopsy of the choroid plexus of the lateral ventricle) using fixed cadaver heads. In the same study, they reported a successful treatment of a patient with obstructive hydrocephalus due to aquedutal stenosis using NeuRobot system.

Zimmermann et al. (41) reported their early experience with six patients with triventricular hydrocephalus submitted to robot-assisted third ventriculostomy using the Evolution 1 robotic device (URS Universal Robots, Scwerin, Germany). No device-related or surgery-related complications occurred in their series. According to the authors' experience, the time for the endoscopic part of the procedure ranged from 17 to 35 min. According to the authors, compared to freehand endoscopy, targeting of small vessels for coagulation can be easier, faster, and more precise, using the guidance of a robotic device (41).

More recently, Calisto et al. (46) expanded the use of ROSA system to endoscopic disconnection of hypothalamic hamartomas. In their series of 20 patients with drug-resistant epilepsy due to hypothalamic hamartomas, conventional disconnection by monopolar coagulation was performed in 13 patients, and thulium laser disconnection in the remaining 7 patients.

Robot-assisted endoscopy has also been applied to skull base approaches (47–55). Lee et al. reported on the feasibility of transoral robotic surgery of craniocervical junction and atlantoxial spine in cadavers using da Vinci robot (Intuitive Surgical, CA, USA)

(55). Also they described their clinical experience with da Vinci robot–assisted odontoidectomy for basilar invagination (54).

Several authors have attempted to verify the feasibility of robotic assistance to commonly performed keyhole intracranial procedures. Hong et al. (56) reported the application of the da Vinci to assist with the supraorbital subfrontal approach through an eyebrow skin incision in a cadaver study. While the authors concluded that such robot-assisted approaches were probably feasible, they noted several drawbacks including the lack of suitable instruments such as bone cutters and the risk of arm collisions. Marcus et al. (57) recently reported their analyses on the suitability of da Vinci robot to a range of keyhole approaches such as supraorbital subfrontal, retrosigmoid and supracerebellar infratentorial in a cadaver study. The authors concluded that da Vinci system is neither safe nor feasible to use in keyhole neurosurgery, mainly due to the lack of haptic feedback (57,58).

Neurosurgical Oncology

Majority of neurosurgical robots have been limited to stereotactic and endoscopic brain procedures (59). The first attempt to incorporate robotic technology in brain tumor surgery was reported by Drake et al. (26) in 1991 using PUMA 200 as a holder and retractor in six patients with brain stem tumor. Later, Goto et al. (43) reported their early experience with NeuRobot as adjuvant in resection of a convexity meningioma.

The first neurosurgical robot effectively incorporated to brain tumor surgery was neuroArm (Figure 14.2) (16,17,60–62). The neuroArm is a teleoperated magnetic resonance–compatible image-guided robot; it incorporates imaging technology with microsurgery and stereotaxy. It comprises two robotic arms capable of manipulating microsurgical tools connected via a main system controller to a workstation with a sensory immersive human–machine interface. One major advantage of this system is that it is equipped with three-dimensional force sensors, thus providing advanced haptic feedback to the surgeon. To date, it is reported that neuroArm has been used in more than 60 patients with brain lesions (62). The first 35 cases were reported by Sutherland et al. (17) in 2013 and included glioma, meningioma, schwannoma, dermoid cyst, abscess, cavernous angioma, meduloblastoma, and radiation necrosis.

Despite this initial advance, robotic technology with haptic feedback is still incipient and not fully integrated to neurosurgical practice.

Spine Surgery

The rationale for the use of robotics in spine surgery is the potential enhancement of the application of minimally invasive procedures by increasing accuracy and reducing radiation exposure for patients and surgeons (63). Since the earliest work on robot-assisted spine surgery in 1992 using the PUMA 260 robot for pedicle screw insertion, several technological developments in robotic technology have been observed in the last years in this field (21).

Besides pedicle screw insertion (14,64–71), robots have been used for puncture-based procedures, such as biopsies (72), vertebroplasties (73,74), and facet blocks (75). Robotic systems are also used for spine tumor ablation (76) and, to a lesser extent, for tumor resection (77). Recently, Beutler et al. (78) reported the use of da Vinci robot for anterior lumbar interbody fusion at L5-S1. Even more ongoing research aims to develop robotized endoscopes capable of exploration and surgery in the subarachnoid space (79).

The use of robotic assistance for pedicle screw placement has been gaining clinical acceptance in select sites throughout the United States and Europe. With this increased utilization, the generation of outcome data has also been accumulating, albeit slowly. Recently, Marcus et al. (80) reviewed the outcomes of robot-assisted pedicle screw placement compared to conventional fluoroscopy-guided technique. They focused on studies using the SpineAssist (Mazor Surgical Technologies Ltd., Caesarea, Israel), the most widely used robot for pedicle screw placement (Figure 14.3). After exclusions, they selected five articles comprising a total of 1,308 pedicle screws: 729 using robot assistance, and 579 using fluoroscopy guidance (14,65–68) (Table 14.2). In general, they observed satisfactory screw placement in 94.1 percent and 92.7 percent of robot-assisted and fluoroscopy-assisted placement, respectively. Regarding radiation exposure, two studies reported radiation exposure to patients and surgeons to be significantly less during robot-assisted procedure compared to fluoroscopy-guided procedures (65,66). Other two studies did not identify statistically significant difference between the techniques regarding radiation exposure (67,68).

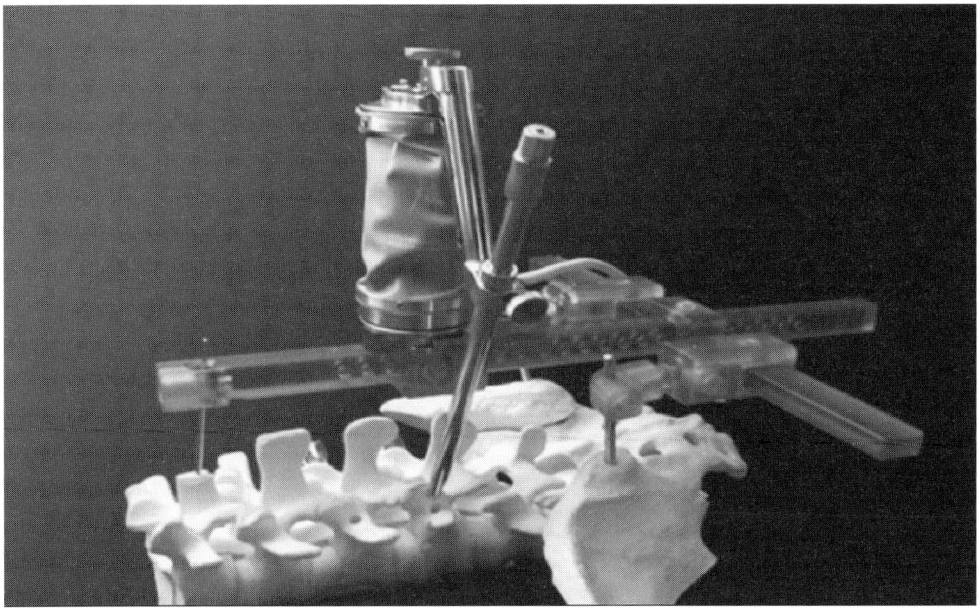

Figure 14.3 Image of the SpineAssist, the only commercial robotic system available for spine surgery. It is a hexapod miniature robotic device that places preoperatively planned trajectories for drilling a screw trajectory. It hovers above the spine via the Hover-T, which might be attached for minimally invasive procedures to a spinous process or the iliac crest. (Reproduced with permission from Stüer C, Ringel F, Stoffel M, Reinke A, Behr M, Meyer B. Robotic technology in spine surgery: current applications and future developments. *Acta Neurochir Suppl*. 2011;109:241–5. doi: 10.1007/978-3-211-99651-5_38.)

More recently, Schatlo et al. (81) reported on their experience with SpineAssist in lumbar degenerative spinal disorders. In a matched cohort analysis, they did not find difference regarding accuracy of screw placement of robot-assisted surgery in comparison with fluoroscopy-guided screw placement. Also, no difference in infection rates was observed between the groups, and only one patient (fluoroscopy group) needed revision surgery due to screw malposition and radiculopathy. No differences in length of hospital stay, cumulative dose of morphine, and mean duration of surgery were identified. Robot-assisted procedures presented significantly less blood loss compared with fluoroscopy group. However, despite demonstrating the utility and safety of robot-assisted screw placement, the authors highlight some technical difficulties that still remain and advocate fluoroscopy backup in the operative room (81).

Peripheral Nerve Surgery

Another possible application of robot-assisted neurosurgery is in the field of peripheral nerve surgery. The improvement of peripheral nerve surgical repair with the use of the robot is possible, thanks to the elimination of the physiological tremor, which perturbs the operating movements, but also thanks to the multiplication of movements, which enhances the precision of such movements (82).

The first attempts to repair the brachial plexus using robot-assisted surgery was described by Mantovani et al. (83) with the da Vinci robot through an endoscopic approach. Results from de Melo et al. (84) also demonstrated the feasibility of endoscopic approach to nerve transfer with da Vinci robot in cadaver.

Miyamoto et al. (85) reported their clinical experience with the use of da Vinci robot in brachial plexus surgery. They described six cases of nerve transfer using the nerve to the long head of the triceps to the axillary nerve with good clinical postoperative results.

Robot-assisted peripheral nerve tumor surgery has also been described. Lequint et al. (86) reported good results in robot-assisted peripheral nerve surgery in a case of intraneural perineuroma. Also, Deboudt et al. (87) demonstrated the feasibility of robot-assisted laparoscopic resection of peripheral nerve schwannomas in two cases.

Other Neurosurgical Applications

Robotic technology is continuously evolving in the field of neurosurgery. Robot-assisted procedures have gained more applications during the

Table 14.2 Systematic review of articles published between 2006 and 2013 comparing robot-assisted pedicle screw placement versus fluoroscopy-guided surgery

Reference	Level of evidence	Study group	Key results	Other
Ringel et al. (67)	Single-center randomized controlled trial (level 2)	60 pts undergoing lumbosacral pedicle screw implantation randomized into two equal groups: 30 pts FG (n = 152 screws), and 30 pts RA (n = 146 screws)	FG: 142/152 (93%) screws satisfactory RA: 124/146 (85%) screws satisfactory ($p = 0.019$)	Ten RA screws required intraoperative revision, one FG screw required postoperative revision. Duration of surgery and radiation exposure was not significantly different with robotic assisted placement.
Roser et al. (14)	Single-center randomized controlled trial (level 2)	37 pts undergoing lumbosacral pedicle screw implantation randomized into three groups: 10 pts FG (n = 40 screws), 9 pts IG (n = 36 screws), and 18 pts RA (n = 72 screws)	FG: 39/40 (98%) screws satisfactory IG 33/36 (92%) screws satisfactory RA: 71/72 (99%) screws satisfactory	Study aims to recruit 30 pts per group. As preliminary results reported here, statistical analysis was not performed.
Schizas et al. (68)	Single-center prospective cohort study (level 3)	34 consecutive pts undergoing thoracolumbar pedicle screw implantation divided into two groups: 23 pts FG (n = 64 screws) and 11 pts RA (n = 64 screws)	FG: 59/64 (92%) screws satisfactory RA: 61/64 (95%) screws satisfactory ($p = 0.71$)	Radiation exposure was not significantly different
Kantelhardt et al. (65)	Single-center retrospective cohort study (level 3)	112 consecutive pts undergoing thoracolumbar pedicle screw implantation divided into two groups: 57 pts FG (n = 286 screws), and 55 pts RA (n = 250 screws)	FG: 262/286 (92%) screws satisfactory RA: 236/250 (95%) screws satisfactory ($p < 0.05$)	Radiation exposure was significantly less in robot-assisted cases ($p = 0.0001$). Duration of surgery was not significantly different.
Lieberman et al. (66)	Cadaveric study	12 cadavers underwent pedicle screw implantation divided into two groups: 2 cadavers FG (n = 37 screws), and 10 cadavers RA (n = 197 screws)	FG: 35/37 (95%) screws satisfactory RA: 194/197 (99%) screws satisfactory ($p = 0.082$)	Radiation exposure was significantly less in robot-assisted cases ($p < 0.001$). Duration of surgery was not significantly different.

Pts, patients; FG, fluoroscopy-guided; IG, image-guided (BrainLab VectorVision); RA, robot-assisted (SpineAssist)
Adapted from Marcus et al. (80).

past years. Besides the indications described above, some authors have reported interesting data of distinct applications. For example, Lollis and Roberts (88,89) have demonstrated good results with placement of ventricular catheters in the setting of small ventricules using SurgiScope. Barua et al. (90,91) have shown the feasibility of accurately and safely delivering small-diameter catheters to the brain for chemotherapy using the NeuroMate robot (Renishaw Plc., Gloucestershire, UK). Finally, Motkoski et al. (92) reported their initial clinical experience with a robot-assisted neurosurgical laser. The authors describe the design, preclinical experiments, and clinical experience with four cases of meningioma resection using a laser tool, specifically designed for NeuroArm robot.

Future Perspectives: Nanorobotics in Neurosurgery

Aside of improvement in visualization techniques and haptic feedback of neurorobots, the future of robotic neurosurgery involves the advancements in nanoneurosurgery – the neurosurgery at the nano level. It involves the use of nanodevices such as nanorobots to be introduced into the vascular system or body cavities, programmed and controlled remotely by the surgeon, in order to perform various diagnostic and therapeutic functions in a very precise and minimally invasive manner leading to faster recovery while communicating with the onsite surgeon through signals (93,94). Various applications have already been investigated in neurosurgery (95–102).

For example, spinal cord injury and nerve damage are areas that certainly will benefit from nanotechnology in near future (103,104). Despite the recent advancements in promoting regeneration of transected nerves and spinal cord via growth factors and enriched scaffolds (105), the difficulties and limitations persist in the ability to target at a small scale such as axons (106). Recently, technological advancements have led to the development of devices on nanoscale that allow manipulation of individual axons. A nanoknife with a diameter of 40 nanometer has been developed and found to be effective for axon surgery (107). Also, the use of dielectrophoresis, which involves the use of electrical fields to manipulate polarizable objects in space, has been found to be effective in achieving controlled movement of axons within a surgical field (108). Following controlled transection of axons and maneuvering them into position using dielectrophoresis, fusion between the two ends can be induced via electrofusion, polyethylene glycon, or laser-induced cell fusion, among other methods. It is certain that the development of cellular level robotic surgery will benefit neurosurgery in the future. The use of nanodevices a new dimension of precision and control with regard to the reconnection of nerves (109).

Another possible application of nanoneurosurgery is in cerebrovascular disorders. Besides applications in ischemic (110,111) and intracerebral hemorrhage (112), nanorobotics can present a potential option for screening of a new aneurysm or closer monitoring of an identified aneurysm. For instance, Cavalcanti et al. have proposed an intravascular nanorobot that can detect brain aneurysm formation by detecting increased levels of nitric oxide synthase protein within the affected blood vessel.

It is imperative that nanotechnology has progressed from a theoretical proposal to an active area of practical research and developments. The improvement in the ability of working in an ever-decreasing scale has been greatly accelerated by advances in manufacturing microelectomechanical systems. These advances may allow manipulation on the scale of individual cells and potentially on the molecular scale in the near future (113). In the future, neurosurgery will benefit from these developments in many areas, including detection of pathology, minimally invasive intracranial monitoring, and pharmaceutical delivery, among many others.

Final Considerations

The future of surgical robotics, in general, will include greater integration with surgical navigation modalities to give surgeons and robots a greater sense of anatomical awareness. Increases in the resolution of navigation systems and patient image data will result in the use of surgical robots in procedures requiring finer movements, such as microsurgery of the brain and spine. The ongoing challenges of surgical robotics are the high cost of technology development, the complexity of recreating human senses, and the limitations of computer processing.

Other areas of medicine have already begun the integration of robotic technologies into clinical practice. However, neurosurgery has been slow to adopt them because of the complexities of brain anatomy and physiology. As technology is continuously evolving, many groups around the world have demonstrated promising results in many robot-assisted neurosurgical procedures. As demonstrated in this chapter, interesting technologies have been developed specifically for neurosurgical use, although one of the current obstacles to widespread adoption is the need to demonstrate benefit in relation to cost. Besides the necessity of further technological development (especially regarding the improvement of haptic feedback and the design of more user-friendly interfaces), future clinical trials are required in order to evaluate the robotic technology in neurosurgical practice as well as to provide a fair comparative analysis of its outcomes in relation to current standard procedures.

References

1. Di Ieva A. Microtechnologies in neurosurgery. *Proc Inst Mech Eng H*. 2010;224(6):797–800.
2. Kwoh YS, Hou J, Jonckheere EA, Hayati S. A robot with improved absolute positioning accuracy for CT guided stereotactic brain surgery. *IEEE Trans Biomed Eng*. 1988;35(2):153–60.
3. Young RF. Application of robotics to stereotactic neurosurgery. *Neurol Res*. 1987;9(2):123–8.
4. Kwoh YS, Reed LS, Chen JY, Shao H, Truong TK, Jonckheere EA. A new computerized tomography aided robotic stereotactic system. *Robot Age*. 1985;7:17–21.
5. Smith JA, Jivraj J, Wong R, Yang V. 30 years of neurosurgical robots: review and trends for manipulators and associated navigational systems. *Ann Biomed Eng*. 2015.
6. Howe RD, Matsuoka Y. Robotics for surgery. *Annu Rev Biomed Eng*. 1999;1:211–40.
7. Barbash GI, Glied SA. New technology and health care costs – the case of robot-assisted surgery. *N Engl J Med*. 2010;363(8):701–4.
8. Bergeles C, Yang GZ. From passive tool holders to microsurgeons: safer, smaller, smarter surgical robots. *IEEE Trans Biomed Eng*. 2014;61(5):1565–76.
9. Gerber N, Gavaghan KA, Bell BJ, et al. High-accuracy patient-to-image registration for the facilitation of image-guided robotic microsurgery on the head. *IEEE Trans Biomed Eng*. 2013;60(4):960–8.
10. Benabid AL, Hoffmann D, Seigneuret E, Chabardes S. Robotics in neurosurgery: which tools for what? *Acta Neurochir Suppl*. 2006;98:43–50.
11. Adler JR, Jr. The future of robotics in radiosurgery. *Neurosurgery*. 2013;72 suppl 1:8–11.
12. Goto T, Hongo K, Yako T, et al. The concept and feasibility of EXPERT: intelligent armrest using robotics technology. *Neurosurgery*. 2013;72 suppl 1:39–42.
13. Kantelhardt SR, Finke M, Schweikard A, Giese A. Evaluation of a completely robotized neurosurgical operating microscope. *Neurosurgery*. 2013;72 suppl 1:19–26.
14. Roser F, Tatagiba M, Maier G. Spinal robotics: current applications and future perspectives. *Neurosurgery*. 2013;72 suppl 1:12–18.
15. Shaikhouni A, Elder JB. Computers and neurosurgery. *World Neurosurg*. 2012;78(5):392–8.
16. Sutherland G. Introduction to virtual reality and robotics in neurosurgery. *Neurosurgery*. 2013;72 suppl 1:7.
17. Sutherland GR, Lama S, Gan LS, Wolfsberger S, Zareinia K. Merging machines with microsurgery: clinical experience with neuroArm. *J Neurosurg*. 2013;118(3):521–9.
18. Alric M, Chapelle F, Lemaire JJ, Gogu G. Potential applications of medical and non-medical robots for neurosurgical applications. *Minim Invasive Ther Allied Technol*. 2009;18(4):193–216.
19. Dogangil G, Davies BL, Rodriguez y Baena F. A review of medical robotics for minimally invasive soft tissue surgery. *Proc Inst Mech Eng H*. 2010;224(5):653–79.
20. Kubben PL, Pouratian N. An open-source and cross-platform framework for Brain Computer Interface-guided robotic arm control. *Surg Neurol Int*. 2012;3:149.
21. Bertelsen A, Melo J, Sanchez E, Borro D. A review of surgical robots for spinal interventions. *Int J Med Robot*. 2013;9(4):407–22.
22. Mattei TA, Rodriguez AH, Sambhara D, Mendel E. Current state-of-the-art and future perspectives of robotic technology in neurosurgery. *Neurosurg Rev*. 2014;37(3):357–66; discussion 66.
23. Zhang Y, Zhao D, Li H, Li Y, Zhu X, Zhang X. Emerging new trends in neurosurgical technologies. *Cell Biochem Biophys*. 2014;70(1):259–67.
24. Mattei TA, Fassett DR. Letter to the editor: The O-arm revolution in spine surgery. *J Neurosurg Spine*. 2013;19(5):644–7.
25. Sakaguchi T. [Percutaneous puncture with a robot]. *Hinyokika Kiyo*. 1985;31(7):1265–8.
26. Drake JM, Joy M, Goldenberg A, Kreindler D. Computer- and robot-assisted resection of thalamic astrocytomas in children. *Neurosurgery*. 1991;29(1):27–33.
27. Lefranc M, Capel C, Pruvot-Occean AS, et al. Frameless robotic stereotactic biopsies: a consecutive series of 100 cases. *J Neurosurg*. 2015;122(2):342–52.
28. Bekelis K, Radwan TA, Desai A, Roberts DW. Frameless robotically targeted stereotactic brain biopsy: feasibility, diagnostic yield, and safety. *J Neurosurg*. 2012;116(5):1002–6.
29. Benabid AL, Cinquin P, Lavalle S, Le Bas JF, Demongeot J, de Rougemont J. Computer-driven robot for stereotactic surgery connected to CT scan and magnetic resonance imaging. Technological design and preliminary results. *Appl Neurophysiol*. 1987;50(1–6):153–4.
30. Haegelen C, Touzet G, Reyns N, Maurage CA, Ayachi M, Blond S. Stereotactic robot-guided biopsies of brain stem lesions: experience with 15 cases. *Neurochirurgie*. 2010;56(5):363–7.

31. Varma TR, Eldridge P. Use of the NeuroMate stereotactic robot in a frameless mode for functional neurosurgery. *Int J Med Robot*. 2006;2(2):107–13.

32. von Langsdorff D, Paquis P, Fontaine D. In vivo measurement of the frame-based application accuracy of the Neuromate neurosurgical robot. *J Neurosurg*. 2015;122(1):191–4.

33. Heuer GG, Zaghloul KA, Jaggi JL, Baltuch GH. Use of an integrated platform system in the placement of deep brain stimulators. *Neurosurgery*. 2008;62(3 suppl 1):245–7; discussion 7–8.

34. Eljamel MS. Robotic neurological surgery applications: accuracy and consistency or pure fantasy? *Stereotact Funct Neurosurg*. 2009;87(2):88–93.

35. Spire WJ, Jobst BC, Thadani VM, Williamson PD, Darcey TM, Roberts DW. Robotic image-guided depth electrode implantation in the evaluation of medically intractable epilepsy. *Neurosurg Focus*. 2008;25(3):E19.

36. Cardinale F, Cossu M, Castana L, et al. Stereoelectroencephalography: surgical methodology, safety, and stereotactic application accuracy in 500 procedures. *Neurosurgery*. 2013;72(3):353–66; discussion 66.

37. Lefranc M, Capel C, Pruvot AS, et al. The impact of the reference imaging modality, registration method and intraoperative flat-panel computed tomography on the accuracy of the ROSA(R) stereotactic robot.*Stereotact Funct Neurosurg*. 2014;92(4):242–50.

38. Gonzalez-Martinez J, Bulacio J, Thompson S, et al. Technique, results, and complications related to robot-assisted stereoelectroencephalography. *Neurosurgery*. 2015.

39. Gonzalez-Martinez J, Vadera S, Mullin J, et al. Robot-assisted stereotactic laser ablation in medically intractable epilepsy: operative technique. *Neurosurgery*. 2014;10 suppl 2:167–72; discussion 72–3.

40. Zimmermann M, Krishnan R, Raabe A, Seifert V. Robot-assisted navigated neuroendoscopy. *Neurosurgery*. 2002;51(6):1446–51; discussion 51–2.

41. Zimmermann M, Krishnan R, Raabe A, Seifert V. Robot-assisted navigated endoscopic ventriculostomy: implementation of a new technology and first clinical results. *Acta Neurochir (Wien)*. 2004;146(7):697–704.

42. Benabid AL, Lavallee S, Hoffmann D, Cinquin P, Demongeot J, Danel F. Potential use of robots in endoscopic neurosurgery. *Acta Neurochir Suppl (Wien)*. 1992;54:93–7.

43. Goto T, Hongo K, Kakizawa Y, et al. Clinical application of robotic telemanipulation system in neurosurgery. Case report. *J Neurosurg*. 2003;99(6):1082–4.

44. Hongo K, Kobayashi S, Kakizawa Y, et al. NeuRobot: telecontrolled micromanipulator system for minimally invasive microneurosurgery-preliminary results. *Neurosurgery*. 2002;51(4):985–8; discussion 8.

45. Takasuna H, Goto T, Kakizawa Y, Miyahara T, Koyama J, Tanaka Y, et al. Use of a micromanipulator system (NeuRobot) in endoscopic neurosurgery. *J Clin Neurosci*. 2012;19(11):1553–7.

46. Calisto A, Dorfmuller G, Fohlen M, Bulteau C, Conti A, Delalande O. Endoscopic disconnection of hypothalamic hamartomas: safety and feasibility of robot-assisted, thulium laser-based procedures. *J Neurosurg Pediatr*. 2014;14(6):563–72.

47. Hanna EY, Holsinger C, DeMonte F, Kupferman M. Robotic endoscopic surgery of the skull base: a novel surgical approach. *Arch Otolaryngol Head Neck Surg*. 2007;133(12):1209–14.

48. O'Malley BW, Jr., Weinstein GS. Robotic skull base surgery: preclinical investigations to human clinical application. *Arch Otolaryngol Head Neck Surg*. 2007;133(12):1215–9.

49. O'Malley BW, Jr., Weinstein GS. Robotic anterior and midline skull base surgery: preclinical investigations. *Int J Radiat Oncol Biol Phys*. 2007;69(2 suppl):S125–8.

50. Cabuk B, Ceylan S, Anik I, Tugasaygi M, Kizir S. A haptic guided robotic system for endoscope positioning and holding. *Turk Neurosurg*. 2015;25(4):601–7.

51. Wirz R, Torres LG, Swaney PJ, et al. An experimental feasibility study on robotic endonasal telesurgery. *Neurosurgery*. 2015;76(4):479–84; discussion 84.

52. Ozer E, Durmus K, Carrau RL, et al. Applications of transoral, transcervical, transnasal, and transpalatal corridors for robotic surgery of the skull base. *Laryngoscope*. 2013;123(9):2176–9.

53. Chauvet D, Missistrano A, Hivelin M, Carpentier A, Cornu P, Hans S. Transoral robotic-assisted skull base surgery to approach the sella turcica: cadaveric study. *Neurosurg Rev*. 2014;37(4):609–17.

54. Lee JY, Lega B, Bhowmick D, et al. Da Vinci robot-assisted transoral odontoidectomy for basilar invagination. *ORL J Otorhinolaryngol Relat Spec*. 2010;72(2):91–5.

55. Lee JY, O'Malley BW, Newman JG, et al. Transoral robotic surgery of craniocervical junction and atlantoaxial spine: a cadaveric study. *J Neurosurg Spine*. 2010;12(1):13–8.

56. Hong WC, Tsai JC, Chang SD, Sorger JM. Robotic skull base surgery via supraorbital keyhole approach: a cadaveric study. *Neurosurgery*. 2013;72 suppl 1:33–8.

57. Marcus HJ, Hughes-Hallett A, Cundy TP, Yang GZ, Darzi A, Nandi D. da Vinci robot-assisted keyhole neurosurgery: a cadaver study on feasibility and safety. *Neurosurg Rev*. 2015;38(2):367–71; discussion 71.

58. L'Orsa R, Macnab CJ, Tavakoli M. Introduction to haptics for neurosurgeons. *Neurosurgery*. 2013;72 suppl 1:139–53.

59. Arata J, Tada Y, Kozuka H, et al. Neurosurgical robotic system for brain tumor removal. *Int J Comput Assist Radiol Surg*. 2011;6(3):375–85.

60. Sutherland GR, Latour I, Greer AD, Fielding T, Feil G, Newhook P. An image-guided magnetic resonance-compatible surgical robot. *Neurosurgery*. 2008;62(2):286–92; discussion 92–3.

61. Pandya S, Motkoski JW, Serrano-Almeida C, Greer AD, Latour I, Sutherland GR. Advancing neurosurgery with image-guided robotics. *J Neurosurg*. 2009;111(6):1141–9.

62. Sutherland GR. Neurorobotics: driving the paradigm shift. *World Neurosurg*. 2014;81(5–6):668.

63. Spetzger U, Von Schilling A, Winkler G, Wahrburg J, Konig A. The past, present and future of minimally invasive spine surgery: a review and speculative outlook. *Minim Invasive Ther Allied Technol*. 2013;22(4):227–41.

64. Devito DP, Kaplan L, Dietl R, et al. Clinical acceptance and accuracy assessment of spinal implants guided with SpineAssist surgical robot: retrospective study. *Spine*. 2010;35(24):2109–15.

65. Kantelhardt SR, Martinez R, Baerwinkel S, Burger R, Giese A, Rohde V. Perioperative course and accuracy of screw positioning in conventional, open robotic-guided and percutaneous robotic-guided, pedicle screw placement. *Eur Spine J*. 2011;20(6):860–8.

66. Lieberman IH, Hardenbrook MA, Wang JC, Guyer RD. Assessment of pedicle screw placement accuracy, procedure time, and radiation exposure using a miniature robotic guidance system. *J Spinal Disord Tech*. 2012;25(5):241–8.

67. Ringel F, Stuer C, Reinke A, et al. Accuracy of robot-assisted placement of lumbar and sacral pedicle screws: a prospective randomized comparison to conventional freehand screw implantation. *Spine*. 2012;37(8):E496–501.

68. Schizas C, Thein E, Kwiatkowski B, Kulik G. Pedicle screw insertion: robotic assistance versus conventional C-arm fluoroscopy. *Acta Orthop Belg*. 2012;78(2):240–5.

69. Shoham M, Lieberman IH, Benzel EC, et al. Robotic assisted spinal surgery – from concept to clinical practice. *Comput Aided Surg*. 2007;12(2):105–15.

70. Sukovich W, Brink-Danan S, Hardenbrook M. Miniature robotic guidance for pedicle screw placement in posterior spinal fusion: early clinical experience with the SpineAssist. *Int J Med Robot*. 2006;2(2):114–22.

71. Lonjon N, Chan-Seng E, Costalat V, Bonnafoux B, Vassal M, Boetto J. Robot-assisted spine surgery: feasibility study through a prospective case-matched analysis. *Eur Spine J*. 2015.

72. Melzer A, Gutmann B, Remmele T, et al. INNOMOTION for percutaneous image-guided interventions: principles and evaluation of this MR- and CT-compatible robotic system. *IEEE Eng Med Biol Mag*. 2008;27(3):66–73.

73. Tovar-Arriaga S, Tita R, Pedraza-Ortega JC, Gorrostieta E, Kalender WA. Development of a robotic FD-CT-guided navigation system for needle placement-preliminary accuracy tests. *Int J Med Robot*. 2011;7(2):225–36.

74. Barzilay Y, Schroeder JE, Hiller N, et al. Robot-assisted vertebral body augmentation: a radiation reduction tool. *Spine*. 2014;39(2):153–7.

75. Cleary K, Watson V, Lindisch D, et al. Precision placement of instruments for minimally invasive procedures using a "needle driver" robot. *Int J Med Robot*. 2005;1(2):40–7.

76. Romanelli P, Adler JR, Jr. Technology Insight: image-guided robotic radiosurgery – a new approach for noninvasive ablation of spinal lesions. *Nat Clin Pract Oncol*. 2008;5(7):405–14.

77. Moskowitz RM, Young JL, Box GN, Pare LS, Clayman RV. Retroperitoneal transdiaphragmatic robotic-assisted laparoscopic resection of a left thoracolumbar neurofibroma. *JSLS*. 2009;13(1):64–8.

78. Beutler WJ, Peppelman WC, Jr., DiMarco LA. The da Vinci robotic surgical assisted anterior lumbar interbody fusion: technical development and case report. *Spine*. 2013;38(4):356–63.

79. Ascari L, Stefanini C, Bertocchi U, Dario P. Robot-assisted endoscopic exploration of the spinal cord. *Journal of Mechanical Engineering Science*. 2010;224(7):1515–29.

80. Marcus HJ, Cundy TP, Nandi D, Yang GZ, Darzi A. Robot-assisted and fluoroscopy-guided pedicle screw placement: a systematic review. *Eur Spine J*. 2014;23(2):291–7.

81. Schatlo B, Molliqaj G, Cuvinciuc V, Kotowski M, Schaller K, Tessitore E. Safety and accuracy of robot-assisted versus fluoroscopy-guided pedicle screw insertion for degenerative diseases of the lumbar spine: a matched cohort comparison. *J Neurosurg Spine*. 2014;20(6):636–43.

82. Nectoux E, Taleb C, Liverneaux P. Nerve repair in telemicrosurgery: an experimental study. *J Reconstr Microsurg*. 2009;25(4):261–5.

83. Mantovani G, Liverneaux P, Garcia JC, Jr., Berner SH, Bednar MS, Mohr CJ. Endoscopic exploration and repair of brachial plexus with telerobotic manipulation: a cadaver trial. *J Neurosurg*. 2011;115(3):659–64.

84. Porto de Melo PM, Garcia JC, Montero EF, et al. Feasibility of an endoscopic approach to the axillary nerve and the nerve to the long head of the triceps brachii with the help of the Da Vinci Robot. *Chir Main*. 2013;32(4):206–9.

85. Miyamoto H, Leechavengvongs S, Atik T, Facca S, Liverneaux P. Nerve transfer to the deltoid muscle using the nerve to the long head of the triceps with the da Vinci robot: six cases. *J Reconstr Microsurg*. 2014;30(6):375–80.

86. Lequint T, Naito K, Chaigne D, Facca S, Liverneaux P. Mini-invasive robot-assisted surgery of the brachial plexus: a case of intraneural perineurioma. *J Reconstr Microsurg*. 2012;28(7):473–6.

87. Deboudt C, Labat JJ, Riant T, Bouchot O, Robert R, Rigaud J. Pelvic schwannoma: robotic laparoscopic resection. *Neurosurgery*. 2013;72(1 suppl):2–5; discussion.

88. Lollis SS, Roberts DW. Robotic catheter ventriculostomy: feasibility, efficacy, and implications. *J Neurosurg*. 2008;108(2):269–74.

89. Lollis SS, Roberts DW. Robotic placement of a CNS ventricular reservoir for administration of chemotherapy. *Br J Neurosurg*. 2009;23(5):516–20.

90. Barua NU, Hopkins K, Woolley M, et al. A novel implantable catheter system with transcutaneous port for intermittent convection-enhanced delivery of carboplatin for recurrent glioblastoma. *Drug Deliv*. 2015:1–7.

91. Barua NU, Lowis SP, Woolley M, O'Sullivan S, Harrison R, Gill SS. Robot-guided convection-enhanced delivery of carboplatin for advanced brainstem glioma. *Acta Neurochir (Wien)*. 2013;155(8):1459–65.

92. Motkoski JW, Yang FW, Lwu SH, Sutherland GR. Toward robot-assisted neurosurgical lasers. *IEEE Trans Biomed Eng*. 2013;60(4):892–8.

93. Saini R, Saini S. Nanotechnology and surgical neurology. *Surg Neurol Int*. 2010;1:57.

94. Freitas RA, Jr. Nanotechnology, nanomedicine and nanosurgery. *Int J Surg*. 2005;3(4):243–6.

95. Elder JB, Liu CY, Apuzzo ML. Neurosurgery in the realm of 10(-9), Part 2: applications of nanotechnology to neurosurgery – present and future. *Neurosurgery*. 2008;62(2):269–84; discussion 84–5.

96. Elder JB, Liu CY, Apuzzo ML. Neurosurgery in the realm of 10(-9), Part 1: stardust and nanotechnology in neuroscience. *Neurosurgery*. 2008;62(1):1–20.

97. Saadeh Y, Leung T, Vyas A, Chaturvedi LS, Perumal O, Vyas D. Applications of nanomedicine in breast cancer detection, imaging, and therapy. *J Nanosci Nanotechnol*. 2014;14(1):913–23.

98. Khawaja AM. The legacy of nanotechnology: revolution and prospects in neurosurgery. *Int J Surg*. 2011;9(8):608–14.

99. Shah S, Solanki A, Lee KB. Nanotechnology-based approaches for guiding neural regeneration. *Acc Chem Res*. 2015.

100. Vidu R, Rahman M, Mahmoudi M, Enachescu M, Poteca TD, Opris I. Nanostructures: a platform for brain repair and augmentation. *Front Syst Neurosci*. 2014;8:91.

101. Leary SP, Liu CY, Apuzzo ML. Toward the emergence of nanoneurosurgery: part III – nanomedicine: targeted nanotherapy, nanosurgery, and progress toward the realization of nanoneurosurgery. *Neurosurgery*. 2006;58(6):1009–26; discussion 26.

102. Leary SP, Liu CY, Apuzzo ML. Toward the emergence of nanoneurosurgery: part II – nanomedicine: diagnostics and imaging at the nanoscale level. *Neurosurgery*. 2006;58(5):805–23; discussion -23.

103. White-Schenk D, Shi R, Leary JF. Nanomedicine strategies for treatment of secondary spinal cord injury. *Int J Nanomedicine*. 2015;10:923–38.

104. Tsintou M, Dalamagkas K, Seifalian AM. Advances in regenerative therapies for spinal cord injury: a biomaterials approach. *Neural Regen Res*. 2015;10(5):726–42.

105. Raspa A, Marchini A, Pugliese R, et al. A biocompatibility study of new nanofibrous scaffolds for nervous system regeneration. *Nanoscale*. 2015;8(1):253–65.

106. Chang WC, Hawkes E, Keller CG, Sretavan DW. Axon repair: surgical application at a subcellular scale. *Wiley Interdiscip Rev Nanomed Nanobiotechnol*. 2010;2(2):151–61.

107. Chang WC, Hawkes EA, Kliot M, Sretavan DW. In vivo use of a nanoknife for axon microsurgery. *Neurosurgery*. 2007;61(4):683–91; discussion 91–2.

108. Sretavan DW, Chang W, Hawkes E, Keller C, Kliot M. Microscale surgery on single axons. *Neurosurgery*. 2005;57(4):635–46; discussion -46.

109. Yang R, Song B, Sun Z, et al. Cellular level robotic surgery: nanodissection of intermediate filaments in live keratinocytes. *Nanomedicine.* 2015;11(1):137–45.

110. Gaurav C, Saurav B, Goutam R, Goyal AK. Nano-systems for advanced therapeutics and diagnosis of atherosclerosis. *Curr Pharm Des.* 2015;21(30):4498–508.

111. Lee HJ, Park J, Yoon OJ, et al. Amine-modified single-walled carbon nanotubes protect neurons from injury in a rat stroke model. *Nat Nanotechnol.* 2011;6(2):121–5.

112. Sang LY, Liang YX, Li Y, et al. A self-assembling nanomaterial reduces acute brain injury and enhances functional recovery in a rat model of intracerebral hemorrhage. *Nanomedicine.* 2015;11(3):611–20.

113. Roy S, Ferrara LA, Fleischman AJ, Benzel EC. Microelectromechanical systems and neurosurgery: a new era in a new millennium. *Neurosurgery.* 2001;49(4):779–97; discussion 97–8.

Chapter 15

Organ Transplant and Robotic Surgery

A Comprehensive Overview

Katherine Stammen, Sudipta Sen, Shilpadevi Patil, Michael Franklin, Gurleen Sidhu, Elyse M. Cornett, Charles J. Fox, and Alan David Kaye

Introduction

Laparoscopy is a minimally invasive surgical technique that incorporates fiberoptic cameras and small ports for access to decrease surgical complications and to improve patient outcomes [1]. The da Vinci surgical system (dVss) (Intuitive Surgical, Sunnyvale, CA, USA), the only FDA-approved surgical robot, is a computer-assisted electromechanical device acting as a remote telepresence manipulator controlled by a surgeon [2]. The dVss provides the operating surgeon with a 3D high-definition view with 10× to 15× magnification, fully restoring hand–eye coordination; it employs wristed instruments, with seven degrees of freedom; and it tracks surgeon's movements 1,300 times per second, providing for tremor filtration and scaled motion. Furthermore, the surgeon simultaneously drives the binocular endoscope, achieving steady view, and toggles between three operative arms [2]. These features translate into significant operative advantages, especially when the operative field is deep and narrow and when fine dissection and microsuturing are required.

Robotic surgery is a refined advancement in classic laparoscopic surgery. It is not a classical robot per se but rather a surgical electromechanical actuator, translating hand movements of the surgeon into wristed instrument actions, which assists in performing complex laparoscopic surgeries requiring fine dissection and microsuturing [3]. The robotic technique was first used for general surgery cases. After gaining enough experience in general surgery cases, it was then extended to organ transplant procedures, kidney transplant (KT) being the first. In 2000, the University of Chicago–Illinois was the first to successfully perform transabdominal hand-assisted robotic donor nephrectomy. Over 700 donor nephrectomies and 70 cases of KT have been performed successfully at the University of Chicago alone using the robotic system. Very few cases of pancreas and liver transplants have been performed worldwide. Robotic-assisted kidney transplantation (RKT) technique has been shown to be feasible and effective for both the donor and the recipient. More case numbers and studies are required to establish similar usefulness in pancreas and liver transplantation [1].

Overall, robotic surgery is a safe technique to accomplish complex surgical procedures in a minimally invasive way for patients with BMI of more than 30 who are more prone to surgical site infection. Additionally, it allows for the ability to manage different pathologies in the same sitting [4]. There is also the benefit of technical ease to the surgeons due to 3D high-definition view, great efficiency in microsuturing through the laparoscopic ports and wristed instruments through seven degrees of freedom, better ergonomics, and decreased surgeon fatigue [4].

Robotic surgery has decreased complication rates in a number of ways. There is a decrease in surgical site infections, which is especially important in organ recipients who are already immune-compromised and in obese patients as compared to classic laparoscopic and open cases [3]. Additionally, patients benefit from a decrease in surgical scarring, decrease in recovery period and early mobilization, increase in patient satisfaction and superior outcomes, smaller incisions with decreased pain and pulmonary complications, and decreased intraoperative blood loss and need for blood transfusion.

There are general concerns in utilizing this type of procedure. Conversions to an open procedure due to complications like intraoperative bleeding from a renal artery or vein, hematoma, chyloperitoneum, and bowel obstruction due to adhesions are all possibilities. Additionally, robotic surgery is costly. Technical failure is always a possibility [5]; a lack of direct contact between the patient and the surgeon, prolonged setup time, difficult instrument exchange with inexperienced surgeons, and need for experienced surgical teams mean that not all hospitals are equipped to handle this type of procedure.

Kidney Transplant

History

Kidney transplant (KT) is the treatment of choice for patients with stage V chronic kidney disease (CKD) as it provides better quality of life, better survival rates, and is cost-effective when compared with other treatment options such as hemodialysis or peritoneal dialysis [6]. Emerich Ullman from Vienna performed the first experimental KT in 1902 when he autotransplanted a dog's kidney from its normal anatomical site to the vessels of the neck, which resulted in urine flow.

Indications and Contraindications

Chronic kidney disease (CKD) is a multifactorial disease and characterized by a decrease in glomerular filtration rate (GFR). End-stage renal disease (ESRD) is established when the GFR falls to less than 15 ml/min [9].

GFR is estimated by the following formula (Modification of Diet in Renal Disease [MDRD] formula)

GFR = 175 × (standardized serum creatinine [mg/dl])$^{-1.154}$ × (Age)$^{-0.203}$ × 0.742(if female) or × 1.21 (if black)

Causes of CKD vary among the world populations. In the developing world, the leading causes of kidney failure include bacterial infection (tuberculosis, streptococcal infection), viruses (HIV, hepatitis B, and hepatitis C), parasites (malaria, leishmaniasis, and schistosomiasis), environmental, and occupational exposure (cadmium, mercury, and lead). In the developed countries, hypertension, obesity, diabetes, smoking, age, and cardiovascular disease are associated with CKD.

Absolute contraindications to renal transplant [11]:

1. Active malignancy
2. Active drug or alcohol addiction
3. Severe ischemic heart disease
4. Severe peripheral vascular disease
5. Severe pulmonary compromise
6. Transplant candidate with cirrhosis
7. Severe cognitive impairment
8. Noncompliance to therapy
9. Deep and persistent infections (e.g., aspergillus, empyema, active CMV, mycobacterial infections)
10. Human T cell lymphotopic virus 1 positivity
11. Pregnancy
12. Cervical and anal intraepithelial neoplasia III, carcinoma in situ associated with HPV infection

HIV type 1 has traditionally been considered as a contraindication for renal transplantation. Survival of HIV-positive patients has increased with lower rates of infection and better control of viral loads with highly active antiretroviral (HAART) therapy.

Box 15.1 KT in humans: timeline of events

Yurii Voronoy, 1933, Ukraine	First human deceased KT. Anastomosed renal vessels to the right femoral vessels in woman with acute renal failure due to mercury poisoning. Graft was rejected due to ABO incompatibly and the patient died after 2 days
Joseph Murray, 1954, Boston, USA	First successful transplant between two monozygotic twins
David Hume, 1954, Boston, USA	First successful deceased transplant
L. E. Ratner, 1995, Baltimore, USA	Laparoscopic donor nephrectomy introduced
J. S. Wolf, 1998, Ann Arbor, USA	Introduced hand-assisted transperitoneal donor nephrectomy
I. S. Gill, 2004, Cleveland, USA	Described single-port transumbilical live donor nephrectomy (natural orifice transluminal endoscopic surgery – NOTES)
E. Renoult, 2006, France	Introduced robot-assisted laparoscopic donor nephrectomy
P. Modi, 2011, India	Introduced laparoscopic KT
P. Giulianotti, 2010, Chicago, USA	Described a technique for RKT

Source: Data taken from [7,8].

Table 15.1 Classification of CKD

Stage	Category	GFR (ml/min/1.73 m^2)
1	Kidney damage with normal or increased GFR	≥90
2	Mild	60–89
3	Moderate	30–59
4	Severe	15–29
5	ESRD	<15 or on dialysis

Source: Data taken from [9].

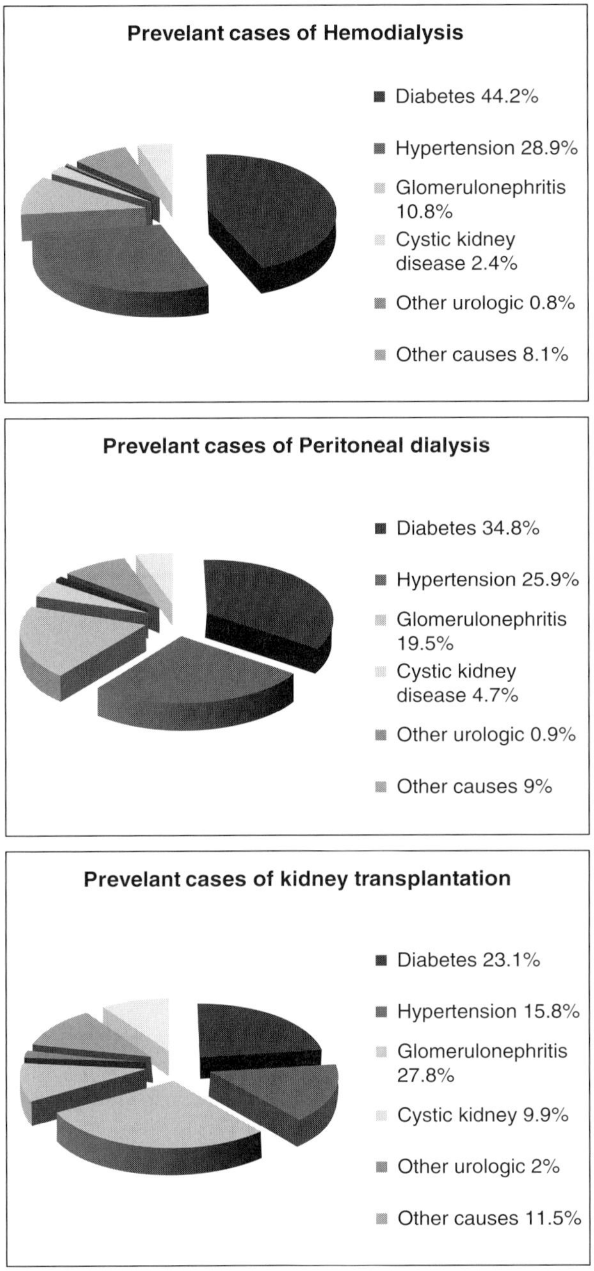

Figure 15.1 Prevalent cases of hemodialysis, peritoneal dialysis, and KT. Original graphs created with data from [10].

Guidelines for renal transplantation in an HIV-infected patient [11]:

1. Life expectancy of at least 5 years
2. Adherence to HAART therapy for at least 6 months
3. CD4 counts of greater than 200 cells/microliter on HAART therapy for at least 6 months
4. HIV viral load of less than 50 HIV-1 RNA copies per milliliter on HAART therapy for at least 6 months
5. AIDS-defining illnesses should be absent

Kidney Donors

There are an increasing number of patients on the KT list. Statistics from the United Network for Organ Sharing from March 2016 indicate about 100,457 candidates are awaiting a KT in the United States alone. Standard criteria donor is defined as one who is 10–39 years old, normotensive with a predonation serum creatinine level of less than 1.5 mg/dl, and cause of death was not due to cerebrovascular accident. In order to expand the donor pool, the expanded criteria donor (ECD) is being used. ECD is used only in those patients who are willing to accept them.

An ECD is defined as:

1. A brain-dead donor aged more than 60 years
2. A donor aged more than 50 years with two additional risk factors:
   a. History of hypertension
   b. Death resulting from cerebrovascular accident
   c. Serum creatinine greater of 1.5 mg/dl or greater

ECD should not be used in patients undergoing retransplantation or those who are less than 40 years, old. Outcome data from use of ECD in patients more than 40 years, especially with diabetic nephropathy or patients who are not diabetic but have a long expected wait time for KT, show better survival rates with an ECD kidney as compared to remaining on dialysis therapy [12].

Live Kidney Donation

Live kidney donation is voluntary, and the best interest of the donor is kept in mind. The Amsterdam forum has established guidelines for live kidney donation (Box 15.2).

A live donor transplant program enables the recipient and donor surgery to be performed simultaneously. A short ischemia time from removal of kidneys from the donor to restoration of blood flow in the recipient results in high-volume urine output, immediate graft function, and initiation of creatinine

Box 15.2 Guidelines for Live Kidney Donation (Data Taken from [13])

1. BP must be less than 140/90 mmHg
2. BMI less than 35 kg/m^2
3. GFR greater than 80 ml/min
4. No proteinuria (urine proteins less than 300 mg/24 hours)
5. Negative urine analysis for erythrocytes
6. Nondiabetic donors
7. Medical renal disease such as urinary tract infection
8. Significant history of renal stones
9. No malignancy
10. Minimal or no cardiovascular and pulmonary risk
11. Obligatory alcohol abstinence and smoking cessation

clearance. Surgical practices have evolved over the years from open lumbotomy and mini-incision muscle splitting open donor nephrectomy to minimally invasive laparoscopic techniques. The introduction of minimally invasive techniques – such as standard laparoscopic, hand-assisted laparoscopic, hand-assisted retroperitoneoscopic, pure retroperitoneoscopic, and robot-assisted donor nephrectomy – has resulted in decreased analgesic requirements, hospital stay, and fewer days off work [13,14].

Robotic Donor Nephrectomy for Live Donor KT

A systematic literature review conducted by Giacomoni et al. out of Italy concluded the benefits of total robotic surgery and hand-assisted robotic nephrectomy. Surgeons' comfort, easier suturing, ease of dissection, and accurate graft preservation were emphasized in this review. Out of the five papers analyzed, no case of donor deaths or complication greater than a Clavien score of 2 were reported [15].

Renoult et al. compared RDN with open donor nephrectomy and reported longer warm ischemic times and operative times with RDN (186 vs. 113 min) and shorter hospital stays with RDN (5.84±1.8 vs. 9.69±2.2 days). The longer warm ischemic times had no adverse effects on short-term graft function. Donor kidneys in both groups started functioning immediately after transplant and serum creatinine levels were equivalent for all donors at 5 days and 1 month after the surgery. Deep venous thrombosis was reported in one patient in the RDN group and one patient in the open group developed acute pyelonephritis [16].

Robotic Kidney Transplant – Surgical Considerations and Outcomes

Giulianotti et al. from Chicago were the first to report a truly RKT in 2009. The surgery took 223 min to perform with a warm ischemia time of 50 min [17]. Case report by Boggi et al. from Europe performed a similar hand-assisted RKT with a warm ischemia time of 51 min [3].

Detailed outcomes after RKT have been reported by three studies. Oberholzer et al. performed RKT on 28 obese patients and compared it to a frequency-matched retrospective cohort of obese patients undergoing open KT. No surgical site infections were noted in the RKT group when compared with the control group (8/28 patients). Only one wound complication of subcutaneous hematoma and wound dehiscence was noted in a patient on Coumadin therapy in the RKT group. Serum creatinine levels and patient and graft survival at 6-month follow-up were comparable between the two groups. These authors pointed out an important issue of enabling obese patients to access KT by reducing complication rates in the high BMI patient population [18].

Tsai et al. described a retroperitoneal approach to RKT in 10 patients with warm ischemia time of 67.4±22.3 min. The average ischemic time was 283.3±51.9 min for live donor transplantation and 630.7±76.6 min from deceased donor. None of the patients in this group experienced any wound complications. The average creatinine at the time of discharge in all 10 patients was 1.31±0.31 mg/dl [19].

Study done by Menon et al. (50 patients) used regional hypothermia during vascular anastomosis with RKT when compared with the previous two studies that were performed under warm ischemia. The donor graft was cooled with an ice jacket, which cooled the kidney and enabled atraumatic handling of the donor organ. The recipient pelvic bed was cooled to 18–20°C with ice slush, and vascular anastomosis was performed under regional hypothermia. Mean warm ischemia time was about 2.4 min and all grafts functioned immediately after surgery. Serum creatinine at the time of discharge was 1.3 mg/dl on an average. No patient was converted from RKT to open KT in this study. No surgical site infections, wound complications, or anastomotic leaks were reported [8].

Initial experience with the use of robotics for KT is beneficial in obese patients. Transperitoneal and extraperitoneal approaches to KT are possible. Regional hypothermia when used has been proven to be beneficial in improving early graft function. Time of anastomosis using robotics depends on the experience of the surgeon. Currently the high cost associated with RKT is the most prohibitive factor for its widespread use.

Anesthesia

Preoprative Evaluation

Patients with ESRD have several risk factors and associated medical diseases. Table 15.2 summarizes common clinical manifestations seen with ESRD.

According to ACC/AHA preoperative guidelines, patients who need emergency surgery such as a KT must proceed to the operating room. Perioperative surveillance, postoperative risk stratification, and risk factor management must continue in the perioperative period. Most patients are on the waitlist before an organ becomes available; as a result, cardiac assessment is recommended in patients with active cardiac conditions. Dialysis, if indicated, is done with 24 hours of the transplant. The dialysis records should be reviewed and pre- and posttransplant weight should be noted as overzealous dialysis resulting in more than 2 kg weight loss can suggest intravascular volume depletion resulting in severe hypotension during the induction of anesthesia. The following routine investigations are reviewed during patient assessment (Box 15.3).

Intraoperative Management

General anesthesia is the preferred technique for KT. Neuraxial anesthesia such as epidural or combined spinal epidural could possibly be performed; however, before choosing this technique, careful consideration must be given to the following in patients with ESRD.

- Altered platelet function
- Uremic bleeding tendency
- Effect of residual heparin after dialysis
- Altered coagulation profile due to coexisting hepatic disease

A large-bore peripheral intravenous line is inserted before induction of anesthesia. Following the induction of anesthesia, a central venous line is placed. Patients with comorbid conditions may require monitoring with an arterial line, pulmonary artery catheter, or transesophageal ECHO. Careful attention must be given to positioning of the patient. Shunts and fistulas for dialysis must be palpated for a thrill.

Administration of normal saline (NS) has been the standard of care for fluid management in patients undergoing KT. The rationale for this practice is

Table 15.2 Clinical manifestations seen with ESRD

Organ system affected	Clinical manifestations
Cardiovascular	Accelerated atherosclerosis, hypertension, left ventricular hypertrophy, congestive heart failure, pulmonary edema, pericarditis, cardiomyopathy, hyperdynamic circulation
Respiratory	Pulmonary congestion, uremic lung characterized by perihilar congestion
Electrolytes	Hyponatremia, hyperkalemia, metabolic acidosis, hyperuricemia, hypercalcemia, hyperphosphatemia, volume expansion
Gastrointestinal	Nausea, vomiting, gastroparesis, pancreatitis, peptic ulcer, bleeding
Hematological	Anemia, platelet dysfunction, B- and T-cell dysfunction
Musculoskeletal	Uremic osteodystrophy (osteomalacia, osteosclerosis, osteitis fibrosa cystica), muscle weakness
Neurological	Fatigue, encephalopathy, dementia, seizures, myoclonus, asterexis, peripheral neuropathy, autonomic dysfunction such as postural hypotension, dialysis disequilibrium syndrome (dehydration, weakness, hypotension, nausea, vomiting, seizures and coma due to changes in ECF volume, electrolyte composition, and cerebral edema)
Endocrine	Vitamin D deficiency, secondary hyperparathyroidism, hypertriglyceridemia, carbohydrate intolerance, diabetes

Source: Data taken from [9].

Box 15.3 Patient Assessment Investigations (Data Taken from [9])

Laboratory

- HLA typing class 1 and 2 and transplant immunology
- ABO
- Complete blood count, platelet, PT, PTT, INR
- Fasting blood sugar
- Calcium, magnesium, phosphate, ALP, AST, LDH, urea, creatinine, uric acid
- Sodium, potassium, chloride, CO_2
- Total bilirubin, direct bilirubin, albumin, total protein
- Total cholesterol, LDL, triglycerides, HDL

Urine

- Urine culture and analysis

Infectious/serology

- Hepatitis B and C
- CMV
- EBV
- HIV
- Varicella

Radiological

- Chest X-ray
- 12-lead EKG

Other

- Mammogram for females more than 50 years of age (within 12 months)
- PSA for men more than 45 years of age
- PAP smear for all adult females (within 6 months)

avoidance of potassium-containing fluids such as Ringer's lactate, which can contribute to intraoperative hyperkalemia. However, the administration of large volumes of NS could result in hyperchloremic metabolic acidosis, which causes an extracellular shift of potassium leading to hyperkalemia. NS administration is attributed to the dilution of extracellular bicarbonate. Chloride content in NS has a greater effect on total body chloride when compared to total body sodium. Potential nephrotoxic drugs must be avoided while administering an anesthetic in patients undergoing KT and in potential kidney donors (Table 15.3).

The use of succinylcholine for rapid sequence intubation must be determined on a case-to-case basis. Patients who present with hyperkalemia or who have uremic polyneuropathy are not ideal candidates for the use of this drug. Vecuronium and Rocuronium are metabolized by the liver and excreted by the kidneys. Active metabolites produced by the liver can accumulate after repeated administration, resulting in prolonged neuromuscular block. Atracurium and Cisatracurium are metabolized by Hoffman elimination and not affected by ESRD. There is a theoretical risk of accumulation of Laudanosine, an active metabolite of Atracurium and Cisatracurium, which can potentially result in convulsions. Laudanosine is partially excreted by the kidneys; however, the concentration found after clinical administration is well below the levels needed for CNS stimulant activity.

Fluoride-induced nephrotoxicity is a potential hazard after administration of volatile anesthetics as inorganic fluoride ions are produced as a metabolic byproduct by these agents. "Rule of 2" helps in determining the amount of anesthetic agent metabolized by the body.

- Desflurane 0.02 percent
- Isoflurane 0.2 percent
- Enflurane 2 percent
- Sevoflurane 2–3 percent
- Halothane 12–20 percent

Subclinical renal toxicity is seen when the concentration of serum inorganic fluoride reaches 50–80 mmol per liter. Clinical nephrotoxicity is seen with levels more than 80 mmol per liter.

Sodium and barium hydroxide lime absorbents react with Sevoflurane and a nephrotoxic byproduct compound A (fluromethyl-2-2-difluoro-1-trifluoromethy vinyl ether) is generated. A fresh gas flow of 1 L/min or more is recommended by the FDA for exposures up to 1 hour and at least 2 L/min when the exposure is greater than 1 hour to avoid accumulation of compound A.

Morphine and meperidine produce active metabolites (morphine 6 glucoronide and normeperidine, respectively), which are eliminated by the kidney and should be, therefore, avoided in patients with ESRD.

Postoperative Management

After extubation, KT patients need specialized nursing care with strict monitoring of urine output and adequate pain control (Table 15.3). Urine output

Table 15.3 Safety profiles of commonly used anesthetic drugs

	Use	Avoid
Volatile anesthetics	Sevoflurane, Isoflurane Desflurane	Enflurane
Induction agents	Propofol, Thiopental	Etomidate
Neuromuscular blockers	Succinycholine (if K <5.5 mEq/l) Cisatracurium Atracurium Rocuronium (±) Vecuronium (±)	Pancuronium
Intraoperative opioids	Fentanyl, Alfentanil Sufentanil, Remifentanil	Morphine, Meperidine
Postoperative analgesics	Morphine, Fentanyl Hydromorphone	NSAIDS COX 2 inhibitors Acetaminophen

Source: Data taken from [20].

is replaced 1:1 during the first 24 hours with NS. Electrolyte replacement is performed separately. Nephrotoxic agents are avoided and immunosuppressant medications are continued postoperatively. Once graft function stabilizes, fluid replacement is decreased to 50 percent of urine output within the next 48 hours and eventually to maintenance IVF. Diet is gradually advanced [21].

Complications in the Early Postoperative Period

Vomiting, pulmonary aspiration, delayed respiratory depression, pulmonary edema, hypertension, or hypotension are possible complications after KT. Mortality after KT is due to cardiac complications in about 33 percent of cases, and this risk is increased in patients with diabetes mellitus (DM), coronary artery disease, and who are more than 60 years.

Major complications such as delayed graft function, graft rejection, and infection are possible. Delayed graft function presents with oliguria, anuria, plateauing, or increase in serum creatinine despite adequate fluid therapy and blood pressure. Surgical causes (venous occlusion, arterial occlusion, bladder obstruction) are ruled out by Doppler and ultrasound evaluation. Dialysis is often needed within the first week of transplantation.

Bacterial infection is commonly seen during the first 4 weeks after transplant. Viral infection (CMV, EBV, HSV, BK polyoma virus) is seen between 4 to 26 weeks especially in patients who are on antithymocyte globulin.

Most cases of graft rejection are reversible. Serum creatinine levels are elevated and diagnosis is established by a renal biopsy [22].

Pancreas Transplant

History

According to the Centers for Disease Control recent diabetes factsheet in 2014, a total of 21 million people, or almost 9 percent of the population, in the United States are diagnosed with DM, with at least 2 million having type 1 DM [23]. Hyperglycemia is the hallmark of both type 1 and type 2 diabetes, but the pathogenesis leading to it differs between the two [24]. Type 1 diabetes occurs when pancreatic beta-cells are destroyed and the patient is insulin-deficient, which is usually the result of an autoimmune process. Type 2 diabetics have defects in both insulin secretion and action [24]. The discovery of exogenous insulin in 1922 changed the treatment of DM type 1 forever, changing it from a rapidly fatal disease to a chronic, incurable illness with long-term sequela that were typical of type 2 DM [25]. These long-term consequences include retinopathy, nephropathy, nephropathy, vasculopathy, and constant monitoring and adjustment of blood glucose levels. Hyperglycemia, especially if exacerbated by hypertension, is the major determinant factor for the development of major complications related to diabetes [26,27]. Tight glycemic control can limit the rate of progression of complications related in DM type 1 as shown by the Diabetes Control and Complications Trial. Although improvements have been made, tight glycemic control is a challenge for a number of patients [28]. Options for tight glycemic control include a constant monitoring of glucose levels and infusion of insulin to counteract hyperglycemia and pancreas transplantation [28]. Pancreas transplantation provides the only proven method to restore intrinsic glycemic control in patients with type 1 DM and some select patients in type 2 DM [29]. The first pancreas transplant took place in the United States in 1966 at the University of Minnesota [24]. Since that time, more than 30,000 pancreas transplants have been reported

Table 15.4 Types of rejection and immune responses

Type of rejection	Time	Immune response
Hyper acute	Immediate	B cells
Accelerated	2–5 days	B cells
Acute	1 week to 3 months	T cells
Chronic	3 months to years	B and T cells

Table 15.5 Contraindications to pancreas transplant

Absolute	Relative
Significant cardiac disease	Age >55 years
Irreversible hepatic or pulmonary disease	Symptomatic peripheral vascular disease
Active infection	Severe aorto-iliac disease
Recent malignancy	
Substance abuse	
Severe psychiatric illness	
Noncompliance	

Source: Data taken from [28].

in the International Pancreas Transplant Registry (IPTR; [29]). There are three main categories of pancreas transplantation: simultaneous pancreas kidney (SPK), pancreas after kidney (PAK), and pancreas-alone transplant (PAT; [28]. Donor sites can be either cadaveric or live donors [24]. Advancements in surgical technique and immunosuppressive agents have improved outcomes with graft survival rates of 85, 72, and 60 percent at 1, 5, and 10 years, respectively, after SPK [30]. Pancreas transplant recipients still have a higher incidence of surgical complications (around 25–30 percent) [29]. This is thought to be possibly related to their primary disease process (DM) and an organ that is highly prone to inflammation and autodigestion [29]. Recently, surgeons have started to use the advantages of robotic surgery to decrease the morbidity related to surgical site infections, fascial dehiscence, late incisional hernias, and possibly decreased length of hospital stay [31]. To date, there are only four groups that have published their experience with robot-assisted pancreatic resection combined with an autologous islet cell transplantation [32].

Indications and Contraindications

The primary indication for a pancreas transplant is the presence of diabetic complications due to hyperglycemia. Progressive secondary complications such as nephropathy, blindness, and vasculopathy leading to amputations are not uncommon. In the infancy of pancreas transplants, the procedure was restricted to those patients only with DM type 1 [28], but it was completed in patients who were considered to have type 2 DM [24]. The patient became insulin dependent even though beta cell function was present, indicated by high C-peptide levels. As with any medical decision, the risk versus benefit needs to be individualized for each patient. Benefits include physiologic insulin regulation, freedom from the daily procedures involved in tight glucose control, and, most importantly, a decrease in morbidity and possible increased mortality of poorly controlled diabetes [5]. The main risks are the inherent risks associated with a major surgical procedure and immunosuppression. It is important also that the patient is able to physiologically withstand the procedure; therefore, patients with significant cardiovascular disease are an absolute contraindication to the procedure. Other relative contraindications include peripheral vascular disease, poorly controlled psychiatric disease, morbid obesity, substance abuse, noncompliance, and any recent malignancy [25].

There are specific criteria for each of the three transplant categories that patients must meet to be considered. For PTA, patients are eligible if they have two or more diabetic complications that have not yet led to end-organ damage, including early nephropathy, microalbuminuria with preserved renal function (normal serum creatinine and creatinine clearance), and labile glycemic control with hypoglycemic unawareness [25]. For patients to qualify for SPK, they must have nephropathy with creatinine clearance <40 ml/min and be on dialysis or near to initiation of dialysis [28]. SPK transplant should be considered the primary option for patients with type 1 DM who do not have an HLA-identical live donor available [25]. Criteria for PAK are the same for PTA, but the renal allograft should be stable and have a creating clearance >40 ml/min.

Surgical Considerations

The allograft to be transplanted can come from either a cadaveric donor or a live donor. Optimal donors are those who are young (<55 years), nondiabetic, normal body weight, and without significant atherosclerotic

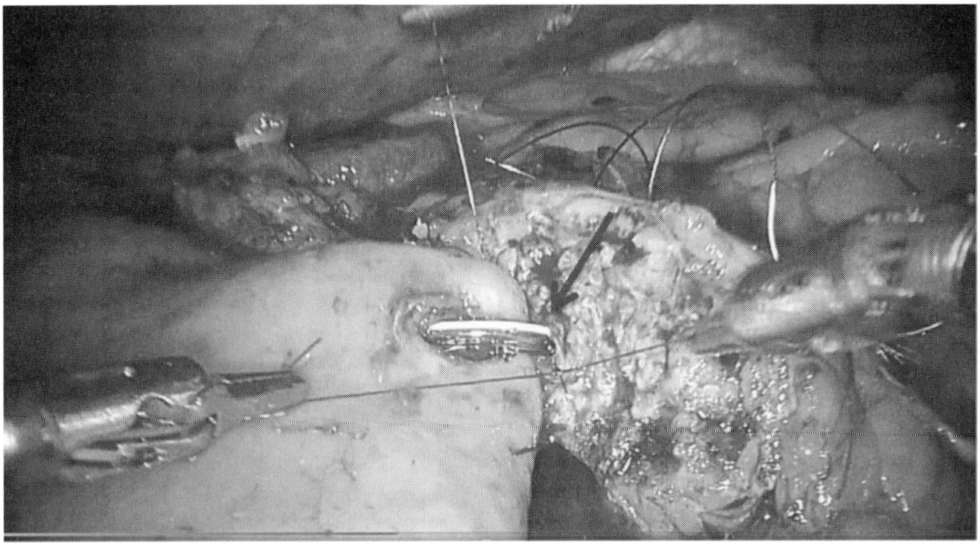

Figure 15.2 Pancreatojejunostomy with pancreatic duct stent (blue arrow) and demonstration of roboticintracorporeal suturing. Permissions from [32].

disease [25]. During removal from a cadaveric donor, the pancreas, duodenum, and spleen are perfused in situ with cold solution and then removed en bloc with the liver. The liver is then separated at 4°C. If a live donor, allografts are taken as segmental grafts from the body and tail of the pancreas [24]. Regardless of which technique is employed – SPK, PTA, or PAK transplantation – the technical aspects are the same. The recipient pancreas is left in place, as it may have some physiologic function. The pancreaticoduodenal allograft is placed in an ectopic location, usually the right iliac fossa as the vasculature is more superficial than the left and the position of the right iliac vessels to not require vascular realignment. It is important that the pancreas allograft is placed intraperitoneally as this is associated with fewer peripancreatic fluid collections and wound complications. If a kidney allograft is being transplanted, it is transplanted in the contralateral iliac fossa [28]. Venous drainage is achieved by anastomosing the donor graft portal vein to the recipient iliac vein or inferior vena cava. An alternative is portal venous drainage through the portal vein of the allograft to the superior mesenteric artery of the recipient, which is debated to have more of a physiologic drainage [28]. Portal venous drainage may result in peripheral hyperinsulinemia, but that is not uncommon in the majority of transplant recipients. The method of venous drainage has not been shown to have any outcome differences and the ultimate determining factor is typically the patient's anatomy [28].

Another variation in transplantation of the pancreas is the drainage of the pancreatic exocrine secretions, which is either completed by bladder drainage (BD) or drainage into the small intestine (enteric drainage – ED), which is determined by where the duodenum is anastomosed [25]. According to the IPTR through 1995, more than 90 percent of all pancreas transplants worldwide were bladder-drained. Comparisons of the benefits and drawbacks of the two can be seen in Table 15.6. Overall, the long-term graft survival, thrombosis, and function rates are similar between the two techniques. Since the mid-1990s, ED has been gaining increasing popularity due to decreased risk of urologic complications and improvements in surgical technique, immunosuppressive therapy, and imaging [24].

As of 2015, only four groups have published their experience with robot-assisted pancreas transplant [30], with the largest case-series of six patients. Preliminary data show that robot-assisted pancreas transplants were well tolerated, where the mean operative time did not change significantly and mean warm ischemia time was comparable to open procedures [29]. The technique by Galvani et al. closely resembled the open technique, but preservation of the vascular supply was kept until the very end to minimize warm ischemia time [30].

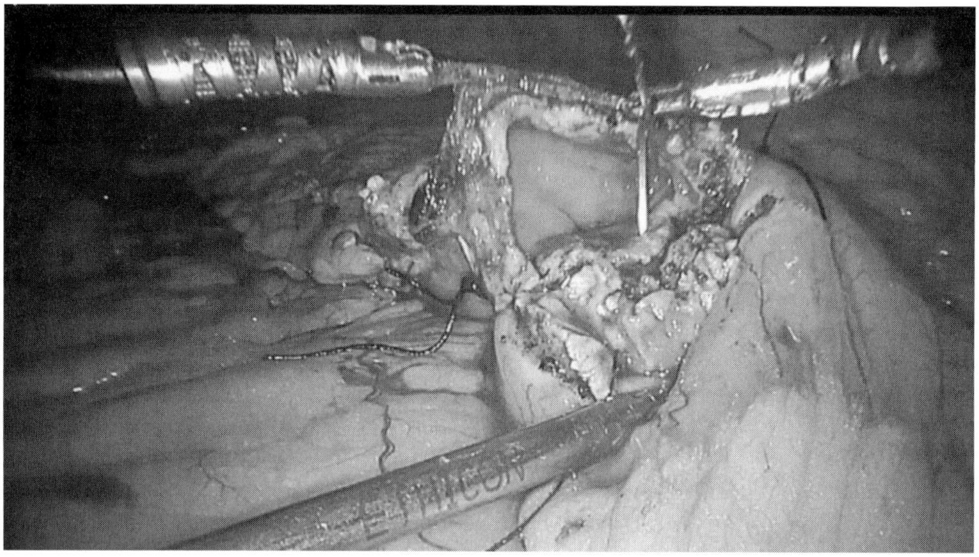

Figure 15.3 Intracorporeal robotic suturing of posterior layer of duodenojejunostomy. Permissions from [32].

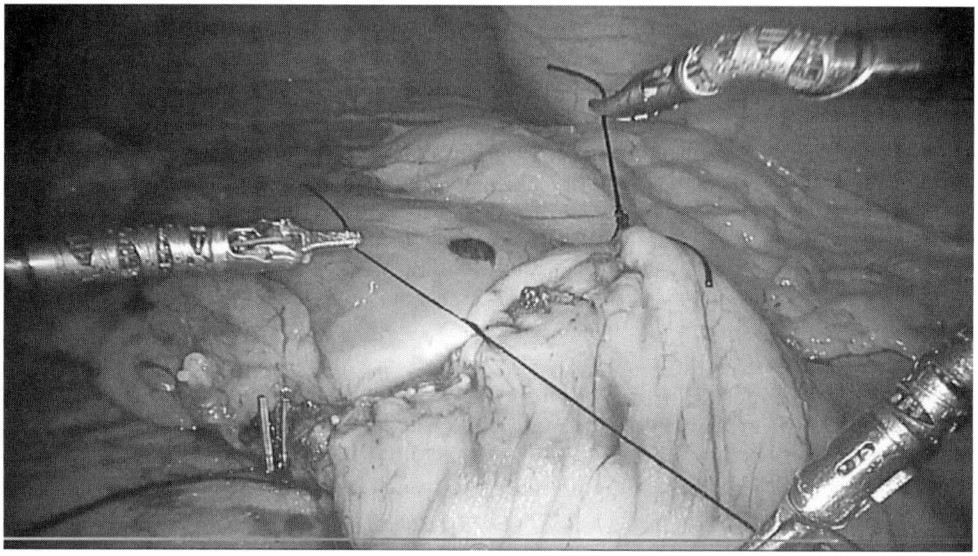

Figure 15.4 Intracorporeal suturing of anterior layer of duodenojejunostomy. Permissions from [32].

Anesthetic Management

Prior to surgery, the patient must be completely evaluated with a history and physical examination. Pertinent laboratory and imaging tests should be reviewed. Attention should be given to patients who have decreased renal function and their current metabolic values. Also, those with renal failure should be within 0.5 kg of their ideal body weight [28]. Also, particular attention should be given to diabetic complications, such as autonomic gastroparesis and orthostatic hypotension [28]. Type and cross should also be sent in anticipation of possibility of the need for transfusion.

Premedication should be administered if pertinent. In patients with significant gastroparesis, premedication with ranitidine, metoclopramide, or even

Table 15.6 Comparison of BD and ED of pancreas exocrine secretions

BD	ED
Intravascular volume depletion	Diabetic enteropathy contraindication
Metabolic acidosis	Increased gastrointestinal bleeding
Increased risk of reflux pancreatitis	Increased incidence of peritonitis
Increased urinary tract complications	Unable to monitor urine amylase
Able to monitor urine amylase for rejection (esp. SPK)	Fewer urologic complications

sodium citrate may be necessary. Anxiolysis should be given if appropriate. Typically a glucose infusion of dextrose 10 percent and insulin infusion are started preoperatively [29].

Routine American Society of Anesthesiologists monitors should always be used. In addition, ST segment analysis is helpful. Invasive arterial pressure monitoring is essential as there is a potential for blood loss, rapid swings in blood pressure, and periodic assessment of acid–base balance and blood glucose [28]. Central venous access is also usually necessary for access, fluid guidance, and use postoperatively as the patient will likely require total parental nutrition for up to 10 days postoperatively. Use of a neuromuscular junction monitoring device is also suggested. During the maintenance phase of anesthesia, a volatile, narcotic-based anesthetic is favored, but total intravenous anesthesia could be used also. Cisatracurium is the common neuromuscular blocker of choice in renal failure patients, but rocuronium and vecuronium have been used without sequelae. For open techniques, epidural anesthesia may be an appropriate adjunct to the maintenance phase, but is likely more commonly used for postoperative pain management, as the procedure typically lasts 3 to 5 hours [28]. An epidural is unlikely to be of benefit to robotic-assisted pancreas transplantation.

After induction, the monoclonal antibody basiliximab is given, as well as methylprednisone. Antibiotic coverage is routinely administered. A nasogastric tube is also placed, which will assist with surgical exposure and a rout for medication administration postoperatively. Tidal volumes of 8–10 mL/kg with low PEEP are preferred. This may need to be adjusted if robotic approach is used as the increased intraabdominal pressures after initiation of pneumoperitoneum and steep Trendelenburg positioning may increase ET-CO_2 without changes in ventilator management [33]. Maintenance fluids should be crystalloids, as colloids may worsen graft edema after surgery. Normovolemia and normotension are the goals during the procedure. Monitoring of blood glucose is especially important during the time of anastomosis, at which time it should be checked every 15 min to monitor for profound hypoglycemia requiring a dextrose infusion [28]. After reperfusion of the allograft, profound hypotension may occur due to the release of iliac vessel clamps. Metabolic abnormalities are often common after reperfusion and treatment of hyperkalemia and academia due to nonperfusion of the lower extremities. It is common to volume-load and correct metabolic abnormalities with either calcium chloride or bicarbonate prior to the release of the cross-clamp to circumvent this hypotension. Ionotropic and vasopressor agents should be readily available at this stage. If a SPK transplant is performed, mannitol and furosemide are commonly given to promote diuresis [28].

Postoperatively, the patient should be cared for in a critical care unit with special attention to acid–base status, oxygenation, respiratory parameters, fluid management, nutritional status, hematologic, and metabolic derangements.

Recovery/Prognosis

Immunosuppression is also a mainstay of transplant surgery. In a review of transplants from 1966 to 2008, the majority of patients received antibody therapy induction followed by a maintenance of Tacrolimus in combination with MMF, with a trend toward Sirolimus-based protocols for maintenance [30].

The goal of transplantation is to have a functional long-term graft survival. Until recently, pancreas transplantation was limited in part to early pancreatic graft thrombosis (3–12 percent) within the first year [25]. Early after transplant, thrombosis is multifactorial but after 2 weeks is mainly due to inflammation [24]. Most centers employ some form of anticoagulation, with aspirin, unfractionated, or low-molecular-weight heparin in patients at higher risk of thrombosis shortly after the procedure. Pancreas transplant recipients are also at higher risk than other types of transplant surgeries to have postoperative complications with an open technique, including wound infections, fascial dehiscence, and postoperative ventral hernias [29]. Preliminary data show that robot-assisted pancreas transplants are well tolerated and may have an effect in mitigating these postoperative complications as techniques are advanced.

Overall, the outcome for pancreas transplantation has improved significantly. Graft survival at 1 year reached 85 percent in SPK, compared to 79 percent in PTA [30]. Patient survival is greater than 95 percent at 1 year and greater than 90 percent at 3 years [30].

Effects of successful pancreas transplantation can provide patients with insulin independence and optimal glycemic control. Cardiovascular effects of this include improved blood pressure, improved lipid profile, and decreased inflammation [5]. Microvascular complications that can be halted or even regressed include improved retinopathy or macular edema, functional improvements in peripheral neuropathy, and possibly autonomic neuropathy improvements. Macrovascular complications include decreased incidence of cerebrovascular accidents, improved cardiac function, and improved peripheral arterial disease [5]. In terms of the effects on diabetes management, successful pancreas transplantation is able to stabilize and even reverse the harmful effects of hyperglycemia, in terms of both macrovascular and microvascular, complications. Robot-assisted pancreas transplant has been shown to be as effective as open procedures and, with continued advances, will circumvent the postoperative complication rates associated with the procedure and allow more diabetics to become insulin-independent.

Liver Transplant

History of Liver Transplantation

The first liver transplantation in a human was performed in 1963, at the University of Colorado, by Dr. Thomas Starzl [34–37]. He described this procedure, as well as two subsequent procedures, in a case-series paper that was published in December that year [37]. Initially, there were a variety of problems associated with this procedure, as none of the first three cases described here survived longer than 22 days, and each of them suffered from irregularities of coagulation. The first patient bled to death on the operating table, and the two subsequent patients' courses were complicated by venous thrombosis and pulmonary emboli [37].

It was not until 1967 that a liver transplant recipient achieved survival longer than 1 year [34–36]. This was described in a case-series published in 1968, which also described other patients with improved survival, and the author attributed these improved results to improvements in donor selection, interim preservation of donor organs, and immunosuppressive agents [38].

In the late 1970s, a pivotal improvement in immunosuppressive therapy for liver transplant patients would prove to be crucial: the replacement of azathioprine with cyclosporine [35,39,40]. The new regimen based on treatment with cyclosporine and prednisone showed significant improvements in long-term mortality. Thanks in large part to this advancement, liver transplantation went from being an experimental treatment to a viable destination therapy for patients with end-stage liver disease [39]. As these procedures became more common, advances in technology, as well as improved surgical technique, would further improve outcomes for these patients. Today, there are a variety of immunosuppressive agents in use for this purpose, allowing for numerous regimens, depending on the circumstances [35,39,41–43].

As outcomes have progressively improved, liver transplantation is now indicated for a variety of both acute and chronic conditions causing liver failure, and is utilized with a high degree of success [34–36,44,45]. There are even dedicated fellowship training programs for liver transplantation for practitioners of both anesthesiology and surgery, and the demand for donor organs is very high [46].

Indications and Contraindications

In 1983, it was officially determined by the National Institutes of Health that the success rate of liver transplantation was high enough that it should no longer be considered an experimental procedure [36]. Today there are a variety of indications for liver resection and transplantation. These include acute liver failure from hepatits A and B viruses, as well as from drug or toxin hepatotoxicity. Also included are chronic diseases leading to cirrhosis, including hepatitis B and C infection, alcoholic liver disease, autoimmune hepatits, cryptogenic liver disease, primary biliary cirrhosis, secondary biliary cirrhosis, and primary sclerosing cholangitis. Additionally, liver failure could result from metabolic diseases such as alpha-1 antitrypsin deficiency, hemochromatosis, Wilson's disease, glycogen storage disorders, type 1 hyperoxaluria, and familial homozygous hypercholesterolemia. Finally, both primary and metastatic cancers causing liver failure, as well as other causes of liver failure such as polycystic liver disease and Budd-Chiari syndrome, may be a reasonable indication for liver transplantation. If untreated, liver failure from these and other conditions can lead to ascites, encephalopathy, dysfunction in the synthesis of important proteins, esophageal varices, portal hypertension, and hepatopulmonary syndrome [36,44].

There are also a variety of contraindications to liver transplantation. Absolute contraindications include brain death, extrahepatic malignancy, active uncontrolled infection or sepsis, active drug or alchohol abuse, noncompliance, any anatomic abnormalities that would make the procedure impossible, or compensated, uncomplicated cirrhosis. Relative contraindications include advanced age, HIV infection, cholangiocarcinoma, portal vein thrombosis, or lack of psychosocial support [35,36].

With continuing advancements in surgical techniques, the next step in this evolution has been the movement toward more minimally invasive methods, such as laparoscopic and robot-assisted liver resection. In theory, the robot-assisted procedure has several advantages over traditional laparoscopy, including improved 3D view, stability, and instrument flexibility. At this point, it has been demonstrated in the literature on a limited basis, but early data suggests that it is at least comparable in safety and success to the same procedure performed with traditional laparoscopy [47–49].

Surgical Considerations

Robot-assisted minimally invasive surgery has been shown to have several advantages when compared to conventional surgical procedures. In some cases, it has been shown to shorten hospital stay, decrease blood loss, and improve patient recovery [49].

To perform a robotic liver resection, general anesthesia is induced and an endotracheal tube placed. The patient will then be positioned by the surgeons, who will then prep and drape the patient in an appropriate fashion. The surgeon will then insert several trochars for the placement of cameras and instruments, as well as an insufflation port for pneumoperitoneum, which provides for better surgical exposure. The placement of these trochars is determined by the part of the liver being resected and the type of exposure needed for a given patient. The robot is then docked and the procedure is performed with the primary operator at the console and an assistant scrubbed in and positioned by the patient to make adjustments to instruments and cameras as needed. The dissection is then performed by the robotic instruments controlled by the surgeon at the console. The resected specimens may then be removed through a small additional incision, which would then be closed by the surgeons, along with the port sites, when the procedure is complete and adequate hemostasis has been demonstrated [47–49].

Robot-assisted liver resection has been described as part of a bridge to liver transplantation, but more data is required to determine its utility for routine use [48]. At this time, there is no case of a complete liver transplantation performed robotically described in the literature, likely due to the size of the organ.

Anesthesia Considerations

Though robotic surgery has numerous benefits for the patient and the surgeon, the anesthetist faces a more challenging perioperative course. Due to the size of the da Vinci robotic surgical system, patient access and patient position are of primary concern. The bed is often rotated 180 degrees away from the anesthetist and the ventilator. The preoperative anesthetic setup should include extensions for all invasive lines, monitors, and the ventilator circuit. Dependent on the operative room size, space and access are often restricted due to the numerous components of the robot. During an emergency, it is essential for an anesthetist to already have invasive access established in the patient. Invasive access is recommended to include a central venous line as well as two large-bore intravenous catheters. The surgery is minimally invasive, but this technique is still relatively "new" to surgeons and often more time-consuming, which can lead to a prolonged intraoperative course. As with any other lengthy procedure, it is ideal to use anesthetics which will not prolong extubation at the conclusion of surgery. Therefore, an epidural is ideal for pain control, along with rapidly metabolized opioids. An inhalation anesthetic, desflurane, and a neuromuscular blocking drug, cisatracurium, would also be ideal

the veno-venous anastomosis is performed first. This anastomosis is completed in an end-to-side fashion with a running suture. Next, the external iliac artery is then clamped between robotic bulldogs, and an oval-shaped window is made in the anterior wall of the artery with the use of robotic scissors. The arterial anastomosis is completed in an end-to-side fashion with 12-cm double-needle 6-0 Gore-Tex suture with a knot in the middle. The ease of fine vascular suturing allowed by the high-definition 3D vision and wrist-like articulation of the robotic system instruments are the most important advantages for this procedure. Upon completion of arterial anastomosis, 100 mg of Lasix and 1g/kg body weight of Mannitol are given intravenously. In some cases, fluid bolus may be required.

After the vascular anastomoses are complete, the clamps on the vein are removed first, followed by removal of the arterial clamps. The reperfusion of the organ and hemostasis are additionally verified and bleeding points secured with 6-0 Prolene suture. At this point, the pressure of pneumoperitoneum is decreased to minimize possible negative effect of high intraabdominal pressure on graft perfusion. This maneuver also allows for better evaluation of hemostasis due to venous bleeding, which could be obscured by high intraabdominal pressure. Vascular reperfusion is the most critical part of robotic transplantation, since significant bleeding could be more difficult to control compared to the open approach. Full attention of the anesthesia team and immediate initiation of adequate resuscitation is of extreme importance.

Adequate reperfusion is verified by a Doppler exam. We routinely use 3 ml of Indocyanine green (ICG) solution given intravenously. The robotic fluorescein camera gives excellent opportunity to observe and document the distribution of the dye into the graft as a surrogate for anastomotic perfusion

Diluted methylene blue solution is introduced into the bladder in order to facilitate its identification. The ureter is anastomosed to the bladder with running 5–0 Monocryl suture. The typical antireflux technique, suturing full thickness of the ureteral wall with the mucosal layer of the bladder, is used. Utilization of ureteral stent is optional.

At the end of the procedure, the mini-laparotomy is closed with running 0 PDS, and the two 12-mm port sites are closed with an endoclosure device and 0 Vicryl suture.

Discussion

The initial experiences shared by centers around the world, applying robotics to transplantation, have demonstrated lower complication rates for RKT in comparison to similar open transplant cohorts [14,15].

Since 2009 the University of Illinois had completed more than 180 robotic-assisted kidney transplants in obese recipients. BMI >30 kg/m^2 has been our only selection criterion, without an upper limit. The mean BMI of the group of patients was 40 kg/m^2. We reported our early experience in a case-control study [13], where the first 28 robot-assisted kidney transplants were compared to a frequency-matched retrospective cohort of obese recipients who underwent kidney transplantation by open technique. At 48 months of follow-up, the GFR was 51.5±30.7 ml/min/1.73 m^2 in the robotic group and 51.9±21.8 ml/min/1.73 m^2 in the control group (p = 0.83). The rate of surgical site infections was significantly higher in the control group compared with the robotic group (28.6 vs. 0 percent, p = 0.004). At 4 years post transplant, eight patients in the control group (28.6 percent) experienced graft loss compared with five patients in the robotic group (17.9 percent). Three (37.5 percent) of eight patients who lost the graft in the control group had concomitant SSI. The patient survival at 48 months was 92.5 percent in the robotic group and 92.4 percent in the control group (p = 0.97). Patients transplanted with minimally invasive approach achieved early mobilization, high patient satisfaction, and an excellent long-term graft function were observed.

Our group conducted a study in which the UNOS registry was reviewed for adult living donor kidney transplant recipients with BMI ≥40 kg/m^2 from September 2009 to December 2014. We compared outcomes in RKT versus standard open kidney transplantation (OKT) at all US centers. Similar patient and graft survival were reported. Renal function, determined by creatinine levels and GFR, was also similar in both groups.

Safety and effectiveness of RKT, which has been proven so far, could be achieved only with perfect collaboration among the different specialty teams during the entire process of transplantation. By providing excellent kidney graft function and minimizing surgical complications, this surgical technique gives the opportunity to the disadvantaged group of obese patients with ESRD to have more realistic access to transplantation.

The robotic approach has been used in different centers for autotransplantation as a means to salvage kidneys with different injuries. The technique published is similar to the one described in literature [16–18].

Surgical Considerations for Robotic Pancreas Transplantation

Even if proven as an effective treatment of insulin-dependent diabetes, pancreas transplantation has the highest rate of surgical complications among solid organ transplants [19]. Constant improvement of the surgical technique and introduction of innovative surgical technology may be one of the most important factors to achieve reduction of post transplant morbidity.

The first robotic pancreas transplants were reported by Boggi et al. in 2012 where they were performed by the assistance of the da Vinci Surgical [20]. Three transplants – one pancreas alone, one pancreas after kidney, and one simultaneous kidney and pancreas – were performed during this endeavor.

Surgical Technique

The patient is positioned supine, with the right flank slightly elevated. The table is then inclined 25 degrees to the left, further elevating the right flank. A 7-cm midline incision is made just above the navel and a GelPort (Applied Medical, Rancho Santa Margarita, CA) device is inserted. Four ports are positioned in the following manner: (1) one 11-mm port is placed within the GelPort to create the pneumoperitoneum, (2) one 11-mm robotic port is placed slightly to the left of the midline a few centimeters below the navel for insertion and use of the laparoscope, (3) two 8-mm robotic ports are placed along the right pararectal line some 5 cm below the costal margin and 3 cm above the pubis, respectively. The da Vinci system is placed to the patient's right side.

After mobilization of the right colon, the common iliac artery and the proximal segment of the inferior vena cava are exposed. To perform the vascular anastomosis, the iliac artery is cross-clamped and the inferior vena cava is partially occluded using bulldog clamps, manually applied through the GelPort. The graft is then introduced and the donor portal vein is anastomosed end-to-side to recipient inferior vena cava. The donor Y graft and recipient common iliac artery are anastomosed also in an end-to-side fashion. Before vascular reperfusion of the graft, the anesthesia team is warned. Occasionally significant bleeding could occur during this phase. Also, the release of a high amount of insulin from the reperfused graft could cause severe hypoglycemia, which in combination with blood loss and pneumoperitoneum could lead to hypotension and shock. The pneumoperioneum is interrupted after graft revascularization, and exocrine drainage is achieved by means of Roux-en-Y duodenojejunostomy.

In the simultaneous pancreas–kidney transplant, the kidney is transplanted in the ipsilateral iliac fossa, according to the technique previously described for RKT. The suprapubic robotic port access is converted into a mini-incision, approximately 3 cm long, and the ureterovesical anastomosis (Gregoir-Lich extravesical anastomosis) is performed manually.

This initial experience showed the safety and feasibility of robotic surgery applied to pancreas transplantation. The graft function observed during follow-up was compatible to standard open pancreas transplants.

Our group at the University of Illinois at Chicago performed three fully robotic pancreas transplants. The first and third ones were pancreas alone and the second simultaneous kidney–pancreas. In all cases the pancreas was transplanted to the left external iliac vessels, which allowed perfect alignment of the vascular anastomosis. In the first case, the exocrine secretions were drained into the urinary bladder through duedenocystoanastomosis. We used an EEA stapler inserted across the stump of the graft. In the second and third cases, we used enteric drainage for pancreatic exocrine secretions. Duodenojejunal anastomosis was completed similarly with EEA stapler. We cannot overemphasize the importance of diligent harvesting of the pancreatic graft and meticulous backbench preparation to avoid disturbing bleeding after graft reperfusion.

Acquisition of more experience in the future will show whether the application of robotic technique for minimally invasive pancreas transplantation could significantly decrease abdominal wall complications, which are quite frequent after pancreas transplants.

Surgical Considerations for Robotics in Living Donor Hepatectomy

Minimal invasive laparoscopic liver resection has evolved greatly during the past few decades. The experience in minimally invasive liver surgery has been steadily increasing [21]. More than 200 robotic-assisted liver resection cases have been published to date, including living donor right hepatectomy [22–24].

Soubrane et al. reported the first clinical series of pure laparoscopic left lateral sectionectomy for living liver donors [25]. For living donor right hepatectomies, the introduction of laparoscopic surgery can be traced back to 2006, when Koffron et al. first reported using the laparoscopy-assisted method [26].

Following the advances in robotic surgical technology combined with the extensive institutional experience with major robotic-assisted liver resections [22], this technology was applied to right living lobe donor hepatectomy. The first robotic living donor hepatectomy was performed in 2012 by Giulianotti et al. at the University of Illinois at Chicago [23].

Since potential liver donors are relatively young and perfectly healthy, extensive testing, besides the standard liver donor work-up, is rarely needed.

Surgical Technique

During the initial dissection of live hilum, the gallbladder is removed. After this, the hepatic artery and the right portal vein are dissected free and hepatic duct is localized. The right lobe is retracted along an upward direction to start the retrohepatic dissection of the inferior vena cava. Consequently, the robotic harmonic scalpel is used to perform transection of the parenchyma. The vascular transections are done using Endo-GIA vascular stapler in the following order: (a) right hepatic artery, (b) right portal vein, and (c) right hepatic vein. The blood loss should be minimal during the transection of live parenchyma. Maintaining the central venous pressure relatively low (3–5 mmHg) is of extreme importance. This approach could potentially increase the chance for developing a CO_2 embolism, if a larger hepatic vein is accidentally opened. Maintaining continous communication and effective collaboration between the anesthesia and surgical teams could not be overemphasized in order to keep the procedure safe.

The main advantages observed with the robotic system, in addition to those previously mentioned, are that it facilitates vascular and biliary dissection all the need of only a smaller subumbilical incision for graft extraction. This incision decreases the pain and risk of pulmonary complications associated with upper midline subcostal incisions.

Conclusion

After accumulating significant experience in different surgical specialties, robotic surgery is here to stay. The necessary skills, acquired with highly complex operations, allowed its introduction in transplantation. The initial experiences are very promising. Constant expansion of the knowledge and abilities of anesthesia, surgery, and medical teams, along with the rapid improvement of the robotic technology, would allow an even broader application of these minimally invasive approaches in transplantation. The candidates for solid organ transplantation, with their long-standing complex medical illness and subject to severe immunosuppression, will continue to benefit the most from this trend and further advancements in surgical techniques.

References

1. Schweitzer EJ, Wilson J, Jacobs S, et al. Increased rates of donation with laparoscopic donor nephrectomy. *Ann Surg*. 2000;232(3):392–400.
2. Horgan S, Benedetti E, Moser F. Robotically assisted donor nephrectomy for kidney transplantation. *Am J Surg*. 2004; 188(4A suppl):45S–51S.
3. Horgan S, Vanuno D, Sileri P, Cicalese L, Benedetti E. Robotic-assisted laparoscopic donor nephrectomy for kidney transplantation. *Transplantation*. 2002;73(9):1474–9.
4. Gorodner V, Horgan S, Galvani C, et al. Routine left robotic-assisted laparoscopic donor nephrectomy is safe and effective regardless of the presence of vascular anomalies. *Transpl Int*. 2006; 19(8):636–40.
5. Horgan S, Galvani C, Gorodner MV, et al. Effect of robotic assistance on the "learning curve" for laparoscopic hand-assisted donor nephrectomy. *Surgical Endoscopy and Other Interventional Techniques*. 2007;21(9):1512–7.
6. Giacomoni A, Di Sandro S, Lauterio A, et al. Robotic nephrectomy for living donation: surgical technique and literature systematic review. *Am J Surg*. 2015.
7. Giulianotti P, Gorodner V, Sbrana F, et al. Robotic transabdominal kidney transplantation in a morbidly obese patient. *Am J Transplant*. 2010;10(6):1478–82.
8. Boggi U, Vistoli F, Signori S, et al. Robotic renal transplantation: first European case. Transpl Int. 2011;24(2):213–8.
9. Doumerc N, Roumiguie M, Rischmann, P, Sallusto F. Total robotic approach with transvaginal insertion for kidney transplantation. Eur Urol. 2015;68(6): 1103–4.

10. Doumerc N, Beauval JB, Rostaing L, Sallusto F. A new surgical area opened in renal transplantation: a pure robot-assisted approach for both living donor nephrectomy and kidney transplantation using transvaginal route. *Transpl Int*. 2016;29(1):122–3.

11. Menon M, Sood A, Bhandari M, et al. Robotic kidney transplantation with regional hypothermia: a step-by-step description of the Vattikuti Urology Institute-Medanta technique (IDEAL phase 2a). *Eur Urol*. 2014;65(5):991–1000.

12. Abaza R, Ghani KR, Sood A, et al. Robotic kidney transplantation with intraoperative regional hypothermia. *BJU Int*. 2014;113(4):679–81.

13. Oberholzer J, Giulianotti P, Danielson KK, et al. Minimally invasive robotic kidney transplantation for obese patients previously denied access to transplantation. *Am J Transplant*. 2013;13(3):721–8.

14. Menon M, Abaza R, Sood A, et al. Robotic kidney transplantation with regional hypothermia: evolution of a novel procedure utilizing the IDEAL guidelines (IDEAL phase 0 and 1). *Eur Urol*. 2014;65(5):1001–9.

15. Tsai MK, Lee CY, Yang CY, Yeh CC, Hu RH, Lai HS. Robot-assisted renal transplantation in the retroperitoneum. *Transpl Int*. 2014;27(5):452–7.

16. Gordon ZN, Angell J, Abaza R. Completely intracorporeal robotic renal autotransplantation. *J Urol*. 2014;192(5):1516–22.

17. Lee J, Ordon M. Innovative applications of robotic surgery: renal allograft and autologous transplantation. *F1000Res*. 2016; 5.

18. Lee JY, Alzahrani T, Ordon M. Intra-corporeal robotic renal auto-transplantation. *Can Urol Assoc J*. 2015;9(9–10):E748–9.

19. Troppmann C, Gruessner AC, Dunn DL, Sutherland DE, Gruessner RW. Surgical complications requiring early relaparotomy after pancreas transplantation: a multivariate risk factor and economic impact analysis of the cyclosporine era. *Ann Surg*. 1998;227(2):255–68.

20. Boggi U, Signori S, Vistoli F, et al. Laparoscopic robot-assisted pancreas transplantation: first world experience. *Transplantation*. 2012;93(2):201–6.

21. Buell JF, Cherqui D, Geller DA, et al. The international position on laparoscopic liver surgery: the Louisville Statement, 2008. *Ann Surg*. 2009;250(5):825–30.

22. Giulianotti PC, Coratti A, Sbrana F, et al. Robotic liver surgery: results for 70 resections. *Surgery*. 2011;149(1):29–39.

23. Giulianotti PC, Tzvetanov I, Jeon H, et al. Robot-assisted right lobe donor hepatectomy. *Transpl Int*. 2012;25(1):e5–9.

24. Lai EC, Tang CN, Li MK. Robot-assisted laparoscopic hemi-hepatectomy: technique and surgical outcomes. *Int J Surg*. 2012;10(1):11–15.

25. Soubrane O, Cherqui D, Scatton O, et al. Laparoscopic left lateral sectionectomy in living donors: safety and reproducibility of the technique in a single center. *Ann Surg*. 2006;244(5):815–20.

26. Koffron AJ, Kung R, Baker T, Fryer J, Clark L, Abecassis M. Laparoscopic-assisted right lobe donor hepatectomy. *Am J Transplant*. 2006;6(10):2522–5.

Chapter 17

Fetal Surgery and Robotic Surgery

Sudipta Sen, Shilpadevi Patil, Elyse M. Cornett, Amit Prabhakar, Matthew Novitch, Alan David Kaye, and Charles J. Fox

Introduction

Fetal surgery involves the treatment of congenital malformations in the developing fetus of a pregnant woman in utero. Fetal surgery, also known as in utero intrauterine or prenatal surgery, dates back to 1963 when the first fetal blood transfusion was performed by Sir A. W. Lilly to a hydropic fetus with Rh disease. The International Fetal Surgical Society was founded in 1982 and was later transformed into International Fetal Medicine and Surgery Society (IFMSS). Directives, policies, and procedures for in utero surgery are laid out by these societies [1].

Over the past few decades, sophisticated imaging such as ultrasonography and magnetic resonance imaging (MRI) have allowed physicians to better identify and define the natural history of congenital malformations. Three-dimensional ultrasound can accurately measure the volume of any fetal organ and is used for detecting surface abnormalities like cleft lip and spina bifida. The central nervous system can be imaged using an echo planar MRI. Open fetal procedures and minimally invasive fetal procedures (fetal endoscopy – FETENDO) have made it possible to correct simple anatomic abnormalities with predictable developmental consequences before birth [1].

Developments in operative techniques and sophisticated anesthesia care have resulted in the treatment of several anatomical abnormalities in utero. Current indications of fetal surgery include treatment of congenital diaphragmatic hernia, cystic adenomatoid malformation of the lung, sacrococcygeal teratoma, obstructive uropathy, twin-to-twin transfusion syndrome (TTFS), twin reverse arterial perfusion (TRAP), amniotic band syndrome, and myelomeningocele.

Historically, surgeons have gained access to the fetus by performing a Pfannesteil incision and a hysterotomy after evacuation of the amniotic fluid. The part of the fetus to be operated upon was extracted out of the uterus and the fetus was washed with warm normal saline to offset drying and cooling when exposed to the external environment. After surgical correction, the fetus was replaced back into the uterine sac and the hysterotomy was closed. This open technique, however, resulted in serious complications to both the mother and fetus. Premature labor, premature rupture of membranes (PROM), maternal bleeding, and infections seen with open procedures led to the development of a minimally invasive procedure, referred to as operative fetoscopy [1,2].

Robotic surgery facilitates operative fetoscopy by magnifying the surgical field, improving ergonomics, and reducing hand tremors. Incorporating the use of robotics into fetal surgery is referred to as “febotics” and has resulted in decreased maternal morbidity and preterm labor by minimizing uterine trauma [2,3].

History of Procedure

Experimental Timeline of Fetal Surgery

In the early sixteenth century, most of the anatomy and physiology of human fetuses were derived from animal models as early observations on human fetus were limited to aborted homunculus. Andreas Versalius, the father of modern anatomy in the sixteenth century, pointed out that the fetus attempts to breathe when exposed to air, and arteries in the umbilical cord pulsate at regular intervals until fetal breathing begins. In the nineteenth century, physiological observations on experimental animal models resulted in better understanding of the living mammalian fetus (Table 17.1).

Fetal Intervention in Humans

Sir Albert William Liley in 1963 conducted the first documented fetal blood transfusion to a hydropic fetus with Rh disease. Using a process similar to amniocentesis, Liley guided a needle through the

Table 17.1 Experimental fetal surgery on animal models

Bichat (1803)	First to study fetal movement
Zunt (1877) and Preyer (1885) [4]	Studied intact fetal guinea pigs and concluded that once a fetus initiates its own breathing, it cannot be returned to its mother
Mayer (1918) [5]	Mayer concluded that several fetal guinea pigs that were removed from the uterus and placed in the abdominal wall cavity of the mother survived
Wolff (1919) [6]	Same results as the study done by Mayer were reproduced in experimental fetal rabbits
Bors (1925) [7]	First reported fetal surgery in animal model: Guinea pig fetus limbs were amputated through a small incision in the uterus. The uterine incision was closed and viable fetuses were delivered after fetal surgery
Nicholas (1925) [8]	Ablated eye, legs, or tails in fetal rats and achieved survival of these fetuses
Hooker (1930) [9] and Nicholas (1925)	Developed technique for spinal cord section
Jost (1946) [10]	Concluded that the removal of fetal rabbit testis influences the subsequent development of sexual organs
Foote and Foote (1949) [11], Domm and Leroy (1951) [12]	Studied the influence of pituitary gland on fetal development by decapitating animals (hypophysectomy)
Louw and Barnard (1955) [13]	Intestinal atresia was reproduced in fetal puppies by ligating the mesenteric vessels
Jackson et al. (1963) [14]	Experimental fetal surgery to simulate coarctation of aorta in a puppy
De Lorimier et al. (1967) [15], Kent et al. (1972) [16], Burington and Olley (1970) [17]	Created diaphragmatic hernia in lamb fetuses early on in gestation to study the physiology and circulation in these fetuses with congenital diaphragmatic hernia
Beck et al. (1970–1973) [18]	Developed sheep models for studying obstructive uropathy

Source: Data taken from [19].

abdominal wall of the pregnant woman and into the abdominal cavity of the fetus. Work on human fetal congenital abnormalities started with the introduction of ultrasound imaging in the 1970s [19].

Michael Harrison, the father of fetal surgery, performed the first successful correction for obstructive uropathy on a human fetus in 1983 at the University of California, San Francisco. Fetal hydronephrosis was a well-understood disease and was easily detected via a sonogram. Michael Harrison (surgeon), Mitchell Golbus (perinatologist), and Roy Filly (sonographer) successfully placed a double-pigtail shunt to relieve the obstruction in this male human fetus [20].

Current work on in utero surgery must adhere strictly to the inclusion criteria laid out by IFMSS (Box 17.1). Currently six fetal congenital malformations (congenital diaphragmatic hernia, sacrococcygeal teratoma, obstructive uropathy, steal syndrome in twin pregnancy, twin reversed arterial perfusion syndrome, and amniotic band syndrome) have been successfully treated by fetoscopic techniques. FETENDO is currently being implemented in the repair of myelomeningocele, pleural fluid collection, premature vascular access, cardiac malformations, congenital high airway obstruction syndrome, and cleft lip and palate [1] (Table 17.2).

Indications and Contraindications

Computer-enhanced robotic surgical systems are being used increasingly to facilitate complex minimal-access surgical procedures. In adult patients, they are being used to perform a wide variety of surgeries, including coronary artery bypass grafting, mitral valve repair, roux-en-Y gastric bypass, colon resection, nephrectomy, and radical prostatectomy [21]. In the area of pediatric fetal surgery, the experience with robotic surgical systems is limited. However, with improvements in robotic technology, the interest and experience of pediatric surgeons with robotic pediatric fetal surgery is growing rapidly. Surgery may offer an alternative to abortion, intrauterine death, or a life with disability for a fetus diagnosed with a severe congenital anomaly.

There are certain prerequisites for a patient to be considered for a fetal surgery. Fetal surgeries are indicated only if there is a true benefit, meaning the benefits outweigh the risks of undergoing a surgery during pregnancy. The fetal condition should be severe enough to warrant the risks associated with in utero treatment. The fetal malformation or condition amenable to fetal surgery must be reliably detectable before birth; the pathophysiology must be reversible

Table 17.2 Milestones in human fetal intervention

Open fetal surgery for uropathy	1983
Open fetal surgery for congenital diaphragmatic hernia	1989
Experimental fetoscopic techniques	1989
First successful human endoscopic vesicostomy	1992
Sacrococcygeal teratoma resection	1992
Ex utero intrapartum treatment (EXIT) procedure developed and used for airway obstruction	1995
First open repair of myelomeningocele in utero	1997
First endoscopic surgery (FETENDO) for tracheal occlusion in congenital diaphragmatic hernia	1998
Radiofrequency ablation in twin reversed arterial perfusion defects	1998
Pericardial tumor resection	2000
Cervical teratoma resection	2001
Treatment of hypoplastic left heart syndrome by balloon septotomy/valve dilation	2004
Treatment of hypoplastic left heart syndrome by laser atrial septotomy	2005
Use of sclerotherapy for congenital cystic adenomatoid malformation	2007

Source: Data taken from [1,20].

Box 17.1 Inclusion Criteria for In Utero Surgery (Data Taken from [1])

1. The congenital abnormality that is being treated must have a well-defined natural history.
2. Associated chromosomal and genetic abnormalities must be ruled out as these impact quality of life and is a contraindication for in utero surgery.
3. The correctable lesion must lead to death or irreversible organ destruction and traditional treatment options are unavailable for the abnormality.
4. Treatment of congenital abnormality must be studied and should be successful in animal models prior to treating human fetuses
5. Procedural risk to the mother must be minimal.
6. The fetal surgical procedure must be technically feasible and performed in a multi-specialized center. The ethics committee of the hospital must offer consultation by practioners not involved with the procedure before obtaining consent for the procedure.

by fetal surgery; and the prognosis following fetal surgery should most likely be improved significantly over postnatal treatment [22]. Selection of appropriate candidates for surgery and optimal timing for intervention continues to be a challenging task for any physician [23].

Indications

Antenatal fetal surgery is currently indicated for life-threatening fetal conditions and congenital malformations that can interfere with normal organ and fetal development such as:

1. Congenital diaphragmatic hernia
2. Obstructive uropathy or antenatal hydronephrosis due to ureteropelvic junction obstruction [22]
3. TTFS and TRAP
4. Myelomeningocele
5. Neck masses occluding the trachea
6. Tumors like congenital cystic adenomatoid malformation of the lung and
7. Sacrococcygeal teratoma [23]

Contraindications

There are some situations or conditions where fetal surgery may be less useful or more unlikely to justify its usefulness.

1. Refusal to treatment and long-term follow-up by the family
2. Inadequate understanding of the natural history of the condition and the efficiency of intervention
3. Mild fetal conditions that can wait for postnatal therapy
4. Severely affected fetus that cannot be saved or have no reasonable benefit with fetal surgery
5. Malformations that do not interfere with normal organ or fetal development
6. Nonaccessibility to a high-risk obstetric unit, neonatal, or pediatric intensive care unit
7. Absence of a multidisciplinary fetal maternal specialist that is experienced in prenatal diagnosis, a pediatric surgeon trained in fetal surgeries, a pediatric anesthesiologist and a neonatologist, bioethical and psychosocial consultation [23]
8. Preterm labor [24] and PROM

Operating Methods

There are various ways that a fetal surgery can be performed. Surgical methods have progressed over the years with advancements in technology. Some of the surgical methods are mentioned below.

Open fetal surgery refers to a hysterectomy that is performed to gain access to the fetus. This method is associated with higher incidence of preterm labor and PROM.

EXIT refers to a method where the delivery of head and shoulders is performed through a hysterotomy incision (uterine incision) while placenta is still providing gas exchange.

Minimally Invasive Surgical Techniques

Closed fetal surgeries are similar to mini-laparotomies without the need for hysterotomy. They have decreased the incidence of preterm labor significantly. The incidence of performing open fetal surgery has decreased and will continue to do so in the near future due to the development and application of newer surgical techniques [22]. Similar to surgeons in many other surgical specialties, pediatric surgeons are increasingly using minimally invasive techniques to minimize patient morbidity. You can minimize uterine trauma by performing procedures fetoscopically, which would decrease maternal morbidity and preterm labor.

Robotic surgery facilitates minimally invasive surgery, possibly making endoscopic fetal surgery more likely to succeed. Surgical robots in use enhance minimally invasive surgery by providing tremor filtration, motion scaling, indexed movement, articulation, and improved ergonomics [25].

Two types of robotic surgical systems have been used:

1. The Zeus robotic surgical system
2. The da Vinci Surgical System (FDA-approved)

These systems have been popularly referred to as surgical robots, but this is a misnomer as robot means "autonomous movement." Neither of the two surgical systems operate without the control of the surgeon, and therefore, the appropriate term for these systems would be "computer-enhanced telemanipulators." In any case, the term "robotic surgery" continues to be used frequently.

Advantages of Robotic Surgery

The da Vinci system offers seven degrees of freedom, including enhanced 3D visualization, articulating instrument grip dexterity, motion scaling, tremor reduction, and better surgical precision, making complex procedures easier to perform. Conventional or standard laparoscopic instruments are only capable of five degrees of freedom (including grip). The Zeus system offers six degrees of freedom (including grip) as compared to the da Vinci system that offers seven degrees of freedom (including grip), thus allowing ease of performance of more complex surgical procedures. Conventional or standard laparoscopic methods require manipulation in the reverse way, whereas the nonreversed instrument control is maintained in the da Vinci robotic system. With the da Vinci system tissue dissection, suture placement is more accurate. Knot tying is more secure than conventional laparoscopic methods [21]. The set-up time and surgery duration decreases as surgeons and nurses become more familiar with the da Vinci system.

Disadvantages

High cost, lack of tactile sensation, additional specialized training for the operating room team, longer surgical times, increased time for setup, and system docking are some of the disadvantages of the robotic system.

Open Operating Techniques

Fetal surgery can only be considered congruous for a certain number of concretely astringent anomalies, and categorical prerequisites for consideration of fetal intervention are strongly defined [26]. Generally, the small size of the fetus and tissue fragility limits surgery to a specific time span, prior to 18 weeks of gestation. After the 30-week mark, the risks of premature labor increase largely and often limit operative measures. This is primarily due to increased reactivity of the uterus with advanced gestation [27]. Perioperatively, a preliminary screening is performed by the attending obstetrician. Review of data, imaging techniques, and amniocentesis to rule out genetic defects and infections are done in the preliminary screening. Medical, social history, and risk factors are reviewed with the mother [27,28].

Anesthetic techniques must include consideration for both the mother and fetus. Prevention of premature labor through tocolytics is used. Halogenated anesthesia may result in uterine relaxation, but it lends the risk of myocardial depression and decreased perfusion for the placenta. Medication use in terms of

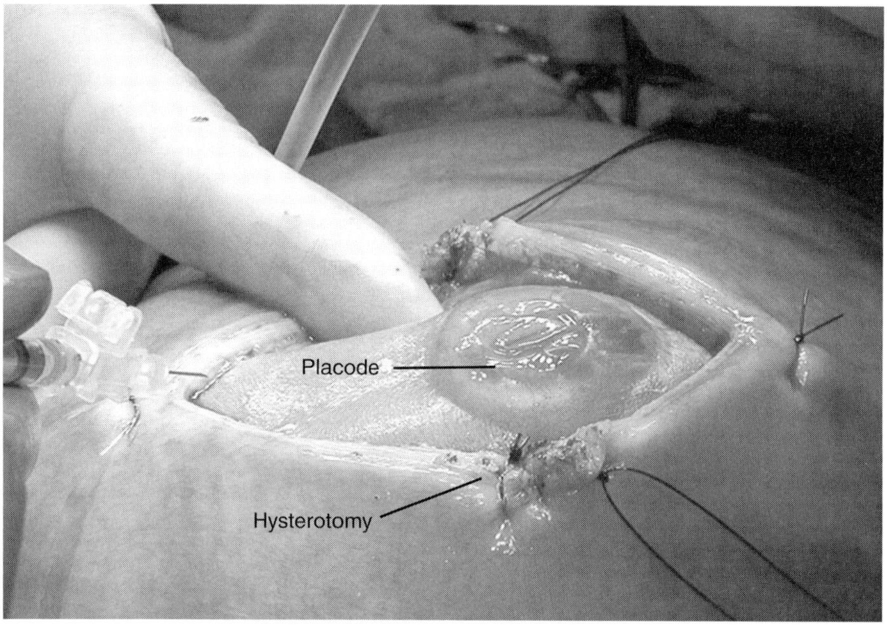

Figure 17.1 The fetus is not removed from the uterus, and the surgery is performed through the hysterotomy opening. Used with permission from [28].

dosage, anesthetics used, and timing of administration are dependent on the healthcare provider and the healthcare institution [28,29]. After skin closure, the anesthetic agents are discontinued and the mother is extubated.

There are two main techniques for open fetal surgery. The first is solely operating through a hysterotomy opening with the fetus still inside the uterus. The second is to remove the placenta from the uterus and perform the procedure on the fetus in this manner, essentially a cesarean section [28,30]. For both options, in order to begin surgery, a hysterotomy is performed on the pregnant woman. Once the fetus is exposed through a low transverse abdominal incision, the fetal and placental positions are determined. The fetus is either removed from the uterus or kept inside the hysterotomy opening [28]. After exposure of the fetus, the respective operative measures take place with care not to compress the umbilical cord and to ensure adequate perfusion for optimal outcomes.

Upon completion, the fetus is either put back inside the uterus and the uterus and abdominal wall are closed up in multiple layers, or the fetus is simply closed in the same manner with the surgeon's choice of sutures. The amniotic fluid is generally replaced before the uterine wall is completely closed. Postoperatively, patients are admitted and observed for an extended period of time. Labor is continuously inhibited via tocolysis until 36 weeks of gestation to prevent preterm labor [31]. Delivery must be performed via a second cesarean section due to the probability of uterine rupture [28]. Following delivery, the infant is followed for an extended period of time using primarily imaging and laboratory techniques. A transparent dressing is used to allow postoperative sonographic monitoring [28].

Possible Side Effects and Complications

The priorities of the surgery are maternal safety, avoiding preterm labor, and achieving the goal of the surgery without complication. For the mother, open fetal surgery has been proven to be reasonably safe [32]. Preterm labor is often the greatest challenge in fetal surgery, as considerable morbidity remains an issue despite recent developments [26]. There are other risks including maternal contraindications to tocolytics and occurrences of preterm labor including vaginal bleeding, fetal distress, and intrauterine infection [28]. Potential maternal complications include extrusion of the entire fetus or a fetal part through the hysterectomy, bowel obstruction, pulmonary edema, placental abruption, and chorioamniitis. Increased rates of cesarean birth, prolonged hospitalization, blood transfusion, and treatment in intensive care have shown to be more common in techniques with hysterectomy as opposed to other methods such as fetoscopy or ultrasound-guided procedures. Endoscopic procedures have shown significantly less morbidity than open operative techniques [33]. Mothers who have undergone any in utero fetal surgery will need a cesarean section with future pregnancies. This issue must be discussed with the mother.

Risk factors for complications increase with multiple gestation, younger age, advanced maternal age, maternal smoking, and a history of preterm labor [34]. It must be considered that premature labor may be appropriate in the case of a hostile uterine environment, and the use of tocolysis may not be warranted, nor the surgical procedure itself. The safety and effectiveness of the surgery is often variable for the fetal participant. Gestational age, pathology, and the procedure itself significantly impact the safety of the procedure. Currently the overall perinatal mortality after open surgery has been estimated to be approximately 6 percent [35]. The major risk to the fetus is uncontrollable labor and premature delivery, thus exposing the child to the well-known risks of low birth weight. The likelihood of preterm labor is proportional to the severity of fetal pathology [36].

Effects on Fertility and Prognosis

The mother carries the majority of risk both during and after fetal surgery. Postsurgical risks and complications are well documented and include, but not limited to, risk of uterine rupture, bleeding, infection, prolonged hospital stay, impaired fertility, and need for future children to be delivered by cesarean section [37]. The relatively small number of cases performed worldwide explains the limited amount of evidence-based data pertaining to postsurgical effects on maternal fertility and overall prognosis. So far, the majority of data has come from retrospective reviews published by designated centers of excellence in maternal–fetal surgery. Sufficient evidence-based data is critical to ensure the mother is able to appropriately make an informed consent [38,39].

Fetal robotic surgery has been shown to have minimal maternal mortality overall [33]. Retrospective analysis of 187 women who had intrauterine fetal intervention resulted in no maternal deaths. However, fetal surgery has been related to significant short-term maternal morbidity. Morbidity has been found to closely correspond to the type of fetal intervention performed. Open procedures are associated with a higher incidence of uterine rupture and dehiscence as compared to less invasive approaches [37]. Overall, the rate of uterine rupture after maternal–fetal surgery is similar to that of classic cesarean sections and ranges from 4 to 9 percent [37]. Additionally, patients who undergo maternal–fetal surgery have not been found to have any long-term detrimental effects on fertility [40]. Cesarean delivery is the intended mode of delivery after hysterectomy because of the potential for uterine rupture with labor [33]. Maternal morbidity and overall risk will likely decline in the future as more advanced technology and techniques are developed.

Ethics

Ethical considerations in medicine are often the most difficult and stressful decisions for both patients and medical professionals. A thorough evaluation of risks versus benefits is a cornerstone for all medical decision making. These considerations help to make up the ethical framework for whether or not a certain therapy, procedure, or surgery is indicated. These ethical issues can become more difficult and convoluted when pertaining to fetal robotic surgery [41]. Healthcare centers that routinely perform fetal robotic surgeries often incorporate insights from multidisciplinary ethics committees to ensure that decision making is reasonable and agreeable for all parties involved [42]. Some of the most important ethical considerations regarding fetal robotic surgery will be discussed below.

The advent of ultrasound dramatically changed obstetric diagnostic medicine [43]. Ultrasound is routinely used throughout the world to assess fetal development during the course of a pregnancy. It can be used to determine a multitude of things ranging from fetal gender to lethal congenital defects [44]. In the event of an abnormal finding in utero, questions immediately arise concerning what can be done. Visualization of the fetal defect by the physician and the family has been associated with evoking stronger feelings when compared to only being cognizant of the fetal defect [45,46]. Ultrasound has necessitated the development of fetal robotic surgery as an attempt to intervene when otherwise no intervention was available.

While ultrasound has helped to increase the utility of maternal fetal surgery, a major issue to consider is who the surgery ultimately benefits. While the obvious answer is the fetus, ethicists have postulated that others involved may also have something to gain [47,48]. Using fetal surgery to act on a known defect in utero can help to alleviate the psychological stress that parents and clinicians may feel compared to waiting for the birth [41]. Any action, regardless of how risky or invasive, is looked upon as a positive action when faced with dire circumstances. Another component to be considered is physician self-interest. Fetal surgery is an extremely specialized subspecialty and any advances in the field have the potential to be met with fame and fortune. A physician should never pursue this type of surgery to fulfill his or her own personal agenda [49].

The concept of patient autonomy is of utmost importance when considering medical ethics. A patient or his or her designated healthcare power-of-attorney should always have the power to decide whether or not to pursue medical treatment. This concept is muddled in fetal robotic surgery as the patient is the unborn fetus and not the mother. The mother is the individual that bears the majority of the risks. The unborn fetus has no choice in the matter. Maternal autonomy should never be overshadowed by fetal interests and thus surgery should only be pursued with the mother's informed consent [49].

While no specific guidelines exist for maternal fetal surgery, several key principles have been proposed to help construct ethical framework worldwide. These have been quoted below from a publication by Lyerly et al. [50].

> First, innovation in maternal-fetal surgery should be conducted and evaluated as research. Second, women must be considered research subjects in these trials. Third, the informed consent process must ensure adequate comprehension and genuine voluntariness in those considering participation. Fourth, discriminatory and fearful attitudes toward individuals with disabilities should be addressed explicitly prior to making a decision to proceed with maternal-fetal surgery in an attempt to correct such disabilities. Fifth, maternal-fetal surgery should not be performed for cosmetic indications unless and until there is reliable evidence that maternal-fetal surgery can be performed safely and that long-term side effects on women and their offspring are minimal. Sixth, centers of excellence should be established for conducting research and providing maternal-fetal surgery. Seventh, funding for research on maternal-fetal surgery should be considered in the context of societal needs.

Reduction of Fetal and Maternal Risk

Reducing both fetal and maternal risk during robotic procedures is of paramount importance. One way to reduce fetal and maternal risk is through the further development of minimally invasive procedures. Ideally, procedures would advance to reduce the risk of fetal surgical complications to near zero. However, treatment-related morbidity is still associated with our current surgical procedures [51–53], and overall, very few surgical procedures are performed fetoscopically [54,55]. The etiology behind the slow development of minimally invasive procedural measures is both technologic and biological in nature. Monetary aspects hinder technological development, and natural fetal physiology limits biological innovations. There is a small market and fiscal benefit to develop new fetal-specific technology, and much of the current hardware used has been developed from laparoscopy, cytoscopy, or other adult and pediatric technologies. It is clear that there are significant impeding agents that prevent the development of fetal surgery, an issue that must be addressed with care if improvement is to be made. In the future, robotics and micro-machines may make procedures more precise and may allow for the completion of increasingly complex operations [56,57]. The use of micro-machines would be less invasive than our current robotic technology [58]. Prototypes for these micro-machines currently exist; however, barriers include new developments needed in the field of imaging technology; safe and effective methods to anesthetize and paralyze the fetus; and, of course, monetary concerns.

Another way to decrease fetal and maternal risk is to predict or prevent the occurrence of preterm delivery after the operation has been completed. One way to address preterm labor is through the use of tocolycits, or anticontraction medications [32]. The severity of fetal pathology is directly proportional to the likelihood of preterm labor [36]; therefore, the prevention of preterm labor in any capacity is beneficial to the fetus and the mother. Further development of new tocolytic agents with less side effects to the mother and fetus would be ideal.

Conclusion

Overall, fetal surgery is a complex, developing procedure with risks and complications, which also exemplifies enormous benefit toward life-threatening fetal conditions. Three percent of babies born in the United States have a complex birth defect, totaling 120,000 per year [59]. Fetal imaging, prenatal testing, and fetal development have all been extensively researched and developed in the last several decades. Since

1963, incredible strides have been made to develop fetal surgery. Contraindications and indications have been well established, as well as the risks and benefits. Information about fetal surgery is becoming more accessible, and providers have become proficient in discussing these factors with families. Operative techniques have been well studied, with open surgeries being the main – although somewhat outdated – method. Currently efforts are being made to enhance fetal surgery by improving the process of holding of preterm labor and by developing minimally invasive procedures.

References

1. P. Wójcicki and P. Drozdowski, "In utero surgery – current state of the art: part I," *Med. Sci. Monit.*, vol. 16, no. 11, pp. RA237–44, 2010.
2. M. Berris and M. Shoham, "Febotics – a marriage of fetal surgery and robotics," *Comput. Aided Surg.*, vol. 11, no. 4, pp. 175–80, 2006.
3. C. G. Knight, A. Lorincz, A. Johnson, K. Gidell, R. Rabah, M. D. Klein, and S. E. Langenburg, "Robot-enhanced fetoscopic surgery," *J. Pediatr. Surg.*, vol. 39, no. 10, pp. 1463–5, 2004.
4. M. Harrison, "Historical perspective." In: M. Harrison, M. Enans, N. Adzick, and W. Holzgreve, eds. *The Unborn Patients: The Art and Science of Fetal Therapy*, 3rd Edition. Philadelphia: Sainders Company; 2001:11–18.
5. A. Mayer, "U bcr die Moglichkeit operativer Eingriffe beim lebenden Saugetierfotus," *Zenh·alb Gynak*, vol. 42, pp. 773–783, 1918.
6. B. Wolff, "Experimentelle Untersuchungen uber die Entstehung extrauteriner Schwangerschaflen und Uber die Moglichkeit operative Eingriffe bcim lebenden Saugetierfetus," *Beitr. Path. Anal.*, vol. 65, pp. 423–432, 1919.
7. E. Bors, "Die Methodik der intcruterinc Operation am uberlebenden Stiugetierfoetus," *Arch. Entwichl-Mech. Org.*, vol. 105, pp. 655–666, 1925.
8. J. S. Nicholas, "Notes on the application of experimental methods upon mammalian embryos," *Anat. Rec.*, vol. 31, no. 4, pp. 385–394, 1925. doi:10.1002/ar.1090310404.
9. D. Hooker, "Spinal cord regeneration in the young rainbow fish, Lebistes reticulatus," *J. Comp. Neurol.*, vol. 56, no. 2, pp. 277–297, 1930. doi:10.1002/cne.900560203.
10. A. Jost, "Sur la différenciation sexuelle de l'embryon de lapin I. Remarques au sujet de certaines operations chirurgicales sur l' embryon II. Expériences de parabiose," *Soc. Biol. Compte. Rendus.*, vol. 140, pp. 461–464, 1946.
11. C. Foote and F. Foote, "Changes in the thyroid gland of hamster embryos hypophysectomized by decapitation," *Anat Rec.*, 1949.
12. L. Domm and P. Leroy, "A method for fotul hypophyscctomy by decupitation in the rat," *Anat. Rec.*, vol. 109, pp. 395–409, 1951.
13. J. Louw and C. Barnard, "Congenital intestinal atresia observations on its origin," *Lancet,* 1955.
14. B. Jackson, G. Piasecki, and R. Egdahl, "Experimental production of coarctation of the aorta in utero with prolonged postnatal survival," *Surg. Forum*, vol. 14, pp. 290–291, 1963.
15. A. DeLorimier, D. Tierney, and H. Parker, "Hypoplastic lungs in fetal lambs with surgically produced congenital diaphragmatic hernia," *Surgery*, vol. 62, pp. 12–21, 1967.
16. G. Kent, P. Olley, R. Creighton, and T. Dobbinson, "Hemodynamic and pulmonary changes following surgical creation of a diaphragmatic hernia in fetal lambs," *Surgery*, vol. 72, pp. 427–433, 1972.
17. J. Burrington and P. Olley, "Experimental diaphragmatic hernias in fetal lambs," *Clin. Res.*, vol. 18, p. 198, 1970.
18. A. Beck, "Intrauterine renal surgery: techniques for exposing the fetal kidney during the last to-thirds of gestation," *Invest. Urol.*, vol. 8, pp. 182–187, 1970.
19. S. J. Han and E. H. Hwang, "The development of fetal surgery," *Yonsei Med. J.*, vol. 42, no. 6, pp. 602–8, 2001.
20. T. Jancelewicz and M. R. Harrison, "A history of fetal surgery," *Clin. Perinatol.*, vol. 36, no. 2, pp. 227–36, 2009.
21. R. Woo, D. Le, T. M. Krummel, and C. Albanese, "Robot-assisted pediatric surgery," *Am. J. Surg.*, vol. 188, no. 4A suppl, pp. 27S–37S, 2004.
22. E. Danzer, F. Schier, B. Paek, M. R. Harrison, and C. T. Albanese, "[Fetal surgery for severe congenital abnormalities]," *Zeitschrift für Geburtshilfe und Neonatol.*, vol. 205, no. 5, pp. 174–88, 2001.
23. K. D. Wenstrom and S. R. Carr, "Fetal surgery: principles, indications, and evidence," *Obstet. Gynecol.*, vol. 124, no. 4, pp. 817–35, 2014.
24. M. Berris and M. Shoham, "Febotics – a marriage of fetal surgery and robotics," *Comput. Aided Surg.*, vol. 11, no. 4, pp. 175–80, 2006.
25. C. G. Knight, A. Lorincz, A. Johnson, K. Gidell, R. Rabah, M. D. Klein, and S. E. Langenburg, "Robot-enhanced fetoscopic surgery," *J. Pediatr. Surg.*, vol. 39, no. 10, pp. 1463–5, 2004.

26. A. W. Flake, "Surgery in the human fetus: the future," *J. Physiol.*, vol. 547, no. 1, pp. 45–51, 2003.
27. N. S. Adzick, "Open fetal surgery for life-threatening fetal anomalies," *Semin. Fetal Neonatal Med.*, vol. 15, no. 1, pp. 1–8, 2010.
28. L. N. Sutton, "Fetal surgery for neural tube defects," *Best Pract. Res. Clin. Obstet. Gynaecol.*, vol. 22, no. 1, pp. 175–88, 2008.
29. K. M. Tran, "Anesthesia for fetal surgery," *Semin. Fetal Neonatal Med.*, vol. 15, no. 1, pp. 40–5, 2010.
30. J. P. Bruner, N. Tulipan, R. L. Paschall, F. H. Boehm, W. F. Walsh, S. R. Silva, M. Hernanz-Schulman, L. H. Lowe, and G. W. Reed, "Fetal surgery for myelomeningocele and the incidence of shunt-dependent hydrocephalus," *JAMA*, vol. 282, no. 19, pp. 1819–25, 1999.
31. M. R. Hüsler, R. D. Wilson, S. C. Horii, M. W. Bebbington, N. S. Adzick, and M. P. Johnson, "When is fetoscopic release of amniotic bands indicated? Review of outcome of cases treated in utero and selection criteria for fetal surgery," *Prenat. Diagn.*, vol. 29, no. 5, pp. 457–63, 2009.
32. R. R. Gaiser and C. D. Kurth, "Anesthetic considerations for fetal surgery," *Semin. Perinatol.*, vol. 23, no. 6, pp. 507–14, 1999.
33. K. Golombeck, R.H. Ball, H. Lee, J. Farrell, D. Farmer, V. Jacobs, M. Rosen, R. Filly, "Maternal morbidity after maternal-fetal surgery," *Am. J. Obstet. Gynecol.*, vol. 194, no. 3, pp. 834–9, 2006.
34. C. V Ananth and A. M. Vintzileos, "Epidemiology of preterm birth and its clinical subtypes," *J. Matern. Fetal. Neonatal Med.*, vol. 19, no. 12, pp. 773–82, 2006.
35. M. P. Johnson, L. N. Sutton, N. Rintoul, T. M. Crombleholme, A. W. Flake, L. J. Howell, H. L. Hedrick, R. D. Wilson, and N. S. Adzick, "Fetal myelomeningocele repair: short-term clinical outcomes," *Am. J. Obstet. Gynecol.*, vol. 189, no. 2, pp. 482–7, 2003.
36. A. W. Flake, T. M. Crombleholme, M. P. Johnson, L. J. Howell, and N. S. Adzick, "Treatment of severe congenital diaphragmatic hernia by fetal tracheal occlusion: clinical experience with fifteen cases," *Am. J. Obstet. Gynecol.*, vol. 183, no. 5, pp. 1059–66, 2000.
37. R. D. Wilson, M. P. Johnson, A. W. Flake, T. M. Crombleholme, H. L. Hedrick, J. Wilson, and N. S. Adzick, "Reproductive outcomes after pregnancy complicated by maternal-fetal surgery," *Am. J. Obstet. Gynecol.*, vol. 191, no. 4, pp. 1430–6, 2004.
38. M. M. S. Noah, M. E. Norton, P. Sandberg, T. Esakoff, J. Farrell, and C. T. Albanese, "Short-term maternal outcomes that are associated with the EXIT procedure, as compared with cesarean delivery," *Am. J. Obstet. Gynecol.*, vol. 186, no. 4, pp. 773–7, 2002.
39. J. A. Farrell, C. T. Albanese, R. W. Jennings, S. J. Kilpatrick, B. J. Bratton, and M. R. Harrison, "Maternal fertility is not affected by fetal surgery," *Fetal Diagn. Ther.*, vol. 14, no. 3, pp. 190–2, 1999.
40. R. D. Wilson, K. Lemerand, M. P. Johnson, A. W. Flake, M. Bebbington, H. L. Hedrick, and N. S. Adzick, "Reproductive outcomes in subsequent pregnancies after a pregnancy complicated by open maternal-fetal surgery (1996–2007)," *Am. J. Obstet. Gynecol.*, vol. 203, no. 3, pp. 209.e1–6, 2010.
41. A. Smajdor, "Ethical challenges in fetal surgery," *J. Med. Ethics*, vol. 37, no. 2, pp. 88–91, 2011.
42. A. W. Flake, "Prenatal intervention: ethical considerations for life-threatening and non-life-threatening anomalies," *Semin. Pediatr. Surg.*, vol. 10, no. 4, pp. 212–21, 2001.
43. M. B. McNay and J. E. Fleming, "Forty years of obstetric ultrasound 1957–1997: from A-scope to three dimensions," *Ultrasound Med. Biol.*, vol. 25, no. 1, pp. 3–56, 1999.
44. K. Burgin, "The tentative pregnancy: prenatal diagnosis and the future of motherhood by Barbara Katz Rothman. New York: Viking Penguin Inc., 1986." *J. Nurse. Midwifery.*, vol. 32, no. 2, pp. 114–15, 1987.
45. D. Kirklin, "The role of medical imaging in the abortion debate," *J. Med. Ethics*, vol. 30, no. 5, p. 426, 2004.
46. E. Jackson, "Regulating reproduction: law, technology and autonomy," *Mod. Law Rev.*, vol. 66, no. 3, pp. 478–81, 2003.
47. S. Zipfel, B. Löwe, T. Paschke, B. Immel, R. Lange, R. Zimmermann, W. Herzog, and G. Bergmann, "Psychological distress in patients awaiting heart transplantation," *J. Psychosom. Res.*, vol. 45, no. 5, pp. 465–70, 1998.
48. E. E. Osuna, "The psychological cost of waiting," *J. Math. Psychol.*, vol. 29, no. 1, pp. 82–105, 1985.
49. L. Doyal and C. Ward, "Fetal surgery: ethical and legal issues," *Semin. Neonatol.*, vol. 3, no. 4, pp. 255–65, 1998.
50. A. D. Lyerly, E. A. Gates, R. C. Cefalo, and J. Sugarman, "Toward the ethical evaluation and use of maternal-fetal surgery," *Obstet. Gynecol.*, vol. 98, no. 4, pp. 689–97, 2001.
51. M. R. Harrison, G. B. Mychaliska, C. T. Albanese, R. W. Jennings, J. A. Farrell, S. Hawgood, P. Sandberg, A. H. Levine, E. Lobo, and R. A. Filly, "Correction of congenital diaphragmatic hernia in utero IX: fetuses with poor prognosis (liver herniation and low lung-to-head ratio) can be saved by fetoscopic temporary tracheal occlusion," *J. Pediatr. Surg.*, vol. 33, no. 7, pp. 1017–22; discussion 1022–3, 1998.

52. J. P. Bruner, W. O. Richards, N. B. Tulipan, and T. L. Arney, "Endoscopic coverage of fetal myelomeningocele in utero," *Am. J. Obstet. Gynecol.*, vol. 180, no. 1, pp. 153–8, 1999.

53. E. Gratacós and J. Deprest, "Current experience with fetoscopy and the Eurofoetus registry for fetoscopic procedures," *Eur. J. Obstet. Gynecol. Reprod. Biol.*, vol. 92, no. 1, pp. 151–9, 2000.

54. J. E. De Lia, R. S. Kuhlmann, and K. P. Lopez, "Treating previable twin–twin transfusion syndrome with fetoscopic laser surgery: outcomes following the learning curve," *J. Perinat. Med.*, vol. 27, no. 1, pp. 61–7, 1999.

55. K. Hecher, W. Diehl, L. Zikulnig, M. Vetter, and B. J. Hackelöer, "Endoscopic laser coagulation of placental anastomoses in 200 pregnancies with severe mid-trimester twin-to-twin transfusion syndrome," *Eur. J. Obstet. Gynecol. Reprod. Biol.*, vol. 92, no. 1, pp. 135–9, 2000.

56. R. D. Howe and Y. Matsuoka, "Robotics for surgery," *Annu. Rev. Biomed. Eng.*, vol. 1, pp. 211–40, 1999.

57. S. Jacobs and V. Falk, "Pearls and pitfalls: lessons learned in endoscopic robotic surgery – the da Vinci experience," *Heart Surg. Forum*, vol. 4, no. 4, pp. 307–10, 2001.

58. S. Roy, L. A. Ferrara, A. J. Fleischman, and E. C. Benzel, "Microelectromechanical systems and neurosurgery: a new era in a new millennium," *Neurosurgery*, vol. 49, no. 4, pp. 779–97; discussion 797–8, 2001.

59. A. W. Flake and M. R. Harrison, "Fetal surgery," *Annu. Rev. Med.*, vol. 46, pp. 67–78, 1995.

Chapter 18

Perioperative Complications of Robotic Surgery

Anesthetic Concerns

Elizabeth A.M. Frost and Clifford M. Gevirtz

Introduction

Robotic assisted surgery (RAS) provides many advantages such as less pain, smaller incisions, decreased blood loss, shorter hospital stay, and greater precision, but it also comes with several complications, many of which impact anesthetic care. Over the past two decades, the number and indications for RAS have increased rapidly. In fact, most major medical centers incorporate this technology, meaning anesthesiologists must have an awareness and understanding of the difficulties that may occur. Problems arise mainly from positioning, creation of a pneumoperitoneum, and restricted access imposed by the robot.[1–3]

Positioning

The most critical part of RAS is patient positioning, which should always be undertaken as a team effort with the surgeon physically present. Compared with other minimally invasive surgery approaches, RAS gives the surgeon better control over the surgical instruments and a better view of the surgical site but only if the patient is in the optimal position. Failure to achieve the appropriate angle results in tedious procedures and even compromise of patient outcome. Moreover, once the robotic arms are docked, little or no change in position can be made.

Surgery in the pelvis and lower abdomen requires a steep Trendelenburg position. Although supine, the position of the robot severely limits access to the airway in head and neck surgery. Generally arms are tucked in the sides, restricting access to intravenous and monitoring devices such as pulse oximetry or arterial cannulae. Changing the table position from supine to Trendelenburg predisposes patients to sliding cephalad and even off the table.[4,5] Various methods have been used including braces, leg suspension, and iliac supports. Shoulder braces and straps are also frequently used. All of these devices can result in nerve injury. An antiskid foam has been suggested as a means to decrease the incidence of neuropathic injury.[6] But prevention requires first of all awareness of the possibility of injury and then meticulous attention to padding.

Steep Trendelenburg position may cause facial, pharyngeal, and laryngeal edema associated with gravitational effects, amount of intravenous fluids given, and/or reduction of venous outflow due to pneumoperitoneum. Restricting fluid administration and reducing the time in the head-down position may limit this complication. The presence of facial and/or conjunctival edema at the end of a case should raise the suspicion of laryngeal edema also and extubation should not be carried out until a satisfactory leak test has been performed.[4,5]

Prolonged periods in steep Trendelenburg position increases intraocular pressure and cerebral blood flow that is not prevented by autoregulation. A recent study of 25 patients undergoing radical prostatectomy in steep Trendelenberg position looked at ultrasonography of optic sheath diameter.[7] The authors demonstrated a significant increase in optic nerve sheath diameter and increases in intracranial pressure (ICP) to >20 mmHg that were significantly associated with increases in blood pressure. While the authors did not feel that these changes were of importance in patients with normal intracranial dynamics, they cautioned that patients with preexisting intracranial pathology may not be candidates for this surgical technique.

Because new surgical skills and training are required to operate the system, the learning curve may be slow and surgeons may need to operate on 12 to 18 patients or more before they adapt. During the training phase, minimally invasive operations can take up to twice as long as traditional surgery, leading to operating room tie-ups and prolonged anesthetic time in abnormal positions that further increase the risk of complications.[8] Patient surveys indicate they chose the procedure based on expectations of decreased morbidity, improved outcomes, reduced blood loss, and less pain.[9] Higher expectations may explain higher rates of dissatisfaction and regret.[8]

Pneumoperitoneum

During RAS for pelvic and gynecologic surgery, patients are placed in the lithotomy position, with arms ticked at the side of the table. Pneumoperitoneum is then initiated with CO_2 as the most frequently used gas. CO_2 is most commonly used as it is noncombustible and safe to use with electrosurgical devices. Its solubility in blood and reactivity with soluble buffering systems minimizes the risk of gas emboli, although that complication may still occur. The patient is then positioned in a 30–45-degree Trendelenburg position. Additional ports are inserted into the abdomen and the robotic arms are docked.

In an attempt to determine the appropriate amount of CO_2 that should be inflated, a dog model was used to measure stepwise increases in intrabdominal pressure (IAP) during inflation. An IAP of 8 was applied to determine the threshold pressure that had minimum influence on hemodynamics.[10] The authors found that at an IAP of 16 mmHg, cardiac output was decreased significantly by 1 hour after the start of insufflation and became progressively lower during the procedure. Systemic vascular resistance was elevated significantly in parallel with the change in cardiac output. Although hepatic arterial blood flow was not decreased significantly, portal venous and superior mesenteric arterial blood flows were diminished significantly, resulting in lower total hepatic blood flow. No significant changes were observed in these parameters at 8 or 12 mmHg. Based on these results, an IAP from 8 to 12 mmHg has been recommended for peritoneal insufflation.

CO_2 is insufflated into the peritoneal cavity at a rate of 4–6 L/min to a pressure of 10–18 mmHg. The pneumoperitoneum is maintained by a constant gas flow of 200–400 ml/min. The raised IAP of the pneumoperitoneum, alteration in patient position, and effects of CO_2 absorption cause changes in physiology, especially within the cardiovascular and respiratory systems. These changes, as well as direct effects of gas insufflation, may have significant effects on the patient, and more so if they are elderly or have associated morbidity. It should be recognized that while the normal IAP is <5 mmHg, it is already increased in obesity and lower amounts of CO_2 may be advisable.

Increased IAP decreases perfusion pressure to all other abdominal organs, especially in the presence of hypotension. The effect, compounded by the action of antidiuretic hormone, is seen especially in the kidneys and is manifest by oliguria. Increasing fluid administration may worsen the situation if extravasated crystalloid enters the gut wall, thereby further increasing IAP and reducing renal perfusion pressure. Prevention requires more liberal use of vasopressor and goal-directed therapy and monitoring of stroke volume indices.

Hemodynamic Effects

Gas insufflation has many hemodynamic effects. Nodal rhythm, sinus bradycardia, and asystole due to vagal stimulation can be initiated by stretching of the peritoneum. Such effects are more pronounced at the beginning of insufflation because of rapid stretching. Systemic absorption of CO_2 can cause metabolic acidosis leading to cardiac arrhythmias, constriction of pulmonary vasculature, and changes in cardiac function such as hypertension and increased cardiac output.[12] As IAP increases, venous return and thus preload is decreased, which decreases cardiac output. The result is that heart rate, mean arterial pressure (MAP), and systemic (SVR) and peripheral (PVR) resistance all increase. Increase in MAP has been shown to be about 25 percent and 20 percent in SVR as IAP increases and compresses the aorta, thus increasing afterload.[13,14] The addition of Trendelenburg position after insufflation does not change the MAP, but SVR returns to baseline.[13] Moreover, insufflation does not appear to have much effect on central venous pressure (CVP), mean pulmonary arterial pressure, and pulmonary capillary wedge pressure. But with change in position to Trendelenburg, all these pressures increase approximately two times from baseline.[13] While these changes may have little effect on a well-hydrated and otherwise healthy individual, in patients with compromised cardiac function, an increased preload may precipitate heart failure.

Respiratory Effects

Steep Trendelenburg position allows the abdominal contents to impinge on the diaphragm, pushing it and all the mediastinal contents cephalad.[15] Functional residual capacity (FRC), and pulmonary compliance are reduced, increasing the risk of atelectasis. These effects are further enhanced by increased pulmonary blood volume and gravitational forces. Also, as peak inspiratory pressures rise, so do the risks of barotrauma. The complication may be reduced by reducing tidal volume while increasing the respiratory rate and allowing a permissive hypercarbia.[16] While small amounts of positive end expiratory pressure may still increase peak pressures, this disadvantage may be offset by improved oxygenation. Pressure-controlled ventilation allows a larger tidal volume at the same inspired pressure.[17,18]

The position required for robotic prostatectomy can also significantly alter the anatomic alignment of the upper (including nasal) airways, a change that may last for several hours into the postoperative period. In a study of 50 patients, forced expiratory volume in 1 second (FEV1) and vital capacity (VC) were significantly reduced for up to 24 hours, and the ratio of maximal mid-expiratory flow to inspiratory flow was increased, indicating increased upper airway resistance.[19] More significant alterations develop in patients with chronic obstructive pulmonary disease when FEV1 and VC may be reduced for up to 5 days.[20] Thus, close attention to adequate oxygenation in the postoperative period is essential.

It is also important to be aware that at any time the endotracheal tube may slip into the right main stem bronchus because of the position. Any change in ventilatory parameters must trigger an immediate high level of suspicion.

Cerebrovascular Effects

Both pneumoperitoneum and/or the Trendelenburg position may increase ICP.[21–24] As IAP increases, venous return from the lumber venous plexus is impaired, thus increasing ICP. Also, the Trendelenburg position allows for increased venous pressure, which blocks cerebral venous return and increases cerebral blood volume. While some of these studies pertain to animal models, more recent work has verified the same effects in humans.[7] For example, one study of 15 neurosurgical patients indicated an average increase in ICP of 5 mmHg when the head was placed in a 30-degree Trendelenburg position.[23] As CO_2 is used for insufflation, hypercarbia may develop and increase cerebral blood flow. To avoid these changes, especially in older people or those with intracranial pathology, maintenance of normocarbia is recommended to preserve cerebral oxygenation levels.[25]

Complications

There are several anesthetic complications that can arise from RAS (Table 18.1).

Subcutaneous Emphysema

One of the commonest complications of RAS is subcutaneous emphysema with an estimated incidence of about 0.3–3.9 percent.[26] The complication usually relates to incorrect positioning of the gas insufflation needle or trocars, anatomical anomalies, or by gas dissecting across weak tissue planes attributable to increased IAP. End-tidal CO_2 levels rapidly become very high, necessitating frequent changes of CO_2 canister. CO_2 may take several hours to dissipate. Risk factors include ET-CO_2 greater than 50 mmHg, the use of six or more ports, longer operative time (>200 min), and older patients. While rarely causing any lasting complications, severe hypercarbia may prove to be life-threatening in patients with intracranial pathology and other comorbidities such as chronic obstructive pulmonary disease.[26] Controlled ventilation should be maintained at the conclusion of surgery until CO_2 has been eliminated.[27] Rarely subcutaneous emphysema may develop in prefascial planes leading

Table 18.1 Anesthetic complications of RAS

Complication	Signs and symptoms	Suggested interventions
Postoperative neuropathy	Dysthesias, paresthesias, paresis	Neurology consult, physical therapy consult, bracing, steroids
Laryngeal edema	Facial edema/scleral chemosis Positive endotracheal cuff leak test (less than 110 ml difference)	Reverse Trendelenberg/steroids
Subcutaneous emphysema	Subcutaneous crepitus	Fasciotomy if respiratory compliance is reduced
Corneal abrasion	Eye pain, excessive tearing, conjunctivitis	Patch the eye, ophthalmology consult

to life-threatening conditions such as pneumothorax, pneumopericardium, and pneumomediastinum.[14,26]

Venous Gas Embolism

Venous gas embolism is a rare but potentially fatal complication. It may occur if CO_2 is insufflated directly into a blood vessel or by gas being drawn into an open vessel by the Venturi effect. The clinical presentation depends on the size of gas bubbles and the rate of entry but may be one of rapidly developing bradycardia and hypotension proceeding quickly to cardiac arrest shortly after insufflation or during dissection of deep dorsal venous plexi during RAS, especially associated with prostatectomy.[28–32] The diagnosis is confirmed by observing gas bubbles on transesophageal echocardiography. Treatment includes rapid deflation of the abdomen and resuscitation of the patient. If severe, the patient may be placed in the left lateral position and the gas aspirated via a central line, as recommended for other gas embolisms. Subclinical embolism has also been described.[31] As CO_2 is very soluble in the presence of erythrocytes, gas embolism during RAS is usually less devastating than air embolism.

Two case reports relate to pneumoperitoneum. In one, transient motor paralysis followed RAS for prostatectomy.[33] Venous air embolism was implicated. In another case, pulmonary edema developed requiring continued intubation and diuretic therapy.[34]

Postoperative Visual Loss

Concerned with an increasing number of patients with postoperative visual loss mainly after spine surgery in the prone position, the American Society of Anesthesiologists (ASA) established a registry in 1999 to gain data and attempt to identify risk factors. Although a single causative factor has not been found and may not exist, several adverse circumstances appear to combine to cause the problem – among them, male gender, obesity, anesthesia duration over 5 hours, prone position, blood loss exceeding 1 liter, head-down position, and administration of excess crystalloids over colloids. In 2005, the ASA appointed a Perioperative Visual Task Force to review and assess the available literature. As a result, several recommendations were made including the need to identify patients at "high risk" (long surgery with substantial blood loss) and informing them of the risk of visual loss, avoiding hypotension, greater use of colloids, and maintenance of a head-up position.[35,36]

While not performed in a prone position, RAS requires very steep, supine, head-down position. Such extreme Trendelenberg position is associated with venous engorgement and edema formation in the head and neck as crystalloids are extravasated and pool by gravitational forces. Also, in a head-down position over time, intraocular pressure increases. In the face of actual or relative hypotension, ocular perfusion pressure is decreased putting the posterior part of the optic nerve, which has a rather tenuous blood supply in the first place, at risk of ischemic injury. Fluid accumulation can combine further to cause a compartment syndrome within the eye. Defective autoregulation and a vascular watershed region in the posterior optic nerve may also be contributing factors. Several cases of postoperative visual loss after robotic prostatectomy have been reported.[35] Given the recommendation by the ASA that patients should be advised of the admittedly small but real risk of postoperative visual loss, discussion should be included in consent. Fluid administration should be kept to a minimum; one author limits his regimen to no more than 800 ml until the surgeon has completed the vesicourethral anastomosis, when a further 700–1200 ml may be given.[3] Not only does this technique minimize head and neck edema but improves the operative view. One retrospective review of 194 patients undergoing RAS found that more restrictive fluid management resulted in overall fewer operative complications.[37] Operative time should also be closely observed and kept as short as possible. Perhaps because of a slower learning curve, it may be prudent to decrease the degree of tilt for a period if at all possible.

Other Complications

The introduction of trocars may cause damage to underlying organs (e.g., liver, spleen, bladder, intestine), which may not be diagnosed immediately at the time of surgery. Damage to blood vessels can also occur and result in massive hemorrhage. An open procedure is likely to be required to curtail hemorrhage. The risk of organ damage can be reduced if trocars are introduced under direct vision.

Corneal abrasions were shown to be increased sixfold over open hysterectomy and significantly more than during laparoscopic hysterectomy.[38] Identifiable preoperative risk factors were increased age and chronic conditions. Risks were decreased in African Americans. Awareness with special attention paid to protecting the eyes is indicated.

Robotic Thoracic Procedures

Surgical procedures commonly performed with the robotic system include thymectomy, pulmonary lobectomy, mediastinal mass excision, esophagectomy, and fundoplications. For thymectomy cases, the patient is positioned with a bean bag in a left or right oblique position. The arm on the elevated side is positioned at the patient's side as far posterior as possible to allow for the insertion of surgical ports. The incisions for the ports are located at the mid-axillary line at the third and fifth intercostal spaces as well as another at the midclavicular line. It is important to avoid overstretching the elevated arm as this may lead to brachial plexus injury as well as being vigilant to prevent crush injuries by the robot arms. Pandey et al. reported a brachial plexus injury after thymectomy where the affected limb was hyperabducted.[39]

In gaining exposure in the thoracic cavity, selective lung deflation is required along with CO_2 insufflation to provide optimum visualization. The anesthesiologist must be aware of the effects of CO_2 insufflation in the thoracic cavity, including obstruction to venous return and hypotension. CO_2 insufflation may also lead to increased peak airway pressures, particularly during one-lung ventilation.

In robotic lobectomy cases, the patient is placed over a bean bag flexed in the lateral decubitus position with the elevated arm slightly extended so that the thoracic cavity can be easily accessed while ensuring the arm is not injured by the robot armatures. In two separate case reports, supraventricular arrhythmias and atrial fibrillation developed in the perioperative period.[40,41] While the exact etiology is uncertain, acidosis from CO_2 insufflation may have played a role.

In esophagectomy cases, a left-sided double-lumen tube is placed and the patient positioned in the left lateral decubitus position with an additional 45-degree tilt to the prone position. Of concern, pulmonary complications appear to occur frequently with pneumonia, and acute respiratory distress syndrome was reported in almost half the cases.[42,43]

Close communication with the surgical team is essential at all times and is the best means to reduce postoperative difficulties.

References

1. Kaye AD, Vadivelu N, Ahuja N, et al. Anesthetic considerations in robotic-assisted gynecologic surgery. *Ochsner J.* 2013;13(4):517–24.
2. Hsu RL, Kaye AD, Urman RD. Anesthetic challenges in robotic-assisted urologic surgery. *Rev Urol.* 2013;15(4):178–84.
3. Gainsburg DM. Anesthetic concerns for robotic-assisted laparoscopic radical prostatectomy.*Minerva Anestesiol.* 2012;78(5):596–604.
4. Phong SVN, Koh LKD. Anaesthesia for robotic-assisted radical prostatectomy: considerations for laparoscopy in the Trendelenburg position. *Anaesth Intensive Care.* 2007;35:281–5.
5. Danic MJ, Chow M, Gayload A, et al. Anesthesia consideration for robotic-assisted laparoscopic prostatectomy: a review of 1500 cases. *J Robotic Surg.* 2007;1:119–23.
6. Klauschie J, Wechter ME, Jacob K, et al. Use of anti-skid material and patient-positioning to prevent patient shifting during robotic-assisted gynecologic procedures. *J Minim Invasive Gynecol.* 2010;17:504–7.
7. Whitely JR, Taylor J, Henry M, et al. Detection of elevated intracranial pressure in robot-assisted laparoscopic radical prostatectomy using ultrasonography of optic nerve sheath diameter. *J Neuro Anesth.* 2015;27(2):155–9.
8. Finkelstein J, Eckersberger E, Sadri H, et al. Open versus laparoscopic versus robot-assisted laparoscopic prostatectomy: The European and US experience. *Reviews in Urology.* 2010;12(1):35–43.
9. Estey EP. Robotic prostatectomy: The new standard of care or a marketing success?. *Canadian Urological Association Journal.* 2009;3(6):488–90.
10. Ishizaki Y, Bandai Y, Shimomura K, et al. Safe intraabdominal pressure of carbon dioxide pneumoperitoneum during laparoscopic surgery. *Surgery.* 1993;114(3):549–54.
11. Perrin M, Fletcher A. Laparoscopic abdominal surgery. *Contin Educ Anaesth Crit Care Pain.* 2004;4(4):107–10.
12. Strang CM, Fredén F, Maripuu E, et al. Ventilation-perfusion distributions and gas exchange during carbon dioxide-pneumoperitoneum in a porcine model. *Br J Anaesth.* 2010;105(5):691–7. doi: 10.1093/bja/aeq211.
13. Lestar M, Gunnarsson L, Lagerstrand L, et al. Hemodynamic perturbations during robot-assisted laparoscopic radical prostatectomy in 45° Trendelenburg position. *Anesth Analg.* 2011;113:1069–75.
14. O'Malley C, Cunningham AJ. Physiologic changes during laparoscopy. *Anesthesiol Clin N Am.* 2001;1:1–18.

15. Baltayian S. A brief review: anesthesia for robotic surgery. *J Robotic Surg.* 2008;2:59–66.

16. Gainsburg DM, Wax D, Reich DL, et al. Intraoperative management of robotic-assisted versus open radical prostatectomy. *JSLS.* 2010;14:1–5.

17. Oğurlu M, Küçük M, Bilgin F, et al. Pressure-controlled vs volume-controlled ventilation during laparoscopic gynecologic surgery. *J Minim Invasive Gynecol.* 2010;17(3):295–300.

18. Stolzenburg JU, Aedtner B, Olthoff D, et al. Anaesthetic considerations for endoscopic extraperitoneal and laparoscopic transperitoneal radical prostatectomy. *BJU Int.* 2006;98(3): 508–13.

19. Groeben HT, Killic O, Boergers A, et al. Lung function and upper airway resistance following robotic radical prostatectomy. ASA Annual Meeting Abstract A1154, October 17, 2011, Chicago.

20. Groeben HT, Killic O, Boergers A, et al. Lung function and upper airway resistance following robotic radical prostatectomy in patients with and without COPDASA. ASA Annual Meeting Abstract A1152, October 17, 2011, Chicago.

21. Halverson A, Buchanan R, Jacobs L, et al. Evaluation of mechanism of increased intracranial pressure with insufflation. *Surg Endosc.* 1998;12:266–9.

22. Doi M, Kawai Y. Mechanisms of increased intracranial pressure in rabbits exposed to head-down tilt. *Jpn J Physiol.* 1998;48(1):63–9.

23. Mavrocordatos P, Bissonnette B, Ravussin P. Effects of neck position and head elevation on intracranial pressure in anesthetized neurological patients. *J Neurosurg Anesthesiol.* 2000;12:10–14.

24. Murthy G, Marchbanks RJ, Wateenpaugh DE, et al. Increased intracranial pressure in humans during stimulated microgravity. *Physiologist.* 1992;35(suppl.):S184–5.

25. Lee JR, Lee PB, Do SH, et al. The effect of gynaecological laparoscopic surgery on cerebral oxygenation. *J Int Med Res.* 2006;34:1–6.

26. Lee DW, Kim MJ, Lee YK, Lee HN. Does intrabdominal pressure affect development of subcutaneous emphysema at gynecologic laparoscopy? *J Min Inv Gyn.* 2011;18:761–5.

27. Harris JA, Gallo CD, Brummett DM, et al. Extra-abdominal pneumodissection after laparoscopic antireflux surgery. *Am Surg.* 2001;67:885–9.

28. Hieber C, Ihra G, Nachbar S, Aloy A, Kashanipour A, Coraim F. Near-fatal paradoxical gas embolism during gynecological laparoscopy. *Acta Obstet Gynecol Scand.* 2000;79:898–9.

29. Cobb WS, F leishman HA, Kercher KW, et al. Gas embolism during laparoscopic cholecystectomy. *J Laparo Endosc Adv Surg Tech.* 2005;15:387–90.

30. Hong JY, Kim JY, Choi YD, et al. Incidence of venous gas embolism during robotic-assisted laparoscopic radical prostatectomy is lower than that during radical retropubic prostatectomy. *Br J Anaesth.* 2010;105:777–81.

31. Hong JY, Kim WO, Kil HK. Detection of subclinical CO2 embolism by transesophageal echocardiography during laparoscopic radical prostatectomy. *Urology.* 2010;75:581–4.

32. Deem S, Davis CR, Tierney JP. Transient paralysis after robotic prostatectomy. *J Robotic Surg.* 2008;2:45–6.

33. Hong JY, Oh YJ, Rha KH, et al. Pulmonary edema after da Vinci-assisted laparoscopic radical prostatectomy: a case report. *J Clin Anesth.* 2010;22:370–2.

34. American Society of Anesthesiologists Task Force on Perioperative Visual Loss. Practice advisory for perioperative visual loss associated with spine surgery: an updated report by the American Society of Anesthesiologists Task Force on Perioperative Visual Loss. *Anesthesiology.* 2012;116(2):274–85.

35. Postoperative Visual Study Group. Risk factors associated with ischemic optic neuropathy after spinal fusion surgery. *Anesthesiology.* 2012;116(1):15–24.

36. Weber ED. Posterior ischemic optic neuropathy after minimally invasive prostatectomy *J Neuroophthalmol.* 2007;27(4):285–7.

37. Piegeler T, Dreessen P, Schlapfer M, et al. Impact of intraoperative fluid management on outcome in patients undergoing robotic-assisted laparoscopic prostatectomy – a retrospective analysis. *Eur J Anaesth.* 2011;28:6AP1–6.

38. Sampat A, Parakati L, Kunnavakkam R, et al. Corneal abrasion in hysterectomy and prostatectomy: role of laparoscopic and robotic assistance. *Anesthesiol.* 2015:122(5):994–1001.

39. Pandey R, Elakkumanan LB, Garg R, et al. Brachial plexus injury after robotic-assisted thoracoscopic thymectomy. *J Cardiothorac Vasc Anesth.* 2009;23:584–6.

40. Park BJ, Flores RM, Rusch VW. Robotic assistance for video-assisted thoracic surgical lobectomy: technique and initial results. *J Thorac Cardiovasc Surg.* 2006;131:54–9.

41. Gharagozloo F, Margolis M, Tempesta B, et al. Robot-assisted lobectomy for early stage lung cancer: report of 100 consecutive cases. *Ann Thorac Surg.* 2009;88:380–4.

42. Van Hilleggersberg R, Boone J, Draaisma WA, et al. First experience with robot-assisted thoracoscopic esophagolymphadenectomy for esophageal cancer. *Surg Endosc.* 2006;20:1435–9.

43. Kerstine KH, DeArmond DT, Shamoun DM, Campos JH. The first series of completely robotic esophagectomies with three-field lymphadenectomy: initial experience. *Surg Endosc.* 2007;21:2285–92.

Chapter 19

Pain Management and Recovery after RAS

Maunak V. Rana and Eric S. Fouliard

Robotic surgery has seen a dramatic increase in use since the initial introduction of the da Vinci system for laparoscopic surgery. One of the purported benefits of the robotic approach is to provide for precise surgical tissue manipulation, access to surgical sites with a minimally invasive approach, and, consequently, less postoperative pain. With the advent of multimodal analgesia, a greater precision in treating pain with the most appropriate technique can be achieved whether by pharmacological agents or neuraxial procedures and nerve blocks.

The most effective way to make surgery less painful may lie in the operative technique utilized rather than the analgesics provided. Thus, the initial question to ponder is whether the robotic surgery platform leads to more comfortable patients. It has been proposed that robotic surgery results in a less painful approach for certain types of surgery and may even be a preferred approach in elderly people and children.[1,2] However, whether a procedure is robotically or conventionally performed, the length and location of the incision mandates the use of neuraxial or regional block.

Anesthesiologists, whether hospital- or outpatient-based, will need to be cognizant of the issues associated with robotic surgery in order to intervene with appropriate pain management strategies. Careful assessment of preoperative, intraoperative, and postoperative considerations is required to formulate a successful plan for pain management of robotic surgery patient.

Preoperative Assessment

The anesthesiologist must be aware of patients at risk for increased postoperative pain during the preoperative evaluation. Obese patients, in particular, may undergo physiological derangements due to steep positional challenges, along with the possibility of conversion to open techniques from the robotic approach. Additionally, those patients with other medical comorbidities, including cardiopulmonary and visceral abnormalities, may be at higher risk for inadequate postoperative pain management.

Surgeon experience also plays a role in pain assessment for robotic surgery patients. Those surgeons who are less experienced with the robotic platform may report longer operating room times and, consequently, increased pain due to the prolonged length of surgery and possibly an increased risk of open conversion. The learning curve for surgeon experience has been evaluated and was noted to be approximately 150 robotic cases before surgeons had routinely reproducible surgical results and a flattening of the learning curve; expert status at robotic surgery was noted to be achieved with at least 250 cases in the urologic literature.[3]

Intraoperative Management

The anesthesia provider must be aware of the indications for the robotic procedure to formulate an appropriate pain management plan. Robotic surgery offers the surgical team the benefit of sharp anatomical visualization. A fundamental tenet of the robotic platform is the allowance of more precision and stability, creating a three-dimensional view for the surgeon to directly appreciate anatomy.[4] Despite this accepted benefit of depth–perception visualization, some have suggested that robotic surgery is no more than a marketing approach and patients are just as well served by conventional surgery.[5]

Robotic surgery has also been reported as being less physiologically disruptive than conventional surgical techniques.[6] The patients who underwent robotic surgical procedures had a shorter operative time, decreased blood loss, and shorter hospital stay as compared to their conventional laparoscopic counterparts. Specific preoperative planning for obese and morbidly obese patients by the anesthesia team should include the cardiovascular/pulmonary and systemic effects of this condition as well as the varied effects of administered pharmacology.

A recent study presented level 2 evidence noting that robotic surgery was an option for staging procedures in obese patients but stopped short of advocating the newer approach over conventional laparoscopic approaches due to the underpowered results. There was no clinically significant benefit for robotic technique over conventional technique in this surgical population. Another study noted that obese and morbidly obese women are good candidates for robotic surgery due to the improved visualization and decreased tissue trespass, which would lead to fewer postsurgical complications.[7]

In the urology literature, robotic surgery has been evaluated extensively from financial, technical, and patient benefit perspectives. Patients have been studied in an effort to analyze the efficacy of robotic prostatic dissection on postoperative pain scores. In a study of 314 patients undergoing radical prostatectomy (159 robotic-assisted versus 154 retropubic radical), patient data was compared regarding analgesic requirements and pain scores. Interestingly, the patients who underwent robotic-assisted prostatectomy did not receive any benefit from a pain management perspective, as patients had similar pain scores in the open retropubic and the robotic prostate groups.[8] This somewhat surprising finding of pain equality despite robotic technique has been suggested to be due to the location of surgical trespass. Lower abdominal incisions are described to be less painful to patients than upper abdominal incisions due to the ease of separation of muscle fibers in the lower abdominal area. Furthermore, the more cephalad the incision in the abdominal musculature, the greater the effect on accessory respiratory muscles, a suggestion that could lead to decreased pulmonary toilet with splinting of involved muscles.

Contrary to this report is the finding of the Vattikutti Urology Institute of Detroit, which has shown benefit in the use of robotic procedures leading to less pain in patients than conventional open procedures.[9] Robotic prostatectomy was also purported to lead to less abdominal surgery as compared to open procedures and laparoscopic approaches due to a more direct visualization of tissues. An example cited was the use of direct peritoneal visualization during the placement of the Verres introducer needle as compared to blind placement during conventional laparoscopy. Theoretically, a direct visualization can lead to less tissue trauma and fewer complications during trocar placement with a decreased risk of umbilical hernia and less morbidity.[10]

A separate group noted in a prospective study, which compared 20 consecutive robotic radical cystectomy patients with those who underwent open radical cystectomy, that the robotic group had similar pain control but less opioid requirements.[11] Daily opiate use along with pain scores were compared between the groups. Other studies have evaluated laparoscopic versus robotic surgery and have not shown a clear benefit for the robotic procedures. A single-center randomized controlled study comparing laparoscopic and robotic sacrocolpopexy surgeries found that robot-assisted surgeries required longer operating room times and patients had increased pain scores at rest and with activity in the first month after surgery.[12]

The anesthesiologist should be vigilant in assessing the preoperative risks of postoperative pain by discussing with the surgeon the risk of converting to an open procedure. While that information may not always be readily provided, anticipating conversion should be part of the anesthesia assessment when planning appropriate pain management techniques. The conversion rate from a purely robotic procedure to open is variably reported in the literature.[13] The risk of converting from robotic to open surgery is increased with a history of multiple prior surgeries combined with anatomically difficult surgical pathology. Depending on the type of surgery, such as an operation that may require a large incision in close proximity to accessory respiratory muscles, neuraxial analgesia and/or nerve blocks may be required and should be planned for.

Regional Anesthesia

In addition to evaluating patient presentation and noting surgical experience, the anesthesiologist must consider the role of regional anesthesia in patients about to undergo robotic surgery and the benefit of this adjunctive analgesic for the type of surgery being performed. A study evaluated the role of transversus abdominis plane (TAP) block in patients undergoing robotic gynecologic oncology surgery.[14] This randomized, placebo-controlled trial placed 64 patients into two groups – the first receiving a single, unilateral TAP block with 30 ml of 0.25 percent bupivacaine with 3 mcg/ml epinephrine adjacent to the robotic assistant port, the second receiving a sham saline injection. Surprisingly, the preoperative TAP block did not decrease opiate use in this population. Another study evaluating the same type of block in gynecologic laparoscopic surgery compared the placement of a preoperative ultrasound-guided TAP block against infiltrating the trocar site intraoperatively with bupivacaine on postoperative pain.[15] The authors presented their findings via this prospective, randomized study and allowed for the observation of subjects initially after surgery and at regular intervals for up to 48 hours postoperatively. The results of this study demonstrated that patients had equal pain scores, regardless of which approach was utilized. While there was a statistically significant improvement in pain scores (on a 10-point scale) at 2 hours and across time with the ultrasound-guided block, clinically significant results were not achieved with this approach.

In patients undergoing robotic-assisted hysterectomy, a prospective, randomized, controlled observer blinded study evaluated the efficacy of bilateral subcostal TAP blocks with bupivacaine against liposomal bupivacaine.[16] Liposomal bupivacaine is a novel preparation of a commonly used local anesthetic encapsulated along with a carrier molecule. The goal of this vesicularly bound bupivacaine is to increase the duration of local anesthetic action by a slow release as compared to plain bupivacaine.[17] During this study, patients were followed for 72 hours after the injection and compared on opioid use, overall satisfaction, and pain scores. Patients were found to have lower opioid use and lower maximal pain scores after the use of liposomal preparation. The results of this study were examined in a pilot study in the urologic population, attempting to compare two different concentrations of the preparation. The prospective evaluation featured the effects of liposomal bupivacaine via a TAP block in robotic prostatectomy in a 20-mL volume (266 mg) versus a 40-mL volume of the same drug. The dilution was performed with 0.9 percent normal saline. Duration of analgesia, time to first opioid, patient-assessed pain scores, opioid use, and adverse events were studied. The median time to the first administration of opioid did not differ between the two groups. Additionally, the secondary outcomes of pain scores, opioid use, and adverse events did not differ based on the volume delivered.

Robotic approaches have been utilized in cardiac surgery.[18,19] Mitral valve repair and replacement is an area that has been studied and performed via a minimally invasive approach. Despite the smaller incisions and theoretical risk of reduced discomfort, patients may still experience discomfort due to surgical trauma and chest tube–induced nerve irritation.[20] Pain scores may not be reduced after the minimally accessed approach as compared to open procedures.[21] Regional anesthesia performed preoperatively has allowed for immediate postsurgical extubation in patients undergoing robotic mitral valve repair. The use of ultrasound-guided paravertebral block in one evaluation provided sufficient analgesia, leading to postprocedure extubation prior to intensive care unit transfer. The advantages of the block are obvious as the possible pulmonary derangements due to mechanical ventilation are avoided.[22–24] Paravertebral block was also evaluated in a randomized, prospective study comparing analgesia and satisfaction for up to 48 hours after surgery.[25] When comparing those patients receiving general anesthesia alone, those patients with paravertebral block had less intraoperative narcotic requirements and less postoperative pain. Satisfaction scores were also higher after paravertebral block. Furthermore, patients were able to be extubated after surgery. A large meta-analysis was conducted reviewing paravertebral blocks in thoracic surgery and found that this approach provided benefits over other forms of analgesia in patients undergoing robotic thoracic procedures.[26]

Neuraxial Techniques

As noted above, robotic surgery is touted as a minimally invasive surgical approach that would allow for intervention without increased analgesia. Typically neuraxial techniques are not required; however, when a procedure is converted from the minimally invasive approach to an open surgery, epidural analgesia may provide relief for surgical pain. The conversion to an open procedure is typically a function of experience of the surgeon and also the difficulty of surgical access and ranges from 4.9 percent for gynecologic oncology surgeries to 15 percent in esophagectomy surgery.[27–29]

Thoracic epidural placement and utilization has been evaluated in robotic surgery and has produced favorable results.[30,31] A prospective randomized trial compared the analgesic effects of thoracic epidural and paravertebral block in patients undergoing robotic coronary artery bypass grafting (CABG) surgery. Despite the fact that robotic surgery entails a small incision compared to traditional midline sternotomy in conventional CABG, thoracotomy does occur with this surgical approach and would, therefore, lead to postoperative discomfort. The patients in the thoracic group had epidural access at C7/T1 with the catheter placed 4 cm beyond the point that loss of resistance was achieved. The paravertebral group had a catheter placed at T4/5 as part of the analgesia for surgery. Patients in both groups received 8 ml of 0.5 percent bupivacaine followed by an infusion of 0.25 percent bupivacaine at 0.1 ml/kg/h. The results indicated that there was no difference in analgesia with the different routes of administration of local anesthetic agents.

Reports exist in the literature on the use of epidural analgesia during robotic surgery with evidence of benefit.[32] Patients undergoing robot-assisted cystectomy received thoracic epidurals for postoperative pain management. In this presentation, patients had the epidural activated during the intraoperative phase to coincide with the ileal conduit portion of the surgery with epidural morphine. The epidural was not activated during the cystectomy portion of the surgery due to the use of steep Trendelenburg position and the risk of hemodynamic aberration.

Improved analgesia with the use of an epidural for robotic surgery may also improve intraoperative pulmonary relationships.[33] As noted previously, robotic-assisted surgeries typically require high-pressure pneumoperitoneum and extreme head-down position for prolonged periods that can lead to ventilation perfusion mismatching. Robot-assisted laparoscopic radical prostatectomy surgery patients have experienced physiologic benefits with the addition of thoracic epidural versus general anesthesia only cohorts. Patients were randomized to receive either T4 thoracic epidural with general anesthesia or general anesthesia alone. The patients in the epidural group were shown to have lower overall peak inspiratory pressure and higher dynamic compliance than the general anesthesia group. The presence of improved pulmonary function would be beneficial to patients in the postoperative arena. Additionally, the epidural group had lower lactate levels and improved oxygenation on arterial blood gas measurements. The presence of lower lactate may have a role in improved analgesia, as lactate can indicate elevated pain states.[34]

Preemptive Analgesia

Preemptive analgesia, the administration of antinociceptive agents prior to a noxious stimulus in an attempt to abolish the development of central sensitization, is a controversial concept in pain management. There are proponents and detractors of this approach to perioperative care. There exists benefit in the selected use of agents to decrease the pain of surgery, especially in the robotic surgery population.[35] In a retrospective analysis, 150 patients who underwent robot-assisted laparoscopic hysterectomy were treated with celecoxib and ropivacaine preemptively against those receiving an opioid-only regimen. The postanesthetic recovery unit time was decreased by 16 min in the multimodal group along with the continued reduced opioid requirements in the first few days after surgery.

Membrane Stabilizers

Membrane stabilizers are a diverse class of agents utilized traditionally as antiepileptic agents in an attempt to decrease or interrupt action potential development across the neuromuscular membrane. Pregabalin is a representative member of this agent class that has shown utility in the pain management of robotic surgery patients. A retrospective study evaluated the use of a multimodal pain regimen on postoperative pain in men undergoing robot-assisted laparoscopic radical prostatectomy.[36] Patients received a pregabalin, acetaminophen, or celecoxib regimen 2 hours prior to surgery and postoperatively, or ketorolac, oxycodone, and acetaminophen. The multimodal group was noted to have a decreased morphine equivalent dose overall and a lower mean postoperative opioid use duration.

A randomized, double-blinded placebo-controlled trial studied the safety and efficacy of pregabalin in robotic thyroidectomy.[37] Patients were divided into two groups, one receiving 150 mg of pregabalin and the other placebo drug 1 hour before surgery and again at 12 hours. Patients were then evaluated for pain and side effects for 48 hours after surgery. Side effects studied included postoperative nausea and vomiting and sedation, which were graded on scales. A particular strength of this study is that patients were followed for 3 months after surgery for the development of postoperative pain. Pain scores were evaluated with a verbal numerical rating scale and compared between the two groups. The pain scores were lower in the pregabalin group and postoperative requirements were lower in this group than controls in the immediate postoperative period. Although suggested as an agent for the prevention of chronic pain, this study showed that there were no differences noted for protection against development of chronic pain with pregabalin administration.[38] The improvement in acute pain scores after perioperative pregabalin administration was also corroborated in a study evaluating patients undergoing laparoscopic cholecystectomy.[39] A dose of 600 mg of pregabalin in divided doses demonstrated pain score improvement and total opioid consumption. This benefit was mitigated by the presence of increased dizziness in patients, despite the improved analgesia.

Intravenous Acetaminophen

Intravenous acetaminophen has been advocated as an agent in the armamentarium of anesthesiologists pursuing multimodal perioperative pain management due to its opioid-sparing effects.[40] The formulation of this agent is 1,000 mg of acetaminophen in 100-mL vials. The cost of this agent may prevent routine use, but it has been evaluated in the robotic surgery population.[41,42] This prospective, randomized, double-blinded study evaluated patients undergoing robotic thyroidectomy, examining the effect of repeat doses of intravenous paracetamol (acetaminophen) on postoperative pain. Patients were randomized to placebo or 1 g intravenous agent 1 hour prior to anesthetic induction and for 6-hour intervals over the following 24 hours. Postoperative pain was noted to be lower in the intravenous paracetamol group, along with less nausea and vomiting. The use of intravenous acetaminophen has also led to an opioid-free perioperative management of patients undergoing robotic prostatectomy. In a study evaluating the opioid requirements after robotic major pelvic surgery, patients were given intravenous acetaminophen during surgery and ketorolac 15 min before the completion of the study. The patients also received acetaminophen and ketorolac in scheduled doses every 6 and 8 hours, respectively. More than half of the patients in the study did not request parenteral opioids during the PACU and postoperative stay. The use of intravenous acetaminophen as part of a multimodal regimen may lead to a paradigm shift in the utility of this agent. While the use of intravenous paracetamol may add to drug costs, improved outcomes and efficiency may result from the inclusion in pain management regimens.[43]

Intraoperative Issues Affecting Pain Management

In addition to various physical factors such as patient habitus, coexisting medical conditions, and surgeon experience, certain factors inherent in robotic surgery deserve consideration in evaluating the pain management of robotic surgery patients.

Patient position is an important consideration for the anesthesiologist to be aware of and to manage appropriately. Typically patients are placed in a steep head-down or Trendelenburg position. Steep Trendelenburg is defined as 30–45 degrees of head-down tilt.[44] Prolonged surgery in this position can lead to an increased risk of thromboembolic episodes due to vascular stasis and pneumoperitoneum.[45] Additionally, with the head-down position, patients can develop elevated central venous pressures, which can cause back pressure increases manifested as increased intraocular pressures (IOP) and intracranial pressure (ICP). Central venous pressure increases three-fold as compared to initial values, with a doubling of mean arterial pressure and pulmonary capillary wedge pressure.[46] A result of this increased pressure translocation to the physiology of the patient is an imbalance in myocardial oxygen supply and demand, thus increasing the oxygen demand. A potential result of this discrepancy may be chest pain and cardiac arrhythmia after surgery. Despite these concerns, heart rate, cardiac output, and mixed venous oxygen content are unaffected.[46]

Another important factor for the anesthesia provider to be aware of is the relationship between pneumoperitoneum and pain risk. The benefit of pneumoperitoneum includes improved visualization and hemostatic tamponade; however, the insufflation of gas, coupled with steep position, can lead to hypotension primarily via decreased venous return. Subsequent hypotension has the potential to lead to decreased urine output and the risk of renal dysfunction. Additionally, pneumoperitoneum has a role in the release of catecholamines, as increased abdominal pressures lead to an increase in catecholamines.[47,48] Increased catecholamines, in addition to stressing patient physiology, can lead to increased postsurgical pain. The end result of this process is the development of oxidative stress and a theoretical release of arachidonic acid, the carboxylic fatty acid constituent of cell membranes that is a key mediator in the inflammatory process and nociception and hyperalgesia.[49,50]

It has been reported in the literature that the combination of a steep Trendelenburg position in addition to high-pressure CO_2 gas insufflation can also lead to shoulder pain due to diaphragmatic irritation.[51] Reduction of high gas flows has shown to decrease the shoulder pain after laparoscopy. Patients were divided into two groups with the first being exposed to 9 mmHg CO_2 versus 12 mmHg for the latter group undergoing surgery. Shoulder pain was found to be less prevalent in the lower pressure group initially after surgery and for 24 hours after ($p < 0.05$).[52]

A consideration for intraoperative pain management for anesthesiologists is to delay utilization of an epidural that has been placed preoperatively due to the steep Trendelenburg position and the ensuing hypotension that may result due to position changes and the effect of local anesthetic sympathectomy.[53] Epidural use should, therefore, be reserved for the portion of operation without Trendelenburg position, during wound closure, or in the postrecovery unit.

Support devices to secure the patient during position changes associated with robotic surgery may also lead to pain issues in the recovery period. Typically a restrictive pad is used in the shoulder area to prevent the patient slipping from the front of the bed during the head-down position. This pad has been associated with brachial plexus stretching and injury, culminating in neuropraxia and risk of neuropathy.[54] The overall incidence of neuropathy in patients undergoing robotic prostate is low with a reported rate of approximately 0.25 percent.[55] The anesthesiologist must be vigilant to patient position as a slight abduction of the upper extremity may lead to brachial plexopathy.[56]

Lower extremity nerves may also be affected with positioning as common peroneal nerve injury may occur with patients placed in the lithotomy position for genitourinary surgeries as the lateral aspect of the leg is compressed with stirrup devices for extended periods.[54] The saphenous nerve is also at risk for injury during surgery, revealing numbness in the medial aspect of the lower extremity due to intraoperative compression.

The development of well-leg compartment syndrome, although not common, is a devastating complication of robotic surgery. As such, this is a risk that the entire operative team needs to be vigilant in preventing.[57] This process has an incidence in 1 in 3,500 operations during major pelvic surgery in the lithotomy position. The risk factors for the development of compartment syndrome in the absence of overt muscle injury include prolonged surgery duration (>4 hours), lithotomy position, steep Trendelenburg position, extended duration ankle dorsiflexion, circumferential wrappings on lower extremities, intraoperative hypotension, hypovolemia, excessive use of vasoconstrictive drugs, peripheral vascular disease, and surgical retraction on major vessels during surgery. Clearly, robotic surgery with a requirement for steep Trendelenburg, possibility of longer surgery times and intraoperative hypotension, can increase the risk of compartment syndrome. Patients can present with paresthesia, which is defined as pain outproportion to degree of overt injury, discomfort on passive stretch of lower extremities, and tightness in the calves. As this process progresses, patients may develop decreased to absent pulses and subsequent ischemia.

Box 19.1 Risk Factors for Well-Leg Compartment Syndrome

Prolonged surgery duration (>4 hours)
Lithotomy position
Steep Trendelenburg position
Prolonged ankle dorsiflexion
Circumferential wrappings on lower extremities
Intraoperative hypotension, hypovolemia
Surgical retraction on major vessels during surgery
Excessive use of vasoconstrictive drugs
Preexisting peripheral vascular disease

Vigilance and active interventions are the best prevention for this dreaded occurrence. Decreasing surgical times, time in the Trendelenburg position, adjusting and removing leg supports every 2 hours for short periods if surgery lasts more than 4 hours would be beneficial in decreasing injury. Ankle dorsiflexion is to be avoided, along with wide blood pressure variations, decreased blood volume, and excessive vasopressor use during surgery (Box 19.1). Treatment involves emergent fasciotomy the pressurized compartments as a delay in treatment can lead to morbidity and mortality.

From an operative management standpoint, aside from increased finance for the hospital, the increased time associated with robotic surgery predisposes the patient to be at risk for increased pain. As the length of surgery increases, there is an increased theoretical use of analgesics as compared to the same operation being performed more quickly.

Surgical Approach Choices and Pain Management

As highlighted above, the location of surgery influences pain management choices for the anesthesiologist in selecting the most appropriate analgesia for the patient. Regarding CABG, the choice of surgical access directly impacts the pain management approach.[58] Sternotomy is typically less painful than thoracotomy, and those approaches requiring sternal approach generally can be treated with intravenous agents in the acute postoperative phase. Surgical approaches requiring analgesic supplementation include thoracotomy for minimally invasive direct CABG (MIDCAB). MIDCAB is a direct approach to CABG on the beating heart. Access is achieved via an incision between the ribs to access the area of bypass. Due to the incision site, supplementation with intercostal nerve blocks and/or regional anesthesia is required for postoperative pain control.

Postoperative Pain Issues

The primary consideration for postoperative pain in robotic surgery patients is: does robotic surgery lend itself to less pain for patients? In select surgical settings, robotic surgery is less painful, but in others, the minimally invasive approach is found to have mixed reviews and does not lead to better postsurgical analgesia.[59] According to a study published in the *Annals of Surgery*, postsurgical pain was found to be less in conventional laparotomy compared to a minimally invasive approach. Additionally, laparotomy patients required one-third less medication in the first 4 hours after surgery compared to their less invasive counterparts.

Effective pain management is reflected by improved pain scores, quicker patient mobility times, and more favorable economics. A cost analysis was performed on postoperative pain management in endometrial cancer patients comparing robotic surgery patients and conventional laparoscopic surgery patients.[60] Patients undergoing laparoscopic surgery were compared to those who underwent robotic surgery and analyzed for postoperative pain requirements in the 24-hour period after reaching the surgical floor. Those patients who underwent robotic surgery had 50 percent fewer nursing interventions for pain control as compared to those patients undergoing traditional laparoscopic surgery. Also, pain scores were lower in the robotic cohort than in the laparoscopic group (2.1 vs. 3.0 on VAS). From a financial perspective, there was a 50 percent decrease in the cost of postoperative pain management in robotic surgery patients ($p < 0.01$).

Ileus is a postoperative event that is a pain issue to be concerned with in abdominopelvic surgery patients. Causative factors of decreased bowel function postsurgery include visceral manipulation and decreased function, opioid-induced decreased motility, and pneumoperitoneum effects.[61] A study evaluated the effects of opioids on postoperative ileus in patients undergoing surgery for bladder carcinoma via open surgery and robotic surgery. Results were evaluated with multivariate analysis of intravenous patient-controlled analgesia (PCA) fentanyl and oral tramadol administrations. Results indicated that robotic surgery reduces the time to flatus and first meal decreasing ileus. In the open surgery group, PCA fentanyl and tramadol increased time to flatus and diet, essentially confirming the slowing and decreased transit time in the gut. The robotic patients had a flatus time increase with tramadol only and no significant increase with PCA fentanyl.

The development of neuropathy is also a pain issue to be focused on, although the incidence of this occurrence is quite low.[62]

Surgical site infections (SSI) have received justifiable importance in the perioperative management of patients by the Centers for Disease Control.[63,64] A known risk factor associated with the development of SSI is longer surgical times. One study reported that infections were more likely to develop in patients who had longer surgery times despite the claim that robotic surgery is associated with less anatomic and physiologic trespass than conventional surgical approaches. Colon surgery, for example, was noted to have a higher infection incidence than genitourinary surgery due to increased length of surgery.

Specific types of pain that anesthesiologists will need to focus on that may be underreported include cephalgia (headache) and ocular pain after robotic surgery. The prolonged steep Trendelenburg leads to an increase in ICP, which can increase the risk for headache.[65,66] Patients may also be at risk for ophthalmic pain after robotic surgery. The steep head-down position coupled with increased ophthalmic pressure and ICP can lead to this phenomenon.[67] IOP reaches peak levels at the end of the steep Trendelenburg position with a level at or around 13 mmHg higher than preinduction levels. Surgical duration and ET-CO_2 were the only predictors of IOP increases in Trendelenburg position. As robotic surgery times may be prolonged in some platforms, patients will be at risk for optic neuralgias. This is a significant consideration for patients with glaucoma and those at risk for ocular hypertension.

Summary

Robotic surgical platforms have advanced the art and science of patient care, allowing for improved visualization and dexterity via a minimally invasive approach beyond conventional laparoscopy. Robotic surgery has also been shown in certain instances to provide quicker recovery and favorable postoperative economics to hospitals. An important consideration for anesthesiologists is pain management of patients undergoing robot-assisted surgery as this format is being utilized with increasing frequency.

As perioperative physicians, anesthesiologists need to consider preoperative, intraoperative, and postoperative issues relevant to the robotic platform. A careful assessment of the patient's history along with detailed analysis of comorbidities begins the process. Review of organ system pathology will help the physician identify patients at risk for increased pain management needs.

Intraoperative concerns, including surgical times, patient position, and pneumoperitoneum, must be followed and carefully scrutinized as factors affecting pain management. The use of neuraxial and regional analgesia has been a noted benefit in surgical settings such as thoracic and cardiac surgery; recovery times have been significantly improved with the robotic approach coupled with a focused regional technique.

Postoperative issues in the robotic surgery patient need to be assessed and followed by the perioperative anesthesiologist as intervention and treatment with the appropriate regimen can decrease pain scores and improve patient recovery (Box 19.2).

Multimodal analgesia, regardless of operative indication, will play an important role in the future pain management of robotic surgery patients as better pain scores and quicker recovery times have been achieved with the addition of membrane stabilizers and selective nonsteroidal antiinflammatory drugs, which have decreased or eliminated opioid requirements in patients. Innovation and less trespass via the robotic approach will continue to progress with improving technology and surgeon/anesthesiologist collaboration. Continued evaluation of the benefits of robotic surgery and the review of protocols via a double-blinded randomized controlled trial approach will enhance and lead to directed, more-focused pain management for superior patient outcome.

Box 19.2 Risks Factors for Increased Pain Requirements after Robotic Surgery

Surgery site/approach
Difficult surgical access
Prolonged surgery
Patient positioning
Surgeon experience
Conversion to open
Medical comorbidity (cardiac disease, diabetes, obesity)
History of preoperative opioid requirements

References

1. R.S. Lee. Pediatric Robot Assisted Laparoscopic Dismembered Pyeloplasty: Comparison with a Cohort of Open Surgery. *J Urol* 2006; 175(2): 683–7.
2. M.L. Knox. Robotic Versus Open Radical Cystectomy: Identification of Patients Who Benefit from the Robotic Approach. *J Endourol* 2013; 27(1): 40–4.
3. S.D. Herrell. Robotic-Assisted Laparoscopic Prostatectomy: What Is the Learning Curve? *Urology* 2005; 66(5), suppl, 105: 7.
4. M. Mack. Minimally Invasive and Robotic Surgery. *JAMA* 2001; 285(5): 568–72.
5. P.T. Ramirez, K.M. Schmeler, J.K. Wolf. Robotic Radical Parametrectomy and Pelvic Lympadenectomy in Patients with Invasive Cervical Cancer. *Gynecologic Oncology* 2008.
6. C.H. Chen. Comparing Robotic Surgery with Conventional Laparoscopy and Laparotomy for Cervical Cancer Management. *Int J Gynecol Cancer* 2014; 24(5): 1105–11.
7. J. Ryu. Retropubic Versus Robot-Assisted Laparoscopic Prostatectomy for Prostate Cancer: A Comparative Study of Postoperative Complications. *Korean J Urol* 2013; 54(11): 756–61.
8. M. Menon. Prospective Comparison of Radical Retropubic Prostatectomy and Robot Assisted Anatomic Prostatectomy: The Vattikuti Urology Institute Experience. *Urology* 2002; 60(5): 864–8.
9. T.G. Costello. Anaesthesia for Robot Assisted Anatomic Prostatectomy. Experience at a Single Institution. *Anaesth Intensive Care* 2006; 34: 787–92.
10. K.A. Guru. Robot-Assisted Radical Cystectomy Versus Open Radical Cystectomy: Assessment of Postoperative Pain. *Can J Urol* 2007; 14(6): 3753–6.
11. M.R. Paraiso. Laparoscopic Compared with Robotic Sacrocolpoplexy for Vaginal Prolapse: A Randomized

Controlled Trial. *Obstetrics and Gynecology* 2011; 118(5): 1005–13.

12. G. Spinoglio. Robotic Colorectal Surgery: First 50 Cases Experience. *Diseases of the Colon and Rectum* 2008; 51(11): 1627–32.
13. B.T. Hotujec. Transversus Abdominal Plane Block in Robotic Gynecologic Oncology: A Randomized, Placebo-Controlled Trial. *Gynecol Oncol* 2015; 136(3): 460–5.
14. L. El Hachem. Randomized Controlled Double-Blind Trial of Transversus Abdominal Plane Block Versus Trocar Site Infiltration in Gynecologic Laparoscopy. *Am J Obstet Gynecol* 2015; 212(2): 182.e1–9.
15. J. Hutchins. Ultrasound Guided Subcostal Transversus Abdominal Plane Infiltration with Liposomal Bupivacaine for Patients Undergoing Robotic Assisted Hysterectomy: A Prospective Randomized Controlled Study. *Gynecol Oncol* 2015; 138(3): 609–13.
16. P. Chahar. Liposomal Bupivacaine: A Review of a New Bupivacaine Formulation. *J Pain Res* 2012; 5: 257–64.
17. S.P. Deshpande. Anesthetic Management of Robotically Assisted Totally Endoscopic Coronary Artery Bypass Surgery (TECAB). *J Cardiothorac Vasc Anesth* 2013; 27(3): 586–99.
18. S.P. Deshpande. Totally Endoscopic Robotic Coronary Artery Bypass Surgery. *Curr Opin Anaesthesiol* 2014; 27(1): 49–56.
19. Y.W. Hsu. Robot-Assisted Mitral Valve Repair. *Journal of Cardiothoracic and Vascular Anesthesia* 2011; 25(4): 721–30.
20. J. Cogan. Pain Levels after Minimally Invasive Cardiac Surgery: Results for the First 7 Days. *Anesth Analg* 2010; 110: 1–101.
21. R.M. Suri. Optimizing Outcomes of Robotic Mitral Valve Repair for All Prolapse Anatomy: The Suri-Burkhart Technique. *Ann Cardiothorac Surg* 2013; 2(6): 841–5.
22. S. Chauhan. Anesthesia for Robotic Cardiac Surgery: An Amalgam of Technology and Skill. *Ann Card Anaesth* 2010; 13: 169–75.
23. J. J. Lynch. Use of Paravertebral Blockade to Facilitate Early Extubation after Minimally Invasive Cardiac Surgery. *Semin Cardiothorac Vasc Anesth* 2010; 14: 7–48.
24. P.J. Neuburger. A Prospective Randomized Study of Paravertebral Blockade in Patients Undergoing Robotic Mitral Valve Repair. *J Cardiothoracic and Vascular Anesthesia* 2015; 29(4): 930–6.
25. D.K. Baidya. Analgesic Efficacy and Safety of Thoracic Paravertebral and Epidural Analgesia for Thoracic Surgery: A Systematic Review and Meta-analysis. *Interactive Cardiovascular and Thoracic Surgery* 2014; 18(5): 626–35.
26. J.R. Lee. Anesthetic Considerations for Robotic Surgery. *Korean J Anesthesiol* 2014; 66(1): 3–11.
27. P.T. Ramirez. Society of Gynecologic Oncology Clinical Practice Robotics Task Force. Robotic-Assisted Surgery in Gynecologic Oncology: A Society of Gynecologic Oncology Consensus Statement. *Gynecologic Oncology* 2012; 124: 180–4.
28. B. Weksler. Robot-Assisted Minimally Invasive Esophagectomy Is Equivalent to Thoracoscopic Minimally Invasive Esophagectomy. *Dis Esophagus* 2012; 25: 403–9.
29. R.A. da Silva Sardenberg. Robotic Thymectomy for Myasthenia Gravis. *J bras pneumol* 2011; 37(5).
30. Y. Mehta. Comparison of Continuous Thoracic Epidural and Paravertebral Block for Postoperative Analgesia after Robotic-Assisted Coronary Bypass Surgery. *Ann Card Anaesth* 2008; 11: 91–6.
31. J. Punj. Anesthesia for Robot Assisted Cystectomy: Our Initial Experience. *The Internet Journal of Anesthesiology* 2007; 16(1).
32. J.Y. Hong. Effects of Thoracic Epidural Analgesia Combined with General Anesthesia on Intraoperative Ventilation/Oxygenation and Postoperative Pulmonary Complications in Robot-Assisted Laparoscopic Radical Prostatectomy. *Journal Endourol* 2009; 23(11): 1843–49.
33. B. Gerdie. Chronic Widespread Pain: Increased Glutamate and Lactate Concentrations in the Trapezius Muscle and Plasma. *Clin J Pain* 2014; 30(5): 409–20.
34. T.M. Shultz. Preemptive Multimodal Analgesia Facilitates Same-Day Discharge Following Robot-Assisted Hysterectomy. *Journal of Robotic Surgery* 2012; 6(2): 115–23.
35. E.J. Trabulsi. Preemptive Multimodal Pain Regimen Reduces Opioid Analgesia for Patients Undergoing Robotic-Assisted Laparoscopic Radical Prostatectomy. *Urology* 2010; 76(5): 1122–4.
36. S.Y. Kim. Perioperative Administration of Pregabalin for Pain after Robot-Assisted Endoscopic Thyroidectomy: A Randomized Clinical Trial. *Surg Endosc* 2010; 24: 2776–81.
37. A. Agarwal. Evaluation of a Single Preoperative Dose of Pregabalin for Attenuation of Postoperative Pain after Laparoscopic Cholecystectomy. *Br J Anaesth* 101(5): 700–4.
38. C. Sarakatsianou. Effect of Pre-emptive Pregabalin on Pain Intensity and Postoperative Morphine

Consumption after Laparoscopic Cholecystectomy. *Surg Endosc* 2013; 27(7): 2504–11.

39. M. Ammar. Intravenous Acetaminophen – Is It Worth the Cost? *Cleveland Clinic Clinical Rx Forum* 2013; 1(2): 1, 5–7.
40. C. Wong. Opioid-Free Analgesia Following Robot-Assisted Laparoscopic Prostatectomy. *J Am Coll Surg* 2013; 217(3): S152.
41. J.Y. Hong. Paracetamol Reduces Postoperative Pain and Rescue Analgesic Demand after Robot-Assisted Endoscopic Thyroidectomy by the Transaxillary Approach. *World J Surg* 2010; 34(3): 521–6.
42. J.S. Jahr. Intravenous Acetaminophen: A Review of Pharmacoeconomic Science for Perioperative Use. *Am J Ther* 2013; 20(2): 189–99.
43. A. Ghomi. Trendelenburg Position in Gynecologic Robotic Surgery. *J Minim Invasive Gynecol* 2012; 19(4): 485–9.
44. A.F. Kalmar. Influence of Steep Trendelenburg Position and Co2 Pneumoperitoneum on Cardiovascular, Cerebrovascular, and Respiratory Homeostasis during Robotic Prostatectomy. *Br J Anaesth* 2010; 104: 433–9.
45. M. Lestar. Hemodynamic Perturbations during Robot-Assisted Laparoscopic Radical Prostatectomy in 45 Degree Trendelenburg Position. *Anesthesia & Analgesia* 2011; 113(5): 1069–75.
46. O. Mikami. High Intra-abdominal Pressure Increases Plasma Catecholamine Concentrations during Pneumoperitoneum for Laparoscopic Procedures. *Arch Surg* 1998; 133(1): 39–43.
47. C. Mann. The Relationship among Carbon Dioxide Pneumoperitoneum, Vasopressin Release, and Hemodynamic Changes. *Anesth Analg* 1999; 89: 278–83.
48. G. Swift. A Prospective Randomised Double-Blind Placebo Controlled Trial to Assess Whether Gas Drains Reduce Shoulder Pain Following Gynaecological Laparoscopy. *Aust N Z J Obstet Gynaecol* 2002; 42: 267–70.
49. H.S. Smith. Arachidonic Acid Pathways in Nociception. *J Support Oncol* 2006; 4(6): 277–87.
50. M. Irvine. Anaesthesia for Robot-Assisted Laparoscopic Surgery. *Contin Educ Anaesth Crit Care Pain* 2009: 1–5.
51. L. Sarli. Prospective Randomized Trial of Low-Pressure Pneumoperitoneum for Reduction of Shoulder-Tip Pain Following Laparoscopy. *Br J Surg* 2000; 87: 1161–5.
52. A.B. de Souza. The Effect of Intra-abdominal Pressure on the Generation of 8-iso Prostaglandin F2A during Laparoscopy in Rabbits. *Human Reproduction* 2003; 18(10): 2181–8.
53. D. Shveiky D. Brachial Plexus Injury after Laparoscopic and Robotic Surgery. *J Minim Invasive Gynecol* 2010; 17(4): 414–20.
54. A. Mattei. Positioning Injury, Rhabdomyolysis, and Serum Creatine Kinase Concentration Course in Patients Undergoing Robot-Assisted Radical Prostatectomy and Extended Pelvic Lymph Node Dissection. *J Endourol* 2013; 27(1): 45–51.
55. R. Pandey. Brachial Plexus Injury after Robotic-Assisted Thoracoscopic Thymectomy. *J Cardiothorac Vasc Anesth* 2009; 23: 584–6.
56. K.Y. Chin. Bilateral Well Leg Compartment Syndrome Associated with Lithotomy (Lloyd Davies) Position during Gastrointestinal Surgery: A Case Report and Review of Literature. *Eplasty* 2009; 14(9): e48.
57. G. Wang. Anesthesia Management for Robotically Assisted Endoscopic Coronary Artery Bypass Grafting on Beating Heart. *Innovations (Phila)* 2010; 5(4): 291–4.
58. P. Ekstein. Laparoscopic Surgery May Be Associated with Severe Pain and High Analgesia Requirements in the Immediate Postoperative Period. *Ann Surg* 2006; 243(1): 41–6.
59. M.A. Martino. A Cost Analysis of Postoperative Pain Management in Endometrial Cancer Patients: Robotic Surgery vs Laparoscopy Surgery. Poster presented at the 2011 Society of Gynecologic Oncology, Orlando, FL
60. K.C. Koo. Analgesic Opioid Dose Is an Important Indicator of Postoperative Ileus Following Radical Cystectomy with Ileal Conduit: Experience in the Robotic Surgery Era. *Yonsei Med J* 2014; 55(5): 1359–65.
61. G. Koc. Lower Extremity Neuropathies after Robot-Assisted Laparoscopic Prostatectomy on a Split-Leg Table. *Journal of Endourology* 2012; 1026–9.
62. D.P. Calfee. Strategies to Prevent Surgical Site Infections in Acute Care Hospitals. *Infection Control and Hospital Epidemiology* 2008; 29(1): 51–61.
63. E.D. Hermsen. Incidence of Surgical Site Infection Associated with Robotic Surgery. *Infection Control & Hospital Epidemiology* 2010; 31(8): 822–7.
64. L.T. Dunn. Raised Intracranial Pressure. *J Neurol Neurosurg Psychiatry* 2002; 73: i23–27.
65. J.R. Whiteley. Detection of Elevated Intracranial Pressure in Robot-Assisted Laparoscopic Radical

Prostatectomy using Ultrasonography of Optic Nerve Sheath Diameter. *J Neurosurg Anesthesiol* 2015; 27(2): 155–9.

66. H. Awad. The Effects of Steep Trendelenburg Positioning on Intraocular Pressure during Robotic Radical Prostatectomy. *Anesthesia & Analgesia* 2009; 109(2): 473–8.

67. Yoshikawa Y, Tsutsumi N, Ohkoshi K, et al. The Effect of Steep Trendelenburg Positioning on Intraocular Pressure and Visual Function during Robotic-Assisted Radical Prostatectomy. *British Journal of Ophthalmology* 2014; 98(3): 305–8.

Chapter 20

Technical Skills Training and Simulation

Jayne Smitten, Fozia Ferozali, Russell Metcalfe-Smith, and John T. Paige

Introduction

Educating healthcare professionals is a process, which requires significant expertise across multiple professions and creative strategies. The advancement of science is bringing about changes in medicine on an almost daily basis. As clinicians, we embrace the need to become life-long learners and continue to provide the best possible evidence-based medicine. We seek to offer better care and implement new techniques. We embrace the clear need to develop. In fact, this need to engage in life-long learning has been codified by certain certifying entities such as the American Board of Surgery's (ABS) Maintenance of Certification (MOC) program.

We need to ensure, therefore, that we embrace this culture of life-long learning and consider the approaches used to develop new professionals, provide continuing professional development (CPD), and consider how we implement the best strategies for reaccreditation. In essence, developing new approaches to how we educate is imperative in an evolving, fast-moving healthcare climate in which medical knowledge doubles in ever-decreasing time cycles. Current approaches to CPD offer many advantages due to the greater availability of technologies, rapid access to information almost anywhere, and a new type of learner who may learn in a different way to how medical education has traditionally been delivered.

Healthcare has additionally been the focus of significant scrutiny with the publication of the seminal Institute of Medicine (IOM) report *To Err Is Human* (Kohn et al., 2000) as well as subsequent reports identifying the high number of deaths and adverse events associated with medical error as a result of poor communication and teamwork (Mazzocco et al., 2009), a problem not isolated to any one region but one seen in health systems globally. Patient safety professionals and patients alike are becoming increasingly interested in accelerating the pace in which CPD and learning is taking place.

Nowhere in the healthcare setting is the pace of change in technology and technique more dramatic than in the operating room (OR). The newly minted surgeon of today who is fresh out of residency is guaranteed to encounter technological and technical developments and innovations that will change the way procedures are performed many times throughout his or her career. Such change is not new: revolutions in surgical care and technique that have transformed surgery in the twentieth century are manifold: vascular surgery developments, improvements in critical care, rise of transplant surgery, and advent of minimally invasive surgery (MIS). The twenty-first century has witnessed the rise of robotic surgery as another potentially transformative development. This latest surgical platform allows surgeons to operate with better visualization and finer control in close cramped spaces, leading to its widespread adoption in urologic, colorectal, and gynecologic procedures within the confined space of the pelvis. As with other new technologies, however, robotic surgery presents new challenges to surgeons such as a complete lack of tactile feedback.

Educational approaches, therefore, need to be developed to help surgeons overcome the learning curve associated with robotic surgery. Meeting the needs of adult learners, individuals who are by definition active participants in learning, and many of those having significant prior experiences that they can relate to during such events is essential in such a situation. Using technology to engage and challenge learners to relate their experience to the reality of the profession in which they engage is critical. Fortunately, traditional and nontraditional educational programs exist to help with CPD related to robotic surgery.

Simulation, experiential education, team-based learning are all approaches with promise related to teaching robotic surgery since they involve engagement of the learner. Of these, simulation-based training (SBT) is particularly attractive because of its proven effectiveness in technical skills acquisition (Willis and van Sickle, 2015) and team training (Amorse et al., 2011). In fact, SBT has been used in healthcare for many years. Nonetheless, SBT has developed to the point that we are now in a position where a significant number of simulators exist that allow for increased realism, and many have a level of fidelity that creates a realistic environment for the development of psychomotor skills. Healthcare educators, therefore, need to develop methodologies to integrate this technology into existing and developing programs.

This chapter will focus on key educational modalities and principles that can be used to help surgeons and surgical teams learn the necessary technical and nontechnical skills (NTS) needed to perform robotic surgery in an efficient, effective, and safe manner. The first section will discuss educational strategies and theories that can be used in the healthcare setting to help decrease the robotic surgery learning curve, including SBT, mastery learning (ML), and interprofessional education (IPE) for team-based learning. The chapter will then focus on specific applications curricula involving SBT, ML, and IPE for robotic surgery.

SECTION 1: EDUCATIONAL STRATEGIES AND THEORIES USEFUL IN ROBOTIC SURGICAL SKILLS TRAINING

Employing a Structured Approach to Simulation-Based Training

Understanding how to implement such SBT programs can be a challenge and really needs champions across professional groups. For a given SBT session, a structured approach should be followed to maximize learning. This approach involves three key steps: (1) the prebrief, (2) participation in simulation-based scenario itself, and (3) the debrief.

The Prebrief

Within the prebrief, the facilitator/teacher delineates both the learning objectives of a simulation session as well as the "ground rules" for the session (Paige et al., 2015). In doing so, he or she is trying to set up the session for success by encouraging participation, eschewing suspicion, and fostering a psychological safety, therby fostering an effective learning environment. Acknowledging to learners that mistakes that occur during the simulation do not have a negative impact on patients and are an opportunity for the whole team to learn is important. The facilitator should emphasize that the session should not be focused on "who is wrong" but instead on "what is wrong" (Rosen et al., 2008). In addition, he or she will alert participants that, while the simulation-based session attempts to reflect reality, limitations do exist to what can be achieved. He or she should explain such limitations and how they should be handled during the SBT session. Ensuring participants acknowledge these limitations and creating a learning environment in which participants feel comfortable to take risks without fear of repercussions helps to create a "suspension of disbelief" in which the learners engage in a "fiction contact" that will drive the team to behave as in a real-life setting, thereby improving learning and behavior adoption.

Lastly, confidentiality is important in achieving psychological safety. If simulation-based activity is formative in nature and not summative, the feedback is designed to improve performance. No consequences outside of the simulation-based environment should exist, and this fact should be stressed to learners. It may, however, be worth considering how to address the apparently incompetent clinician if patient safety may be at risk.

Participation in the Simulation-Based Activity Itself

The actual simulation-based acitivity can focus on any number of learning objectives such as team-based training, technical skills acquisition, or conflict management. A key concept to remember is that *simulation is a tool, not a curriculum.* Thus, learning objectives for the educational intervention should be established first. From them, the appropriate types of simulation-based or other educational modality can be chosen to ensure that these objectives are achieved. and then determining what simulation-based or other educational modality should be employed. These steps are part of the curriculum development process. Several models exist for helping to create and evaluate a curriculum and its effectiveness (Chauvin, 2012). One such example is the ADDIE (Analyze, Design, Develop, Implement, and Evaluate) method of curriculum development. The model chosen, however, is not as important as taking a structured approach based on sound educational principles.

The concept of fidelity in simulation is worth discussing and considering when developing training activities, since it is often erroneously associated with the degree of technology of a simulator (Paige, 2012). Fidelity in simulation can be broken down into three main dimensions. Equipment fidelity reflects the degree to which a simulator/simulation looks like the real-life setting. Environment fidelity reflects the degree to which a simulator/simulation acts as in a real-life setting. Finally, psychological fidelity is the degree to which learners are made to feel like they are in the real setting (so-called "suspension of disbelief"). The more a simulator/simulation reflects reality, the higher the fidelity. The degree of fidelity is *not synonomous with* the degree of technology of a simulator/simulation. For example, a computer-operated manikin may have high equipment fidelity since it can mimic physiologic signs and responses. Its use to help someone learn physical exam, however, might result in low psychological and environment fidelity, since it cannot move or talk appropriately. Thus, choosing what works best to achieve one's desired learning objectives can help match the simulator and degree of fidelity required for a successful educational intervention. In many cases, simple, cheap approaches work well in creating believable environments and procedures (i.e., high fidelity). Hybrid simulation is another strong approach in which real people paired with partial task trainers can create strong fidelity across all three dimensions.

The Debrief

The debrief is, without question, the most important component of a SBT session in terms of optimizing retention of key knowledge, skills, and atttitudes (KSAs) by the learner. Unfortunately, it is often overlooked and treated as an afterthought. Usually, a great deal of effort is placed into creating the ideal simulation-based scenario or training activity in lieu of honing debriefing skills. The process of active reflection and conceptualization after simulation-based experience is key to helping learners engage completely in the Kolb cycle of experiential learning (i.e., concrete experience, reflective observation, abstract conceptualization, and active experimentation). Such reflection often takes more time than the simulation-based activity itself. As a rule of thumb, the debrief should last almost twice as long as the scenario itself (Paige et al., 2015).

Debriefing, when applied well, can often result in a learner-centered experience in which the learners guide themselves to observations and conclusions related to their experience. In this ideal setting, the debriefing facilitator acts a guide, providing input on a limited basis as the learners identify their own learning gaps and determine solutions to them. At other times, the debriefer might have to play a more active role. In fact, the debriefer must wear many hats in order to optimize learning in the debriefing: facilitator, cognitive detective, time keeper, co-learner. No matter what role the debriefer adopts, his or her job during the debrief is threefold: (1) make it safe (i.e., create a psychologically safe learning environment), (2) make it stick (i.e., ensure that learning objectives are attained and practice gaps identified), and (3) make it last (i.e., engage learners to commit to applying KSAs learned to their actual clinical practice) (Paige, 2012).

Mastery Learning to Achieve Learner Milestones in Surgical Simulation-Based Education

Mastery learning (ML), developed and subsequently refined by Benjamin Bloom in 1968 and 1971, is a pedagogical approach that is being integrated into medical and surgical simulation-based curricula with the potential for more realistic and cost-effective results (Bloom, 1968, 1979, 1985; McGaghie, Issenberg, Cohen, Barsuk, & Wayne, 2011). Although ML has demonstrated effectiveness in a diversity of subject areas (Fox, 2004; Guskey, 2010; Schellhase, 2008), much debate exists related to its benefits. Nonetheless, ML has particular merits and advantages related to its use in simulation-based surgical education (Table 20.1).

Core to the ML concept in surgical education is the combination of group-based teaching with individual mentoring in order to achieve mastery in a particular skill, task, or procedure. ML learners are required to demonstrate successful completion of progressively more complex tasks as they progress along the various stages to ML that Bloom described (Bloom, 1985). ML essentially involves teaching a topic or procedure in a logical sequence of steps/lessons, starting with simple tasks and progressing to more complex maneuvers. At each step/lesson in the learning process, overt demonstration of mastery is required prior to moving forward to the next step/lesson (Anderson, 2000). Simulation-based learning events, no matter

Table 20.1 Considerations for ML effectiveness in surgical healthcare simulation-based education

Consideration	ML adaption and modification for learner
Teacher/learner-improved affective health	Increases confidence, EQ improvement, improved potential for win-win situation, readiness to teach and learn
Ability differentiation	Assists learners with less aptitude in certain skills (i.e., suturing psychomotor ability)
Maturity	Allows for adjustments for generational differences (i.e., younger learners may be less motivated or disciplined)
Diversity of simulator devices	Requires creative, innovative assortments of teaching devices and approaches for increasing competencies
Flexibility of timing	(CON) Costs increase with additional time for "enrichment" learning activities with practice autonomies. (Autonomous, peer-reviewed practice time could alleviate this challenge.) (PRO) Mastery-level opportunities eventually leads to achieving success of skill/milestones
Reaching ML	Positive effects on academic achievements; improves knowledge retention

what degree of fidelity involved, allows for customization of ML by tailoring the sessions/lessons that the learner must complete. Thus, ML is a methodology that focuses on feedback within the experiential learning cycle. Ideally, such ML would be fully integrated into the training curricula, allowing for ML opportunities at anytime. By incorporating the appropriate simulation-based technologies into a curricula, instructors are able to adapt the educational environment to reach a curriculum's learning objectives for a mixture of learners. In addition, ML instructors allow for tailored instruction and assignments for learners based on formative assessment with feedback and coaching. This form of just-in-time instruction allows learners to progress at their own rate along the curriculum and focus on learning gaps particular to an individual. Thus, learners can work toward *being the best they can be* to achieve learning objectives in following their own unique surgical skills. The outcome of such individual, learner-centered feedback and coaching results in all learners attaining the minimal level of mastery as set by the learning objectives of the curriculum.

ML in technical skills acquisition draws on two key learning theories. The first is Ericsson's theory of expertise that focuses on *deliberate practice* (Ericsson, 2004). Such practice involves repeated practice of specific skills with immediate feedback and ample time for drilling. In this manner, learners are pushed just beyond their comfort zone in order to attain the next level of mastery. The second is the Fitts-Posner three-stage theory of motor acquisition (Fitts & Posner, 1967). This theory postulates that motor skills are learned over a three-stage process in which the skill is initially understood (cognition), its mechanics are honed (integration), and then finally mastered and refined (automation). Thus, the ML process involves deliberate practice of skills and tasks to the point of precision and fluidity in a stepwise manner to ultimately master a procedure in its entirety. A useful dictum for such learning can be summed as follows:

> Don't practice until you get it right. Practice until you can't get it wrong
>
> (Unknown)

The design of simulation-based ML programs has shown promise in surgical skill development and improved patient outcomes (Barsuk, McGaghie, Cohen, O'Leary, & Wayne, 2010; Zendeias, Cook, Bingener, Huebner, Dunn, Sarr, & Farley, 2001). The key focus is on surgical clinical competencies and patient safety, which appears to ultimately prove positive patient outcomes. A research study by Zendeias et al. (2011) on simulation-based ML curriculum for totally extraperitoneal laparoscopic inguinal hernia repair demonstrated decreased operative time, improved surgical trainee skill performance, decreased surgical complications, and decreased patient overnight stays. Another interesting study from a school of medicine in Chicago involving central venous catheter subclavian and internal jugular insertion skills in an intensive care unit (Barsuk et al., 2010) revealed that ML improved clinical and patient outcomes. The study presented significantly less arterial punctures and insertion failure rates. In addition to an 85 percent reduction in catheter-related bloodstream infections, the research concluded that there were also significant cost savings (Cohen, Feinglas, &

Barsuk, 2010). In essence, like the enduring and successful MasterCard "*priceless*" campaigns of the past, the savings alluded to for patients are *priceless*! In this particular study, the improvements in surgical skills accounted for better patient outcomes, thus implying best practices and excellence as in the famous "*priceless*" slogan.

Team-Based Education and Learning: The Importance of Interprofessional Education

The traditional approach to CPD and medical education has been to educate each profession in isolation. This traditional approach fails to train the professional to work with other individuals from different professions in a complex healthcare environment. The education of professionals in isolation builds on the lack of appreciation of the manifold skills and abilities held by each member of a multiprofessional care team. Furthermore, such training reinforces the silo mentality (Bleakley, 2006) often encountered in the OR and the tendancy toward tribalism (Gillespie et al., 2010) among the different professions, creating a viscious cycle in which these attitudes and postures destructive to team interaction and collaboration are passed on to the younger generation of clinicians. Such an educational approach also neglects the reality of the OR. While surgeons perform their procedures, a whole team, all with specific and distinct roles, supports them to achieve their operative goals. Thus, surgery is inherently a team sport, and, consequently, training and teaching teams as a unit are important. By applying these concepts to the educational environment, surgical teams are able to train one another, honing communication and collaboration as well as disproving misconceptions and biases that one profession might have for another.

Inter-professional education (IPE), therefore, is an essential component for any educational curricula focusing on surgeons and surgical procedures. This fact is especially true since the Inter-Professional Education Collaborative (IPEC) has defined four key domains of competency that every healthcare professional should possess in order to work effectively in today's dynamic clinical environment: (1) values/ethics for interprofessional practice, (2) roles and responsibilities, (3) teams and teamwork, and (4) interprofessional communication (IPEC, 2011). Defined by the World Health Organization as an activity that brings together two or more professionals to learn with, from, and about each other (WHO, 2015), IPE is a powerful tool that can be used in helping to build highly reliable, effective teams.

The use of IPE can help teamscome together in the most emergent situations and draw on important principles related to leadership and followership to adapt to the changing environment and successfully treat a critically ill patient. Key to such success, however, is to recognize the need for team training using IPE to become an expert team. In professional sports, a team may train for many days prior to competitions. Members learn how to achieve a goal and understand how they each perform a part in achieving that goal. The more they work together, the more efficient team performance becomes. The pit crews in Formula One racing are an excellent example of how concerted, continual practice can hone a team's cohesiveness such that a complete set of tires can be replaced in seconds during a pit stop. In essence, a whole team works together to allow one driver to succeed. Such exceptional skill takes training, teamwork, and much practice.

One approach is to incorporate team training into a high-fidelity simulation environment. Every simulation scenario should incorporate key learning objectives. Often, they will involve teaching the team-based competencies and coordinating mechanisms described above – the NTS. Focusing purely on NTS often leads to a lack of success in engaging some clinicians. The reality is, however, that 80 percent of adverse events are the result of failures in the use of NTS. Not addressing these skills in SBT, therefore, would be a disservice to the learner.

SBT offers a great opportunity to incorporate IPE to help teams develop KSAs related to leadership, followership, and communication (Paige et al., 2009). Taking clinical teams away from their daily work environment and exposing them to various events offers the team a chance to reflect on their performance. This experience should not be as individual professions but as a team of professionals – the same team that delivers care to patients on a daily basis. Such training of the team as a whole unit, in lieu of its individual members, will help in the development of team-based competencies essential for highly reliable team function: leadership, mutual performance monitoring, backup behavior, team orientation, and adaptability (Salas et al., 2005). Such an approach not only enhances performance but creates a greater appreciation of each team member's abilities and roles.

In addition to teaching team-based competencies related to highly reliable team function, SBT should also focus on three important coordinating mechanisms that enhance team collaboration: shared mental model, mutual trust, and communication (Salas et al., 2005). Communication in healthcare is a key coordinating mechanism that requires practice and development outside of the clinical environment in order to hone and improve. Fortunately, many tools exist to help ensure that, in stressful, dynamic surgical environments, messages are communicated and understood unambiguously. For example, the Situation, Background, Assessment and Recommendation tool can be used to communicate an event and provide the recipient with clear information on what is being requested. Other tools include the CUS terms that are used to convey concern realted to a patient safety issue. The use of these agreed-upon terms (e.g., "I am *concerned*, I feel *uncomfortable*, *stop*") should serve as a red flag to the recipient and trigger a huddle to address the issues. Thus, the CUS terms provide a format for emergency communication during an actual critical event. These communication tools, as well as others, are part of the Agency for Healthcare Research and Quality's TeamSTEPPS™ curriculum, a program designed to promote teamwork and team collaboration. Team training in these and other communication tools is necessary to ensure that everybody understands their responsibilities, thereby recognizing when these techniques should be applied.

Summary

When based on sound educational principles, effective curricula can be developed to assist surgeons and their teams in mastering the use of the robot in the OR. Useful modalities include SBT for both technical and team-based KSAs, ML techniques used in a stepwise fashion to teach robotic surgery's intricacies, and team-based training using IPE. These modalities draw on key educational theories related to Knowles, Bloom, Ericsson, as well as Fitts and Posner, and curricula should be developed using educationally sound methods such as the ADDIE model. By employing these techniques, educators can develop interventions that will allow learners to attain mastery in robotic surgery at their own pace. Fortunately, much work has already been done related to the use of SBT in team-based training and ML in skills acquisition in healthcare in general and robotics surgery in particular, which will be discussed in the next section.

SECTION 2: APPLICATIONS OF SBT CURRICULA TO ROBOTIC SURGERY

Skill Sets Required for Robotic Surgery

In the United States, robotic surgery was introduced around the turn of the millineum (Liu & Curet, 2015). Its development was, in part, a response to the MIS revolution and the psychomotor difficulties that it created for surgeons who had practiced open surgery their entire careers. By pairing a surgical console with three-dimensional vision to robotic arms holding multiarticulated instruments, the developers of robotic surgery were attempting to restore the natural hand movement, visual depth, and articulation of instruments that had been lost with the introduction of MIS. By doing so, they saw five distinct advantages to the use of robotic surgery over MIS surgery: (1) three-dimensional vision, (2) seven degrees of freedom of movement of instruments, (3) elimination of instrument tremors, (4) loss of fulcrum effect, and (5) better precision and accuracy using downscaled instrument movements (Foote & Valea, 2015). Nonetheless, by creating a console that is removed from the patient at which the surgeon performs the procedure, they introduced new challenges related to the console's technical operation and the OR team interaction during a procedure.

The development of a specialized console from which the surgeon operates the instruments used in robotic surgery has resulted in the introduction of several new technical skills that a surgeon must master in order to perform robotic surgery effectively. In their review, Curet and Liu (2015) identified a core set of skills that were required to operate the console in robotic surgery that was independent of both the type of procedure performed and the surgical specialty involved. Five of these skills involved interfacing with the console controls themselves: (1) bimanual wrist manipulation, (2) camera control, (3) master clutching to manage hand position, (4) use of the third arm instrument, and (5) activation of energy sources.

Two other core skills that were identified were related to psychomotor features of robotic surgery: (1) appropriate depth perception and (2) awareness of force applied to instruments. The former of these two skills may seem surprising since three-dimensional vision is reportedly a benefit of robotic surgery. This skill may be a legacy of MIS surgery and related to the work done on earlier models of robotic trainers that may not have been as effective in rendering three-dimensional vision. It may also be related to the interaction between surgeon, eye ports, and the console. The latter of these two skills is directly related to the complete loss of tactile feedback that results from remotely controlling the instruments. It is an important consideration for surgeons performing robotic surgery, since basic surgical tasks in which tactile feedback is employed (e.g., suturing, dissection, cutting, retraction) require attention to visual cues in robotic surgery to ensure that the application of undue force is avoided.

In addition to the core set of technical skills unique to the operation of the console used in robotic surgery, several technical skills common to MIS and open surgery have also been identified in the literature (Liu & Curet, 2015). They include suturing, knot tying, needle manipulation, dissection, cutting, and retraction. Also, certain NTS have been identified as important, given the unique setup of robotic surgery in which robotic arms need to be "docked" to the patient by a bedside assistant who changes out instruments and assists with retraction. Thus, team communication, patient side cart positioning, and instrument docking have been identified as important to successful use of the robot.

Thus, the implementation of robotic surgery into a surgeon's clinical practice is accompanied by the need to acquire new psychomotor skills unique to a remote console setup as well as to hone traditional technical and nontechnical skills needed for effective surgical practice. Fortunately, many groups from diverse surgical specialties have worked to develop training curricula to address these issues. In fact, several multiinstutional efforts have been undertaken that have provided useful simulation-based curricula in both domains, as the subsequent sections will describe.

Technical Skills Training in Robotic Surgery

Robotic surgery's unique console design (i.e., in which the surgeon is physically removed from the patient and conducts the operation via an interface) makes it especially conducive to using simulation-based virtual reality (VR) constructs for teaching technical skills. Thus, several different VR robotic simulators have been developed and commercially introduced (Table 20.2). Each one has specified tasks for training, has undergone varying degrees of validation by research groups, and some have even been used as a platform for developing curricula for teaching and training in robotic surgery. Of note, the surgical education platform does not have three-dimensional imaging, uses a computer screen in lieu of a simulated robotic console interface, and has limited core robotic skills. The da Vinci Surgical Simulator was developed in conjunction with Mimic Technologies and can be used for practice in the OR and outside of it. Three simulators currently offer procedural training: the Robotic Surgical Simulator (RoSS) via their Hands-On Surgical Training (HOST) system, the dV Trainer using the Maestro AR system, and the da Vinci Surgical Simulator with its Robotix Mentor.

In addition to the development of commercial VR robotic simulators, several groups, at both the single institutional and the multisocietal collaborative levels, have developed proficiency-based curricula using mastery ML learning principles to help surgeons develop both core robotic skills and surgical skills employed in robotic surgery (Table 20.3). These curricula have been developed for use on VR simulators or on the da Vinci robot itself and have demonstrated effectiveness in most cases. Notable large-group collaboratives that have succeeded in developing comprehensive technical skills curricula include the multiinstitutionally developed Fundamental Skills of Robotic Surgery and the Fundamentals of Robotic Surgery created by a large consortium involving multiple surgical specialties that use the robot in clinical practice. Walliczek et al. (2015) have also demonstrated that increased frequency of training helps with skill acquisition in robotic surgery.

Although all VR simulators have in-built metrics for assessment and some of these have demonstrated evidence of validity for training learner groups, research has been undertaken to develop other assessment instrument tools to assess skill levels in robotic procedures and tasks. The Global Evaluative Assessment of Robotic Skills (GEARS) is one of the best known examples (Goh et al., 2012; Sanchez et al. 2016). This global scale rates operative performance in six domains using a 5-point Likert scale. The domains

Table 20.2 Current VR simulators in commercial use for training in robotic surgery technical skills

Simulator	Manufacturer	Skills modules	Evidence for validity	Evidence for transfer of training	Major curricula incorporated into simulator	Estimated cost
RoSS		Core robotic skills: bimanual wrist manipulation, camera movement, master clutching, third arm manipulation, energy source use Surgical skills: suturing, tying, vessel clipping, suture cutting	Content validation skills exercises No construct validation of performance metrics	Transfer of training to dry lab exercises, inanimate models	Fundamentals Skills of Robotic Surgery	$100,000–125,000
Surgical Education Platform	SimSurgery AS, Oslo, Norway	Core robotic skills: bimanual wrist manipulation Surgical skills: suturing, tying, needle manipulation, instrument manipulation	Limited content validation skills exercises Construct validation of performance metrics	None	None	$40,000–45,000
dV Trainer	Mimic Technologies, Seattle, WA	Core robotic skills: bimanual wrist manipulation, camera movement, third arm manipulation, energy source use, needle manipulation, suturing, knot tying, dissection	Content validation skills exercises Construct validation of performance metrics	Transfer of training to dry lab exercises, inanimate models	Fundamentals of Robotic Surgery	$85,000–100,00
da Vinci Skills Simulator	Intuitive Surgical, Sunnyvale, CA	Needle manipulation, suturing, knot tying, dissection Core robotic skills: bimanual wrist manipulation camera movement, third arm manipulation, energy source use, suturing, tying, vessel clipping, suture cutting	Content validation skills exercises Construct validation of performance metrics	Transfer of training to dry lab exercises/inanimate models, tissue models, and supracervical hysterectomy	Fundamentals of Robotic Surgery	$85,000–90,000

Source: Curet and Liu (2015); Moglia et al. (2015); Cumar, Smith, and Patel (2015); Lallas and Davis (2012); Bric, Lumbard, Frelich, & Gould (2016).

include depth perception, bimanual dexterity, efficiency, force sensitivity, autonomy, and robotic control. This tool has been used to evaluate robot-assisted radical prostatectomy (Goh et al., 2012). In addition, it has been demonstrated to be effective at differentiating expert, intermediate, and novice performance (Sanchez et al., 2016). GEARS holds potential as an evaluative tool for both formative and summative

Table 20.3 Robotic surgery technical skills curricula

Curriculum; institution/group	Targeted skills/ procedures	Platform	Components	Effectiveness
Fundamental Inanimate Robotic Skills Tasks; Methodist Institute for Technology, Innovation, and Education, Houston, TX (2010, 2015)	Basic core robotic and surgical skills	da Vinci robot with inanimate models	Modular with four inanimate exedrcises	Significant differentiation between novice, intermediates, and expert users
University of Texas Southwestern curriculum, Dallas, TX (2012, 2012)	Basic core robotic and surgical skills	da Vinci robot with inanimate models	Online tutorial, ½ day interactive session, proficiency-based training on nine inanimate exercises	Significant improvement in pre- to postintervention scores
Fundamental Skills in Robotic Surgery – multiinstitutional (2013, 2014)	Basic core robotic and surgical skills	RoSS VR simulator	Sequential, modular, proficiency-based divided into four modules	Significant improvements in robotic surgical skills
Medical College of Wisconsin curriculum, Milawaukee, WI (2014, 2014)	Basic core robotic and surgical skills	da Vinci VR surgical simulator	Sequential, proficiency-based training on five exercises	Significant improvements on performing simulated tasks on da Vinci platform
Dunlan, Rege, Hogg, Gilberg-Fisher, Tesfay, & Scott (2012); Fundamentals of Robotic Surgery, multisocietal (2014)	Cognitive, psychomotor, and team skills	da Vinci robot with inanimate models da Vinci VR Surgical Simulator dV VR Trainer	Sequential, modular, proficiency-based modules with online components	Multiinstitutional randomized controlled trial underway
European Association of Urology Robotic Training Curriculum; EAU Robotic Urologic Section	Robot-assisted radical prostatectomy (RARP)	da Vinci VR Surgical Simulator; animal and cadaveric platforms	E-learning; week of simulation-based practice using VR, animal, and cadaveric models, modular training in RARP	Improvement in da Vinci VR tasks; 8 out of 10 fellows deemed ready to perform RARP independently

Source: Goh et al. (2015); Dunlan et al. (2012); Dunlan et al. (2012); Stegemann et al. (2013); Bric et al. (2014); Raza, Froghi, and Chowriappi (2014); Smith, Patel, & Satava (2014); Volpe, Ahmed, and Dasgupta (2015).

assessment of residents and surgeons performing robotic procedures in the clinical setting.

Nontechnical Skills Training in Robotic Surgery

As alluded to earlier, the introduction of robotic surgery into the OR increases the complexity of not only the technical aspect of a procedure but the team communication and collaboration as well. The surgeon no longer is in close proximity with the surgical team (i.e., surgical assistant, scrub technician, anesthesia provider). Instead, he or she is unscrubbed, not facing the team, physically removed, and seated at a console that occupies his or her full attention. Furthermore, the potential consequences of certain complications, such as uncontrolled hemorrhage, are magnified with the surgeon separated from the operative field, since reaction times are inherently longer. Thus, training in team communication and interaction becomes even more essential in order to overcome these new realities brought about by the technology. Fortunately, several authors have begun to employ simulation-based techniques to address team-based learning and dynamics related to robotic surgery.

Examples of simulation-based team training for robotic surgery run the gamut of scenarios and employ a variety of technologies. The FRS curriculum includes a team training component focusing on the interprofessional team, use of a robotic surgery checklist, robotic-specific communication techniques, post-operative debriefing, and crisis management (Smith, Patel, & Satava, 2014). Essential principles identified for successful team interaction and training were manifold: inclusion, empowerment, person-specific, reiterative, "just in time," ownership, and closed-loop communication. Existing team-based curricula such as TeamSTEPPS have been identified by the FRS group as appropriate for application to robotic surgery. Such introductory team-based training provides a foundation on which further NTS training can be undertaken that focuses on more complex aspects of team interaction in robotic surgery.

In addition to the FRS overviews of team-based aspects of robotic surgery, other groups have focused on more specific components of team interaction in robotic surgery. Mimic Technologies have developed the Xperience Team Trainer to help train bedside assistants with demomstrated effectiveness (Xu et al., 2015). Urologists at the Mayo Clinic in Jacksonville, Florida, have developed a three-phase curriculum for teaching first assistants taking part in a robot-assisted prostatectomy (Thiel et al., 2013). Phase 1 of this curriculum involved hands-on training on the robot related to its functionality, such as docking. Phase 2 focused on the key steps of a RARP using video review. Phase 3 emphasized simulation-based practice of drills for spatial orientation, cutting, and bimanual dexterity. In a small pilot of this curriculum, participants found that it improved their spatial orientation intraabdominally. Such crew-based (i.e., focusing on one or several members/professions of an interprofessional team) SBT is valuable in robotic surgery because it allows each crew to hone skills and communication related to its particular duties in a robotic surgery case. Once such training has been completed, full team exercises can be undertaken to address issues that may arise during a robotic procedure.

Robotic surgery's complexities relate to instrument arms, docking, altered team dynamics, and robotic-specific communication with surgical assistants from whom the surgeon is separated and line of sight can in and of itself create additional stresses on surgical teams and their interaction and collaboration. Suh et al. (2016) have demonstrated that even the simplest of distractions (such as having to acknowledge a change in heart rate or answering a question) can increase surgeon workload and stress, leading to technical errors. Adding into this mix, an intraoperative crisis and an unprepared team might quickly become overwhelmed and unable to respond properly. Huser et al. (2014) have addressed such concerns by creating an in situ team SBT scenario in which a computer-based mannequin attached to a robotic system undergoes myocardial fibrillation. Interprofessional teams consisting of nurses, an anesthesiologist, and surgeons (i.e., urologists and gynecologists) underwent training initially and again 7 weeks later. Such distributed training resulted in a significant improvement in the restoration of stable circulation from an average of almost 7 min to 3.5 min. Clearly, regular training in crisis management that may arise during a robotic surgical case has value in helping to prepare operative teams in rapid, efficient response.

Implementing a SBT Curriculum for Robotic Surgery

Given the many examples of both technical and non-technical skills–based curricula available for training in robotic surgery, a comprehensive SBT program should be implemented to prepare both surgeons and OR team members in its use. Kumar et al. (2015) have suggested a stepwise approach for such a program in which preclinical training begins with didactic lectures related to robot function followed by dry lab technical skills practice using a proficiency-based curriculum incorporating VR simulators or inanimate models on a robot. Dry lab work would then progress to practice on animal tissue models and/or cadaveric procedural practice. Concomitantly, SBT of crews/teams in routine docking and robot use would then be undertaken for a particular targeted procedure with crisis management training using a computer-based mannequin for potential serious complications or events related to the procedure. Clinical training would then be undertaken with observation, dual console use, and mentoring. In this manner, surgeons and teams can learn to use robots in practice in a safe, simulation-based learning environment without risk to the patient.

Conclusion

The introduction of robotic surgery in the OR has presented surgeons and OR personnel alike with new skills and dynamics to learn in order to use it effectively. The surgeon–console interface to control instruments located at a distance has resulted in a new core set of robotic surgery skills that must be learned: (1) bimanual wrist manipulation, (2) camera control, (3) master clutching to manage hand position, (4) use of the third arm instrument, (5) activation of energy sources, (6) appropriate depth perception, and (7) awareness of force applied to instruments. In addition, team interaction is different due to the seclusion of the surgeon from the rest of the operative team and his or her loss of line of sight with other team members. Fortunately, through the application of sound educational principles related to such things as ML and IPE, simulation-based curricula have been developed to teach both the technical and nontechnical skills needed to practice safe, effective robotic surgery. A comprehensive program for teaching robotic surgery should include both these skill sets and should focus on the individual surgeon/team member as well as the team as a whole. It can borrow from existing curricula with evidence of effectiveness in the literature, can be built from the ground-up, or can be a combination of the two. Whatever the case, when based on sound educational principles, such a program will prepare the OR robotic team for challenges that may arise during one of these complex cases.

Footnote: (*Citing Cohen et al., 2010. Total annual estimated savings: $820,000, 139 patient hospital days, and 120 MICU days. Compared with the intervention cost analysis ($112,000), the net savings was $708,000.)

References

Agency for Healthcare Research and Quality. www.ahrq.gov/.

American Board of Surgery. www.absurgery.org/

Murphy M, Redding S, Twyman J, eds (2013). *Handbook on innovations in learning*. www.centeril.org/handbook/resources/fullchapter/Handbook_on_Innovations_in_Learning.pdf. Retrieved May 15, 2016

Anderson JR (2000). *Learning and memory: An integrated approach* (2nd ed.). New York: John Wiley and Sons.

Armour Forse R, Bramble JD, McQuillan R (2011). Team training can improve operating room performance. *Surgery*. 150(4):771–8.

Barsuk JH, McGaghie WC, Cohen ER, O'Leary KJ, Wayne DB (2009). Simulation-based mastery learning reduces complications during central venous catheter insertion in a medical intensive care unit. *Critical Care Medicine*. 37:2697–01.

Barsuk, JH (2012). Use of simulation-based mastery learning to improve patient outcomes for central venous catheter insertion.

Bleakley A (2006). You are who I say you are: the rhetorical construction of identity in the operating theatre. *J Workplace Learning*. 18(7–8):414–25.

Bloom BS (1968). Learning for master. *UCLS-CSEIP Evaluation Comment*. 1(2):1–12.

Bloom BS (1971). Mastery learning. In JH Block (Ed.). *Mastery learning: Theory and practice*, pp. 47–63. New York: Holt, Rinehart, & Winston.

Bloom BS (1979). Mastery learning – does it work? *Educational Leadership*. 37(2):110–13.

Bric J, Connolly M, Kastenmeier A, Goldblatt M, Gould JC (2014). Proficiency training on a virtual reality robotic surgical skills curriculum. *Surg Endosc*. 28:3343–8.

Bric JD, Lumbard DC, Frelich MJ, Gould JC (2016). Current state of virtual reality simulation in robotic surgery training: a review. *Surgical Endoscopy*. 30:2169–78.

Chauvin SW (2012). *Educational principles in simulation in radiology*. New York: Oxford University Press.

Cohen ER, Feinglass J, Barsuk JH (2010). Cost savings from reduced catheter-related bloodstream infection after simulation-based education for residents in a medical intensive care unit. *Simulation in Healthcare*: 98–102.

Kumara A, Smithb R, Patela VR (2015). Current status of robotic simulators in acquisition of robotic surgical skills. *Curr Opin Urol*. 25:168–74.

Damavandi ME, Shekari KZ (2010). Effect of mastery learning method on performance, attitude of the weak students in chemistry. *Procedia – Social and Behavioral Sciences*. 5:1574–9.

Dulan G, Rege RV, Hogg DC, Gilberg-Fisher KK, Tesfay ST, Scott DJ (2012). Content and face validity of a comprehensive robotic skills training program for general surgery, urology, and gynecology. *American Journal of Surgery*. 203:535–9.

Dulan G, Rege RV, Hogg DC, et al. (2012). Developing a comprehensive, proficiency-based training program for robotic surgery. *Surgery*.152:477–88.

Ericsson KA (2004). Deliberate practice and the acquisition and maintenance of expert performance in medicine and related domains. *Acad Med*. 79;suppl 10:S70–81.

Fitts PM, Posner MI (1967). *Human performance*. Belmont, CA: Brooks/Cole.

Foote JR, Valea FA (2015). Robotic surgical training: where are we? *Gynecologic Oncology*.

Fox, EJ (2004). The personalized system of instruction: a flexible and effective approach to mastery learning. In D. Moran & R. Malott (Eds.), *Evidence-based educational methods* (pp. 201–21). San Diego: Elsevier.

Gillespie BM, Chaboyer W, Wallis M, Fenwick C (2010). Why isn't "time out" being implemented? An exploratory study. *Qual Saf Health Care*. 19:103–6.

Goh AC, Aghazadeh MA, Mercado MA, et al. (2015). Multi-institutional validation of fundamental inanimate robotic skills tasks. *Journal of Urology*. 194:1751–6.

Goh AC, Goldfarb DW, Sander JC, Miles BJ, Dunkin BJ (2012). Global evaluative assessment of Robotic skills: validation of a clinical assessment tool to measure robotic surgical skills. *Journal of Urology*. 187:247–52.

Guskey, TR (2010). Lessons of mastery learning. *Educational Leadership: Interventions That Work*. 68(2):52–7.

Guskey, TR (2005). Formative classroom assessment and Benjamin S. Bloom: theory, research, and implications. Paper presented at the Annual Meeting of the American Educational Research Association, Montreal, Canada.

Huser A-S, Muller D, Brunkhorst V, Kannisto P, Musch M, Kropfl D, Groeben H(2014). Simulated life-threatening emergency during robot-assisted surgery. *Journal of Endourology*. 28.

Interprofessional Education Collaborative Expert Panel (2011). *Core competencies for interprofessional collaborative practice: report of an expert panel*. Washington, DC: Interprofessional Education Collaborative.

Kohn LT, Corrigan JM, Donaldson MS, eds (2000). *To error is human. Building a safer health system*. Washington, DC: National Academy Press.

Kumar A, Smith R, Patel, VR (2015). Current status of robotic simulators in acquisition of robotic surgical skills. *Current Opinion in Urology*. 25:168–74.

Lallas CD, Davis JW (2012). Robotic surgery training with commercially available simulation systems in 2011: a current review and practice pattern survey from the Society of Urologic Robotic Surgeons. *Journal of Endourology*. 26(3):283–93.

Liu M, Curet M (2015). A review of training research and virtual reality simulators for the da Vinci surgical system. *Teaching and Learning in Medicine*. 27(1):12–26.

Mazzocco K, Petitti DB, Fong KT, et al. (2009). Surgical team behaviors and patient outcomes. *Am J Surg*. 197:678–85.

McGaghie WC, Issenberg SB, Cohen ER, Barsuk JH, Wayne DB (2011). Medical education featuring mastery learning with deliberate practice can lead to better health for individuals and populations. *Academic Medicine*. 86(11):e8–e9.

Moglia A, et al. (2015). A systematic review of virtual reality simulators for robot-assisted surgery. *Eur Urol*, doi:10.1016/j.eururo.2015.09.021

Paige JT,(2012). *Principles of simulation in radiology*. New York: Oxford University Press.

Paige JT, Arora S, Fernandez G, Seymour N (2015). Debriefing 101: training faculty to promote learning in simulation-based training. *Am J Surg*. 209(1):126–31.

Paige JT, Kozmenko V, Yang T, et al. (2009). High-fidelity, simulation-based, interdisciplinary operating room team training at the point of care. *Surgery*. 145(2):138–46

Rosen MA, Salas E, Wu TS, et al. (2008). Promoting teamwork: an event-based approach to simulation-based teamwork training for emergency medicine residents. *Acad Emerg Med*. 15:1190–8.

Raza SJ, Froghi S, Chowriappa A, et al. (2014). Construct validation of the key components of fundamental skills of robotic surgery (FSRS) curriculum –a multi-institution prospective study. *JSurg*. 71:316–24.

Salas E, Sims DE, Burke CS (2005). Is there a big five in teamwork? *Small Group Res*. 36:555–99.

Sánchez R, Rodríguez O, Rosciano J, et al. (2016). Robotic surgery training: construct validity of Global Evaluative Assessment of Robotic Skills (GEARS). *J Robot Surg*.

Schedllhase KC (2008). Mastery learning reconsidered. *Review of Educational Research*. 57(2):175–213.

Smith R, Patel V, Satava R (2014). Fundamentals of robotic surgery: a course of basic robotic surgery skills based upon a 14-society consensus template of outcomes measures and curriculum development *Int J Med Robotics Comput Assist Surg*. 10:379–84.

Stegemann AP, Ahmed K, Syed JR, et al. (2013). Fundamental skills of robotic surgery: a multi-institutional randomized controlled trial for validation of a simulation-based curriculum. *Urology*. 81:767–74.

Suh IH, LaGrange CA, Oleynikov D, Siu K-C (2016). Evaluating robotic surgical skills performance under distractive environment using objective and subjective measures. *Surgical Innovation*. 23(1):78–89.

Thiel DD, Lannen A, Richie E, et al. (2013). Simulation-based training for bedside assistants can benefit experienced robotic prostatectomy teams. *Journal of Endourology* 27(2).

Volpe A, Ahmed K, Dasgupta P, et al. (2015). Pilot validation study of the European Association of Urology Robotic Training Curriculum. *European Urology*. 6(8):292–9.

Xu S, Perez M, Perreno C, et al. Face, content, construct, and concurrent validity of a novel robotic surgery patient-side simulator: the Xperience team trainer. *Surg Endosc*. doi:10.1007/s00464-015-4607-x

Willis RE, Van Sickle KR (2015). Current status of simulation-based training in graduate medical education. *Surg Clin North Am*. 95(4):767–79.

World Health Organization (2010). *Framework for action on interprofessional education & collaborative practice*. Geneva: World Health Organization. http://whqlibdoc.who.int/hq/2010/WHO_HRH_HPN_10.3_eng.pdf. Accessed February 3, 2015.

Zendeias B, Cook DA, Bingener J, et al. (2011). Simulation-based mastery learning improves patient outcomes in laparoscopic inguinal hernia repair: a randomized controlled trial. *Ann Surg*.254(3):502–9, discussion 509–11.

Chapter 21

Understanding the Market Forces and Opportunity Costs of Robotic Surgery

Aaron A. Laviana and Jim C. Hu

Introduction

With greater national focus on efficient resource utilization with the Acountable Care Organizations and the Affordable Care Act, there is greater emphasis on understanding the true cost of care.[1] Concomitantly, novel medical technologies have been rapidly adopted without fully weighing the evidence. Against this backdrop, the da Vinci (Intuitive Surgical, Sunnyvale, CA) robotic surgery platform has rapidly and broadly disseminated to treat the gamut from urologic disease and benign hysterectomies in the pelvis to mitral valve prolapse in the chest.[2] Research on cost-effectiveness of robotic surgery remains sparse as it competes with and replaces gold standard open and conventional laparoscopic approaches.[3] In the United States alone, robot-assisted laparoscopic surgery increased more than 400 percent between 2007 and 2011, with some reports of 1000 percent growth for benign hysterectomy.[4–7]

Current pragmatists argue robot-assisted surgery may be costlier than conventional, open techniques due to longer operative times, higher costs of disposable equipment, and the higher upfront purchase acquisition costs and training associated with robotic technology. Nevertheless, there are many potential advantages, including improved magnification, reduced blood loss, and shorter hospital stay, as well as a shorter learning curve compared to convetional laparoscopy for procedures such as partial nephrectomy.[8,9] Ultimately, there remains a dearth of strong evidence for clear overall superiority of robotic surgery over conventional approaches for perioperative and long-term outcomes. This issue becomes more salient given the numerous studies that demonstrate wide differences in costs between surgical approaches.[10]

The rapid adoption of robot-assisted surgery is likely multifactorial with aggressive direct-to-consumer marketing by surgeons, hospitals, and the surgical robot manufacturer stoking demand.[11] Additionally, the short learning curve compared to laparoscopy and increased magnification may decrease the risk of significant bleeding, potentially attracting less experienced surgeons to robot-assisted surgery. This disruptive technology, thus, has surgery practice patterns while affecting the delivery and total costs of treating surgical disease.[12–14]

With life expectancy continuing to increase, the probability of individuals being diagnosed with a disease amenable to surgical treatment and possible robotic surgery is increased as well. Resultantly, the shift to more expensive treatments has important public health implications. Nguyen et al. demonstrated an increasing cost for prostate cancer care caused by technological changes in the management of prostate cancer.[15] Furthermore, economic considerations are increasingly important for appropriate resource allocation in an era shaped by inflationary pressures and fiscal constraints. In the United Kingdom, for instance, the National Institute for Health and Clinical Excellence requires high-level evidence for novel treatments before providing it to patients and agreeing to pay for it.[16] As a result, healthcare systems need to weigh the costs of robotic equipment against the costs of alternatives, also taking into consideration the quality of each treatment option in order to determine the overall value of each modality. As such, demand for cost comparisons and comparative effectiveness research to determine the economic efficacy of newly introduced surgical technologies is required and, for the most part, lacking in evidence-based literature.[17,18] Nevertheless, there has been a movement to apply the costing principles learned in the private industry and government sector to reveal hidden sources of cost, unveiling the lack of transparency and true costs of care.[19] As such, the remainder of this chapter focuses on what we know regarding the costs of robotic surgery in different surgical subspecialties and ends by highlighting novel costing mechanisms to help us better understand the costs of robotic technology. This latter focus also alludes to costing paradigms that may be used to determine true costs across healthcare systems, while also arguing whether the robotic platform should be centralized or available to all providers.

Urologic Surgery

Among the vanguard in robotic surgery, urologic surgeons used the robotic platform to perform the first robot-assisted laparoscopic prostatectomy (RALP) in 2000.[20] Resultantly, there is more robust literature describing the costs of robotic surgery for urologic disease, although how these costs are derived remains largely unclear. Pate et al. examined variation in the open market cost of a RALP in US hospitals for an uninsured patient, identifying a cohort of 100 hospitals.[21] Of these hospitals, 70 responded with facility pricing estimates averaging $34,720 and ranging from $10,100 to $135,000, all for the same procedure. These estimates were significantly higher at academic centers. Across the spectrum of private and academic centers, surgeon and anesthesia fees averaged $8,280 without a significant difference by practice setting. In another study examining the comparative effectiveness of robot-assisted versus laparoscopic and open urologic surgery, Yu et al. used data from the Nationwide Inpatient Sample and found the estimated cost of RALP to be $10,804 versus $10,082 and $9,693 for laparoscopic and open prostatectomy, respectively.[8] Similarly, radical nephrectomy costs were $13,894, $11,153, and $12,548 for robotic, laparoscopic, and open approaches, respectively, while partial nephrectomy estimates were $15,724, $12,401, and $11,817 for the robotic, laparoscopic, and open techniques, respectively. The authors concluded that in the absence of demonstrable cost-effectiveness, fiscal responsibility for the incremental cost of robotic surgery might shift from insurers to patients, as is the case in China.

Selective referral may attenuate healthcare costs associated with robotic surgery, as volume outcomes research demonstrates that higher provider volume is associated with decreased morbidity and mortality.[22,23] Similarly, higher hospital volume is associated with decreased morbidity for colon and breast cancer surgeries.[24,25] Moreover, hospital volume is inversely related to in-hospital mortality and length of stay after RALP.[26] Despite the known advantages of high-volume hospitals, surgeon volume appears to be the primary driver of radical prostatectomy outcomes, as intensive care admissions and length of stay have declined over the past 20 years.[27,28] As a result, many favor the centralization of RALP to hospitals demonstrating "performance excellence" with the goal of continued process refinement to minimize morbidity, mortality, and healthcare costs.[29,30] Given the majority of RALP are performed by low-volume surgeons performing less than 10 cases a year, selective referral of radical prostatectomies to high-volume surgeons may lead to improved oncologic and functional outcomes with significant cost savings.[31]

Several studies analyzed radical prostatectomy provider effects on costs, with higher surgeon and hospital volumes associated with a reduction in costs. Williams et al. estimated that selective referral to high-volume surgeons at intermediate and high-volume hospitals nationally for radical prostatectomy would reduce healthcare costs by more than $28.7 million.[32] This amount exceeds the $19 million the National Cancer Institute allocated to funding surgery-related research in 2010 for prostate cancer.[33] Others have shown that higher surgeon volume is associated with lower hospital charges, suggesting that as radical prostatectomy surgeons gain experience and move further along the learning curve, they become more efficient, achieving better outcomes at lower costs.[29,34,35]

Transoral Robotic Surgery

In December 2009, the FDA approved the use of the da Vinci system to perform transoral robotic surgery (TORS) for all benign disease and select malignant lesions of the throat and voice box.[36] Since that time, there have been a multitude of head and neck diseases treated with robot-assisted surgery, but whether there is an economic advantage to TORS remains to be elucidated. Recently, two cost-effectiveness studies have been published assessing the role of robotic surgery in oropharyngeal carcinoma. Hammoudi et al. compared TORS for squamous cell carcinoma of the upper aerodigestive tract and a matched group conventional surgery for the same indication, assessing 26 subjects in each group.[37] Altogether, there was no significant difference in disease-specific survival at 3 years ($p = 0.76$), although mean durations of feeding by nasogastric tube and hospitalization were shorter for the TORS group ($p = 0.001$, respectively). Mean treatment cost was $7,124 lower for the TORS group ($p = 0.03$).

In a similar analysis, de Almeida et al. presented an economic evaluation comparing TORS to (chemo) radiotherapy for the management of early-stage oropharyngal cancer.[38] Treatment for TORS and (chemo) radiotherapy were modeled using decision analysis with recurrences modeled over a 10-year period via a Markov model. TORS demonstrated a $1,366 cost savings and an increase of 0.25 quality-adjusted life years (QALYs) per case in comparison to (chemo)radiotherapy. TORS was sensitive to variations in adjuvant therapy, costs, utilities, complications, and recurrence rates in deterministic and probabilistic sensitivity analysis. The cost-effectiveness was reduced with increasing adjuvant therapy for TORS and decreasing concurrent chemotherapy for radiotherapy.

Gynecologic Disease

Similar to other fields, the true economic advantage for robotic surgery in gynecologic disease remains unknown, with most data suggesting the robotic platform is costlier without a known improvement in outcomes. In an economic analysis of robotic versus laparoscopic surgery for endometrial cancer, Venkat et al. collected data from hospital billing records, physician professional group billing records, tumor registry, and medical records on operations performed by a single surgeon.[39] These were matched based on age, histology, and stage of disease over the same period. Of 54 subjects, 27 underwent robotic and the rest laparoscopic surgery. Hospital charges for robotic versus laparoscopic surgery were $64,266 versus $55,130 ($p= 0.036$). Nevertheless, the reimbursement to the hospital was not statistically different at $13,003 for robotic and $10,245 for laparoscopic surgery ($p = 0.28$). The operating suite, room and board, anesthesia, postanesthesia care unit, and pathology accounted for over 90 percent of the hospital charges. Meanwhile, the surgeon charges were similar, with estimates of $6,824 and $6,327 for robotic and laparoscopic surgery, respectively ($p = 0.033$). Differences in anesthesiologist charges were only slightly more pronounced between robotic and laparoscopic surgery with charges estimated at $4,049 and $2,985, respectively ($p= 0.001$). Therefore, while the direct costs and charges associated with robotic surgery were higher compared to laparoscopic surgery, actual reimbursements to the hospital, surgeon, and anesthesiologist were not significantly different when added together. Part of the reason for this difference likely stems from the fact that there is no specific Current Procedural Terminology code assigned for robotic surgery, meaning providers often use a laparoscopic surgery code to bill. Institutions, nonetheless, may vary in what they ultimately charge patients.

With regard to benign hysterectomy, robotic surgery has gained relatively rapid acceptance. A noteworthy study by Wright et al. reported that robotic hysterectomy increased almost 1,000 percent between 2007 and 2010, from 0.5 to 9.5 percent of all hysterectomies, while rates of laparoscopic hysterectomy increased from only 24.3 to 30.5 percent.[7] Most importantly, however, the authors concluded that robotic hysterectomy was being adopted faster than the literature supports. Unlike robot-assisted laparoscopic prostatectomy, the benefits of robot-assisted hysterectomy are not necessarily as pronounced. Complications were equivocal across the board for robotic versus laparoscopic hysterectomy with the only appreciable difference being a minor difference in hospital length of stay: 20 percent of robotic hysterectomy subjects stayed longer than 2 days compared with 25 percent of laparoscopic surgery subjects. Despite similar perioperative outcomes, the robotic approach is associated with an increased cost of approximately $2,200, an increment that is difficult to justify in an era of value-based care and cost containment.[7] Even the past president of the American Congress of Obstetricians and Gynecologists, James T. Breeden, was quoted as saying, "There is no solid proof that robotic gynecologic surgery is even as good as existing minimally invasive measures."[40] Altogether, if rapid adoption of robotic surgical technology continues, this must be matched by high-level evidence.

General Surgery

Debate over the value of robotic surgery also extends to general surgeons. Given the higher costs, it remains unclear whether robotic surgery can become cost-efficient and thus whether the general surgery community will justify its use. Breitenstein et al. performed one of the first robotic cost-effectiveness studies in general surgery comparing the safety and costs of robotic versus laparoscopic surgery for cholecystectomy in patients with symptomatic cholecystolithiasis.[41] A prospective case-matched study was performed on 50 consecutive subjects, matched according to age, gender, surgical experience, histology, and American Society of Anesthesiologists score. Skin-to-skin operation time (55 vs. 50 min) and hospital stay (2.6 vs. 2.8 days) were not statistically different

($p > 0.05$). Overall, hospital costs were significantly higher for robot-assisted cholecystectomy ($7,985.40 versus $6,255.30, $p < 0.001$) with an absolute difference of $1,730.10. Thus, while robotic surgery appears to be a safe approach, the cost of robotic technology did not support adoption for this indication.

More recent literature by Park et al. assessed the surgical outcomes of robot-assisted colectomy (RAC) versus laparoscopically assisted colectomy (LAC) in treating right-sided colonic cancer.[42] Seventy-one subjects were randomized to both groups. RAC was associated with longer operative time (195 versus 130 min, $p < 0.001$) and higher hospital costs ($12,235 versus $10,320, $p = 0.013$). The increased costs were attributed primarily to the surgical costs of the robotic platform, including the costs of all the disposable equipment.

In another assessment using the Nationwide Inpatient Sample to assess short-term outcomes for robot-assisted colorectal surgery, lower volume was associated with significantly more overall complications and higher costs (all $p < 0.001$) at the hospital and surgeon level.[43] Similar to other studies, this argues that robotic surgery may be better suited to high-volume surgeons and hospitals in order to achieve high-quality outcomes.

Cardiothoracic Surgery

Robot-assisted surgery was first used for primary lung cancer resection in 2002, although two of the first five procedures were converted to open thoracotomy due to safety concerns.[44] Since then, the safety profile of robotic surgery for cardiothoracic surgery has improved dramatically with multiple studies demonstrating that robotic thoracic surgery can be performed with perioperative morbidity similar to video-assisted thoracospocic surgery (VATS) and open thoracotomy approaches. Nevertheless, whether the robotic platform adds significant benefit at a reasonable cost remains unknown.[45] In a retrospective study by Park et al. comparing robotic, VATS, and thoracotomy for lobectomy, robotic surgery was found to add additional direct OR costs compared with conventional VATS or thoracotomy, without additional indirect costs.[46]

A more recent study by Swanson et al. assessed the impact of robot-assisted thoracic surgery (RATS) lobectomy on clinical and economic outcomes by comparing hospital costs and clinical outcomes for VATS versus RATS lobectomies and wedge resections, matching for comorbidities, demographics, and hospital characteristics.[47] After analyzing 15,502 subjects, robotic surgery was associated with higher average hospital costs with the average cost of RATS lobectomy estimated at $25,040.70 versus $20,476.60 for VATS lobectomy ($p < 0.001$). Similarly, RATS versus VATS wedge resection was costlier at $19,592.40 versus $16,600.10 ($p < 0.001$), respectively. Inpatient operating times were also longer for RATS versus VATS wedge resection (3.26 vs. 2.86 hours, $p < 0.001$) and lobectomy (4.49 vs. 4.23 hours, $p = 0.096$), although not statistically significant in the latter. Length of stay and perioperative adverse events were similar.

Similar to thoracic surgery, there are also very few direct comparisons between different approaches for cardiac surgery. Hassan et al. compared minimally invasive mitral valve repair or replacement (mini-MVR) versus robotic MVR from a cost–benefit perspective in a meta-analysis.[48] The authors found only three prior studies to compare costs in the literature. Furthermore, on a per-case basis, robotic MVR exceeded the cost of conventional MVR by $2,064.90 and by $271 for mini-MVR. Thirty-day mortality rates were similar between mini-MVR and robotic MVR groups (1.24 vs. 0.55 percent, respectively, OR 2.27, $p = 0.052$). Nevertheless, the conversion rate to conventional MVR was 0.77 percent in mini-MVR and 1.83 percent in robotic MVR (OR 0.32, $p < 0.001$). Mean cardiopulmonary bypass time was longer in mini-MVR (137.4 vs. 130.4 min), whereas cross-clamp time was shorter (82.2 vs. 96.7 min), and it is unknown whether this was significantly different.

Most recently, the direct costs and 30-day morbidity and mortality of robotic coronary artery bypass graft (CABG) versus conventional CABG were also compared at a single institution based on hospital, clinical, and financial records.[49] After analyzing 2,088 consecutive patients from 2007 to 2012, robotic CABG was associated with shorter operative times (5.61 vs. 6.6 h, $p < 0.001$), lower blood transfusion rate (12.8 percent vs. 22.6 percent, $p = 0.04$), shorter length of stay (6 vs. 7 days, $p = 0.0001$), and a lower NY state complications composite rate (4.26 vs. 13.48 percent, $p = 0.01$). Nevertheless, the cost of robotic procedures was not significantly different from matched conventional cases ($18,717.35 vs. $18,601, $p = 0.13$), except 26 hybrid coronary revascularizations in which angioplasty was performed on the same admission (hybrid $25,311.1 vs. conventional $18,966.13, $p = 0.02$).

Time-Driven Activity-Based Costing

Although understanding the cost of producing services and products is a fundamental part of business management, accurately measuring healthcare costs remains a challenge, as inferred from these previous studies. In traditional fee-for-service models, the insurer is accountable for as physicians and health systems are incentivized toward quantity rather than quality.[50] Resultantly, traditional accounting methods often involve significant cost shifting from low reimbursing service lines to more profitable ones, obscuring the true cost of any one structure. Furthermore, busy physician practices often lack the resources necessary to evaluate cost across services, focusing instead on more readily available data such as revenue or reimbursement.[17] Not surprisingly, large interhospital variability is often found for the same procedure with metrics failing to explain why these differences exist.[21] As society moves toward accountable care organizations and bundled payments as mechanisms to mitigate our growing healthcare expenditures, health systems must become proficient at systematically bending their cost curves.[51] The first step in accomplishing this goal is understanding costs on a detailed level.

Time-driven activity-based costing (TDABC) is a well-described costing paradigm used in a variety of industries.[52] When used in healthcare, it allows the actual expense of providing care to be calculated by aggregating costs over the full cycle of care for a patient's medical condition.[19] This cost is dependent upon the actual use of resources involved in the care process and incorporates the proportion of time devoted by each resource as well as the cost of each resource per unit time.[53] TDABC allows all personnel, equipment, facility, and support costs to be directly attributed to the organization's output of patient care, illuminating areas of inefficiency and highlighting opportunities for rational cost reduction.[54] Work performed by the Department of Urology at UCLA has spearheaded the utilization of TDABC and detailed the true costs of care for treating small renal masses (SRM) and localized, low-risk prostate cancer.[55,56]

With regard to SRM, defined as less than 4 cm in size, our healthcare team at UCLA traced the path of a patient throughout the episode of care for treatment of a SRM.[55] This involved identifying the cost of care for every resource used in treatment, including space, materials and equipment, and personnel in both the outpatient and inpatient settings, and also calculating the average time a patient spends with each resource. The episode of care was then defined as the summation of the quantity of resource units multiplied by the price per unit time of that resource.[57]

Robot-assisted laparoscopic partial nephrectomy represented the most expensive treatment for SRM, 69.7 percent more costly than the least costly inpatient treatment – laparoscopic radical nephrectomy ($17,841.79 vs. $10,514.05).[55] Robot-assisted laparoscopic radical nephrectomy and open partial nephrectomy were the second and third most expensive treatments at $15,819.24 and $12,610.30, respectively, while active surveillance was the least costly treatment modality at $1,018.50. Although equipment costs were greater for laparoscopic radical nephrectomy than open partial nephrectomy, faster operating room times (195.2 vs. 217.3 min, $p = 0.001$) and shorter length of stay (2.4 vs. 3.7 days, $p = 0.13$) were the primary drivers in lowering costs. Robot-assisted laparoscopic partial nephrectomy was 12.7 percent more costly than robot-assisted laparoscopic radical nephrectomy, largely due to instrument costs.

In a similar fashion, TDBAC has also been used to detail the costs of localized, low-risk prostate cancer, tracing the episode of care for a patient with prostate cancer from the initial visit with a urologist for elevated prostate-specific antigen through 12 years of follow-up given previously reported results of prolonged long-term survival among all treatment arms.[56] Across the spectrum of care for low-risk prostate cancer, there was substantial variation in cost, ranging from $7,298 for active surveillance to $23,565 for intensity-modulated radiation therapy (IMRT) at 5 years of follow-up. Radiation costs varied considerably due to the number of treatments delivered and fixed costs of the equipment. For example, whereas the cost of each treatment session was similar between stereotactic body radiation therapy and IMRT ($479.31 vs. $297.84), the total number of treatments (5 vs. 45) largely drove the differences in cost at 5 years ($11,665 vs. $23,565).

RALP was the second most expensive modality at $16,946 at 5 years, with its most significant costs fueled by equipment costs and an inpatient stay, which was estimated at 1.28 days (mean cost $2,306, $n = 65$). Total operative costs were $11,839, of which 83.2 percent ($9,855) were fixed costs attributable to staff, space, equipment purchase fees, and depreciation/maintenance, and 16.8 percent ($1,984) were disposable costs from the robotic instruments.

With numerous treatment modalities currently available for prostate cancer and notable long-term survival regardless of intervention, the individual value of each treatment cannot be defined until we have a better understanding of the true cost of care.[58,59] This includes not only the diagnostic and in-hospital costs but the cost of care over time. Unfortunately, current costing mechanisms lack transparency and can appear arbitrary. This can be especially important in the case of uninsured patients, who face substantial and unpredictable hospital and physician bills.

Conclusion

In an era where robot-assisted surgical technology is rapidly adopted, there is a pressing need for high-level evidence in the form of prospective randomized trials or device registries to assess whether robotic technology can be cost-effective in high-volume centers in the hands of experienced surgeons. TDABC methodology evaluates costs at the specific resource level, allowing further examination into the relative contribution of materials, personnel, and space toward each task. TDABC may improve return on investment in healthcare and facilitate a sustainable healthcare system. As our healthcare system continues toward bundled payments for surgical subspecialties, the onus is on surgeons to analyze costs and reduce inefficiencies. This costing paradigm provides analytic data to improve the organizational structure of clinical departments, reducing waste. Additionally, this infrastructure has the ability to transcend multiple service lines across an institution, greatly improving its economy of scale. Altogether, the robotic platform is here to stay, but refining patient selection and improving efficiency remain vital to scaling the value proposition.

References

1. Frank I, Blute ML, Cheville JC, Lohse CM, Weaver AL, Zincke H. Solid renal tumors: an analysis of pathological features related to tumor size. *J Urol.* 2003;170:2217–20.
2. Barbash GI, Glied SA. New technology and health care costs – the case of robot-assisted surgery. *NEJM.*2010;363(8):701–4.
3. Cha EK, Wiklund NP, Scherr DS. Recent advances in robot-assisted radical cystectomy. *Curr Opin Urol.* 2011;21(1):65–70.
4. Cooper MA, Ibrahim A, Lyu H, Makary MA. Underreporting of robotic surgery complications. *Journal for Healthcare Quality.*2015;37(2):133–8.
5. Ghani KR, Sukumar S, Sammon JD, et al. Practice patterns and outcomes of open and minimally invasive partial nephrectomy since the introduction of robotic partial nephrectomy: results from the nationwide inpatient sample. *J Urol.* 2014;191(4):907–12.
6. Sivarajan G, Taksler GB, Walter D, et al. The effect of the diffusion of the surgical robot on the hospital-level utilization of partial nephrectomy. *Med Care.* 2015;53(1):71–8.
7. Wright JD, Ananth CV, Lewin SN, et al. Robotically assisted vs laparoscopic hysterectomy among women with benign gynecologic disease. *JAMA.* 2013;309(7):689–98.
8. Yu HY, Hevelone ND, Lipsitz SR, et al. Use, costs and comparative effectiveness of robotic assisted, laparoscopic and open urological surgery. *J Urol.* 2012;187(4):1392–8.
9. Smith JA, Jr, Herrell SD. Robotic-assisted laparoscopic prostatectomy: do minimally invasive approaches offer significant advantages? *J Clin Oncol.* 2005;23(32):8170–5.
10. Bolenz C, Gupta A, Hotze T, et al. Cost comparison of robotic, laparoscopic, and open radical prostatectomy for prostate cancer. *Eur Urol.* 2010;57(3):453–8.
11. Pappas TN, Jacobs DO. Laparoscopic resection for colon cancer – the end of the beginning? *NEJM.* 2004;350(20):2091–2.
12. Trinh QD, Sammon J, Sun M, et al. Perioperative outcomes of robot-assisted radical prostatectomy compared with open radical prostatectomy: results from the nationwide inpatient sample. *Eur Urol.* 2012;61:679–85.
13. Barbash GI, Glied SA. New technology and health care costs – the case of robot-assisted surgery. *NEJM.* 2010;363(8):701–4.
14. Hu JC, Wang Q, Pashos CL, et al. Utilization and outcomes of minimally invasive radical prostatectomy. *J Clin Oncol.* 2008;26(14):2278–84.
15. Nguyen PL, Gu X, Lipsitz SR, et al. Cost implications of the rapid adoption of newer technologies for treating prostate cancer. *J Clin Oncol.* 2011;29(12):1517–24.
16. House of Commons Health Committee. National Institute for Health and Clinical Excellence. Eighth Report of Session 2012–13, Volume II. 2013: 1–135.
17. Porter ME, Lee TH. The strategy that will fix health care. *Harvard Business Review.* October 2013: 1–19.
18. Filson CP, Hollingswoth JM, Skolarus TA, et al. Health care reform in 2010: transforming the delivery system to improve quality of care. *World J Urol.* 2011;29(1):85–90.

19. Kaplan RS. Improving value with TDABC. Time-driven activity-based costing presents significant opportunities to enhance quality of care and outcomes while reducing costs- and provides a foundation for value-based payment. *Healthcare Financial Management Association.* 2014;68(6);76–83.
20. Abbou CC, Hoznek A, Salomon L, et al. Remote laparoscopic radical prostatectomy carried out with a robot. Report of a case. *Prog Urol.* 2000;10:520–3.
21. Pate SC, Uhlman MA, Rosenthal JA, et al. Variations in the open market costs for prostate cancer surgery: a survey of US hospitals. *Urology.* 2014;83(3):626–30.
22. Birkmeyer JD, Finlayson SR, Tosteson AN, et al. Effect of hospital volume on in-hospital mortality with pancreaticoduodenectomy. *Surgery.*1999;125(3):250–6.
23. Patti MG, Corvera CU, Glasgow RE, Way LW. A hospital's annual rate of esophagectomy influences the operative mortality rate. *J Gastrointest Surg.* 1998;2(2):186–92.
24. Schrag D, Cramer LD, Bach PB, et al. Influence of hospital procedure volume on outcomes following surgery for colon cancer. *JAMA.* 2000;284(23):3028–35.
25. Roohan PJ, Bickell NA, Baptiste MS, et al. Hospital volume differences and five-year survival from breast cancer. *Am J Public Health.* 1998;88(3):454–7.
26. Ellison LM, Heaney JA, Birkmeyer JD. The effect of hospital volume on mortality and resource use after radical prostatectomy. *J Urol.* 2000;163(3):867–9.
27. Hu JC, Gold KF, Pashos CL, Mehta SS, Litwin MS. Role of surgeon volume in radical prostatectomy outcomes. *J Clin Oncol.* 2003;21(3):401–5.
28. Hu JC, Gold KF, Pashos CL, et al. Temporal trends in radical prostatectomy complications from 1991 to 1998. *J Urol.* 2003;169(4):1443–8.
29. Wilt TJ, Shamliyan TA, Taylor BC, et al. Association between hospital and surgeon radical prostatectomy volume and patient outcomes: a systematic review. *J Urol.* 2008;180(3):820–8; discussion 828–9.
30. Barocas DA, Mitchell R, Chang SS, Cookson MS. Impact of surgeon and hospital volume on outcomes of radical prostatectomy. *Urol Oncol.* 2010;28(3):243–50.
31. Savage CJ, Vickers AJ. Low annual caseloads of United States surgeons conducting radical prostatectomy. *J Urol.* 2009;182(6):2677–9.
32. Williams SB, Amarasekera CA, Gu X, et al. Influence of surgeon and hospital volume on radical prostatectomy costs. *J Urol.* 188(6):2198–202.
33. Nowroozi MR, Pisters LL. The current status of gene therapy for prostate cancer. *Cancer Control.* 1998;5(6):522–31.
34. Ramirez A, Benayoun S, Briganti A, et al. High radical prostatectomy surgical volume is related to lower radical prostatectomy total hospital charges. *Eur Urol.* 2006;50(1):58–62; discussion 62–53.
35. Begg CB, Riedel ER, Bach PB, et al. Variations in morbidity after radical prostatectomy. *NEJM.* 2002;346(15):1138–44.
36. FDA clears transoral robotic surgery – developed at Penn – for tumors of mouth, throat and voice box. *Penn Medicine News Release* 2009. www.uphs.upenn.edu/news/News_Releases/2009/12/tors-robotic-head-neck-surgery/ Accessed January 4, 2016.
37. Hammoudi K, Pinlong E, Kim S, et al. Transoral robotic surgery versus conventional surgery in treatment for squamous cell carcinoma of the upper aerodigestive tract. *Head Neck.* 2015;37(9):1304–9.
38. de Almeida JR, Moskowitz AJ, Miles BA, et al. Cost-effectiveness of transoral robotic surgery versus (chemo)radiotherapy for early T classification oropharyngeal carcinoma: a cost-utility analysis. *Head Neck.* 2016;38(4):589–600.
39. Ran L, Jin J, Xu Y, et al. Comparison of robotic surgery with laparoscopy and laparotomy for treatment of endometrial cancer: a meta-analysis. *PLoS One.* 2014;9(9):e108361.
40. Kirkner RM. Rush to robotic surgery outpaces medical evidence, critics say. *Managed Care.* May 2014. http://www.managedcaremag.com/archives/2014/5/rush-robotic-surgery-outpaces-medical-evidence-critics-say≥ Accessed January 4, 2016.
41. Breitenstein S, Nocito A, Puhan M, et al. Robotic-assisted versus laparoscopic cholecystectomy: outcome and cost analyses of a case-matched cohort study. *Ann Surg.* 2008;247(6):987–93.
42. Park JS, Choi GS, Park SY, et al. Randomized clinical trial of robot-assisted versus standard laparoscopic right colectomy. *Br J Surg.* 2012;99(9):1219–26.
43. Keller DS, Hashemi L, Lu M, et al. Short-term outcomes for robotic colorectal surgery by provider volume. *J Am Coll Surg.* 2013;217(6):1063–9.
44. Melfi FM, Menconi GF, Mariani AM, et al. Early experience with robotic technology for thoracoscopic surgery. *Eur J Cardiothorac Surg.* 2002;2(5):864–8.
45. Park BJ. Cost concerns for robotic thoracic surgery. *Ann Cardiothorac Surg.* 2012;1(1):56–8.
46. Park BJ, Flores RM. Cost comparison of robotic, video-assisted thoracic surgery and thoracotomy approaches to pulmonary lobectomy. *Thorac Surg Clin.* 2008;18:297–300.
47. Swanson SJ, Miller DL, McKenna RJ Jr, et al. Comparing robot-assisted thoracic surgical lobectomy with conventional video-assisted thoracic surgical

lobectomy and wedge resection: results from a multihospital database (Premier). *J Thorac Cardiovasc Surg.* 2014;147(3):929–37.

48. Hassan M, Miao Y, Lincoln J, et al. Cost-benefit analysis of robotic versus nonrobotic minimally invasive mitral valve surgery. *Innovations.* 2015;10(2):90–5.
49. Leyvi G, Schecter CB, Sehgal S, et al. Comparison of index hospitalization costs between robotic CABG and conventional CABG: implications for hybrid coronary revascularization. *J Cardiothorac Vasc Anesth.* 2016;30(1):12–8.
50. Kaplan RS, Porter ME. How to solve the cost crisis in health care. *Harvard Business Review.* 2011:46–64.
51. Porter ME. What is value in health care? *NEJM.* 2010;363(26):2477–981.
52. Stout DE, Propri JM. Implementing time-driven activity-based costing at a medium-sized electronics company. *Management Accounting Quarterly.* 2011; 12(3):1–11.
53. Kaplan RS, Anderson SR. Time-driven activity-based costing. *Harvard Business Review.* 2004:131–8.
54. McLaughlin N, Burke MA, Setlur NP, et al. Time-driven activity-based costing: a driver for provider engagement in costing activities and redesign initiatives. *Neurosurg Focus.* 2014;37(5):E3.
55. Laviana AA, Kundavaram CR, Tan H-J, et al. Determining the true costs of treating small renal masses using time-driven activity-based costing. *Urology Practice.* 2016. Epub ahead of print.
56. Laviana AA, Ilg AM, Veruttipong D. Utilizing time-driven activity-based costing to understand the short- and long-term costs of treating localized, low-risk prostate cancer. *Cancer.* 2016;122(3):447–55.
57. Kaplan RS, Anderson SR. Time-driven activity-based costing. *Harvard Business Review.* November 2004:131–38.
58. Ubel PA, Asch DA. Creating value in health by understanding and overcoming resistance to de-innovation. *Health Aff (Millwood).* 2015;34(2):239–44.
59. Daskivich TJ, Fan K-H, Koyama T, et al. Effect of age, tumor risk, and comorbidity on competing risks for survival in a U.S. population-based cohort of men with prostate cancer. *Ann Intern Med.* 2013;158(10):709–17.

Chapter 22

The Past, Present, and Future of Robotics

A Surgical and Anesthetic Perspective

Maunak V. Rana and Aladino De Ranieri

Origins

There has been a significant increase in the volume of robotic surgical procedures in the last decade. Robotic surgery was born in 1985 with the Programmable Universal Machine for Assembly (PUMA 560) robot arm, which was used in a CT-guided neurosurgical biopsy procedure. Since that fateful use of adjunctive technology, robotic surgery has increasingly been utilized for surgery. The first laparoscopic surgery, a cholecystectomy, was performed in 1987. The PUMA system was subsequently used to perform a robotic transurethral resection. In 1990, the AESOP system, developed by Computer Motion, became the first system approved for endoscopic robotic surgery. The new millennium saw the da Vinci system approved by the FDA as the first robotic system for laparoscopic surgery.[1] This development was a particularly momentous event in the history of robotic surgery because this was the first time the regulatory agency approved an entire system, including instruments and cameras, for robotic surgery. In essence, this heralded the transition from robotic tools to an entire robotic platform. The three-dimensional screen and image allowed for better visualization, coupled with the introduction of miniaturized arms that decreased tissue trespass and ergonomic wrist movement led to a virtual representation of surgery, controlled by a surgeon at a remote controller system.

Innovation in surgical technology coupled with exposure of anesthesiologists to keep abreast of these changes will allow for surgical teams to progress toward newer vistas, allowing for as real as experience as possible, regardless of the virtual approach to surgery.

Financial Considerations

As surgical advancement is considered, direct and hidden costs are to be considered, when evaluating the benefits of innovation. Currently, the da Vinci system has initial equipment costs in the arena of $2 million. Coupled with this is a service contract of at least $100,000 per year, and $200 per-case single-use equipment. An estimate is that a typical robotic procedure costs $1,000–2,000 more than a corresponding laparoscopic procedure.[2]

Additionally, surgical and operating room time factors into cost considerations for future development. The innovation in robotic equipment has led to improved visualization and technique with improvements in equipment. Operating room costs are variable, which range from $15–20 per operating room minute for a basic surgery versus $30–80 per operating room minute for more complex cases.[3] When analyzing the cost–benefit ratio, centers should ask whether advancement in the robotic platform leads to faster operating times and, therefore, less costs.

Surgical and Anesthetic Considerations

Robotic surgery has advanced the progress of virtually every surgical subspecialty. There has been a rapid development and incorporation of robotics in surgery over the past three decades, resulting in numerous benefits and, at the same time, several challenges. The laparoscopic approach rapidly became a preferred technique to many open procedures due to decreased perioperative comorbidities, decreased length of stay, decreased trespass on tissues with smaller physical footprint of equipment, and increased patient satisfaction.[4,5] The trend and demand for minimally invasive surgery fueled a subsequent generation of robotics

In order to keep up with the addition of robotic surgery into the realm of training programs, consensus statements have been developed by a multidisciplinary group of experts. A gradual-stepped approach is advocated to guide a new robotic surgeon to proficient and expert levels.[6] Innovation in medicine leads to improvements in patient safety. With advancement in robotic surgery, enhancement of the surgical platform would lead to improvement in visualization and a decrease in iatrogenic injury that can result from the surgical technique. Vascular and visceral injury can be decreased, as manipulation of tissues and surgical dissection can be improved. Surgeon experience will also improve as newer technologies are embraced and utilized. Currently, the risk of iatrogenic injury has been reported to be 0.4–5 per 10,000 cases. This spread of injury would potentially trend downward with greater experience and improved technology.[7]

Alongside the surgical enhancements to the robotic world, vigilance and considerations from anesthesiologists involved in these operations can lead to safer operations.[8,9] Anesthesia providers have a limited patient access due to the physical layout of the robotic platform and equipment.[10] Currently, for robotic abdominopelvic surgery, a steep degree of Trendelenburg position is required to optimally visualize the pelvis and lower abdomen. This has obvious ramifications on patient position as a patient improperly secured may be in danger of falls and potential damage from surgical instruments and access devices. Additionally, neuropathic injuries may occur with inadequate and improperly positioned shoulder braces. This effect leads to a decrease in the FRC, leading to an altered V/Q mismatch, further challenging the anesthetic management of patients who may be obese and at risk for respiratory compromise. From a strictly mechanical perspective, migration of the endotracheal tube may occur, leading to a mainstem translocation of the tube, compounding atelectasis and pulmonary compromise. Furthermore, vital organ edema may develop, particularly in the brain, upper airways, and lungs. The result of this increased fluid aberration is an increase in intracerebral and ophthalmic pressures.

The physical presence of the pneumoperitoneum applied for visualization during robotic surgery can lead to deleterious effects that anesthesiologists need to be cognizant about. The development of increased peak airway pressure, hypercarbia, atelectasis, with potentiality for gas embolism and pneumothorax are additive with the positioning concerns highlighted above.

Anesthesiologists also need to be vigilant for the risk of occult blood loss, as visualization is not as global as with open procedures. Hemodynamic along with cardiac changes in physiologic parameters can clue in the perioperative physician on alterations.

Due to the fact that robotic surgeries can be longer procedures than similar open approaches, the concern of hypothermia may develop as patients are exposed to more gas via peritoneal insufflation along with anesthetic gas. As surgical technology improves, these risks would be decreased, leading to fewer theoretical iatrogenic concerns.

A significant enhancement that can lead to improvement in visualization is the use of augmented reality surgery. Augmented reality serves to enhance the visualization of a surgical target with a superimposed image, leading to an improvement in complex surgical dissections.[11,12] The concept of adding and improving on spatially visualized objects, once the brainchild of science fiction, has a role in the advancement of robotic surgery. The improvement involves the concept of registration, which is the process of placing two images in the same coordinate system, effectively aligning corresponding points.[12] A clear example of this enhancement is having a preprocedure ultrasound or CT scan superimposed on a visualized surgical space.[13] The benefit of this added reality is the overlaying of ultrasound anatomy over the visualized image. This addition assists the surgeon in appreciating the nuances of surface anatomy, an ability particularly suited for surgical encounters requiring fine dexterity, such as tumor resection surgery.[14] Augmented reality will have a role not only in the education of established surgeons but also those physicians in graduate medical training programs.[15]

Anesthetic Considerations

Robotics has also been utilized in anesthesia, which includes manual and pharmacologic robots. Manual robots assist anesthesiologists in performing an increasing number of procedures to a differing degree.[16] Patient intubation is being evaluated in a robotic platform as is the placement of nerve blocks for regional anesthesia.[16–18] The Kepler robotic system has been utilized for intubation in humans.[17,18] This system was tested in ASA I patients with a platform made up of a joystick, the JACO robotic arm, a video laryngoscope, and a software control system (Figure 22.1). A webcam was used to provide live video feed of the entire process. The median intubation time was 21 s. There were no reported dental injuries, esophageal intubation, mucosal/lip bleeding or damage. One intubation was abandoned due to laryngoscope fogging.

Pharmacological robots are those technologies that are involved in the administration of anesthetic agents to surgical patients. An early robotic

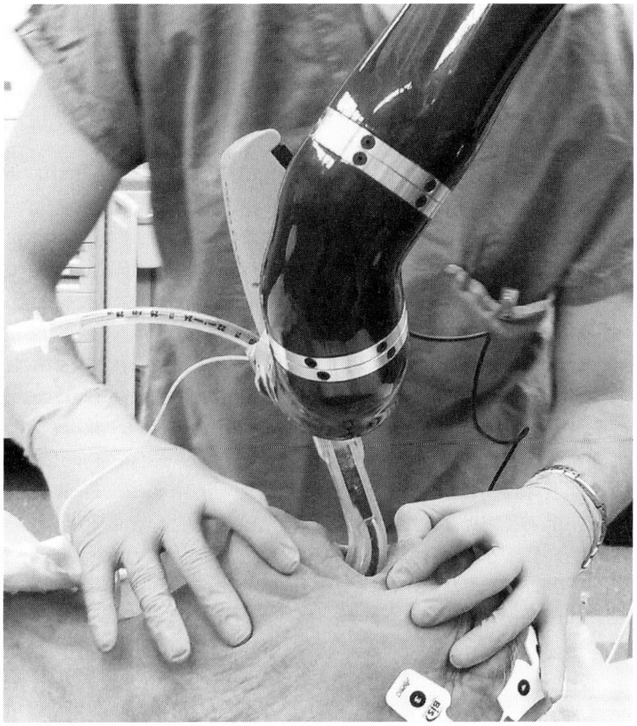

Figure 22.1 The Kepler intubating system (edited image from McGill University Medical Center. Accessed November 28, 2015 from https://muhc.ca/sites/default/files/news/DrHemmerling_KIS_closeup_20avril2011.jpg). Courtesy of Montreal General Hospital MUHC.

anesthesia provider, McSleepy, was developed at McGill University. The device is a closed-loop system that has been used to deliver IV sedation, narcotic, and muscle relaxant.[19] Closed-loop systems integrate patient data and calculate and administer anesthetic agents for surgical patients. The McSleepy system monitors patient consciousness and movement and then delivers agents based on patient characteristics and algorithmic programming. Additionally, surgeon and anesthesiologist preference can be incorporated into the platform's delivery of medication via artificial intelligence technology. Further robotic technology has been developed to assist in procedural sedation. A robotic "team" was tested in 2010 with McSleepy and da Vinci surgical robotics in a patient undergoing prostatectomy.[20] The SEDASYS system (Ethicon) has recently been approved by the FDA as a computer-assisted sedation delivery system to administer Propofol during gastrointestinal procedures, including esophagoduodenoscopy and colonoscopy.[21] The device utilizes standard ASA monitors and delivers Propofol and oxygen based upon patient responsiveness measured as grip strength to an audible cue. This technique is known as an automated responsiveness monitor (ARM). SEDASYS was presented to reduce the risks of oversedation as patients had less oxygen desaturation than control patients. These target-controlled infusion devices have raised controversy as to their imprecision in achieving and maintaining the desired drug concentration.[22]

Pain Management Robotics

Robotic platforms are also being tested for use in pain management procedures. In one study, a robotic needle arm driver was used to place twelve 22-gauge needles in a cadaveric lumbar paraspinal target.[23] The robotic arm was from URobotics Laboratory at Johns Hopkins based on a platform for accessing kidney targets via a fluoroscopic percutaneous approach. The system consisted of a robotic arm/needle driver, a mounting base, a touch screen, and a joystick controller. The motion of the robotic arm included multiple degrees of freedom with the ability to rotate for theoretical accuracy with needle placement. The physician operator controlled the robotic arm via a joystick and was able to retain manual control as required. Target points were a nerve root and the parafacet region. Biplanar fluoroscopic guidance was used after needle placement to gauge accuracy. The results were fairly precise as the needles were within 3 mm of predetermined targets, with the average at 1.44 mm. Time for needle placement and fluoroscopic exposure was not reported in this feasibility study.

Another feasibility study was performed on patients comparing operator-controlled robotic blocks and manual blocks, each in 10 patients in the L3–S1 levels. One patient in the robotic group required to be converted to the manual approach due to malfunction as the needle was slipping from the driver during placement. In this study, robotic-assisted interventions were deemed feasible.[24]

Moreover, robotic platforms utilizing flexible needles and trajectories to target tissues, thereby avoiding iatrogenic injury of neurovascular structures, have been tested and are under development.

Robotic-assisted procedures are also being tested for regional anesthesia and peripheral nerve blockade.[25] In this study, the da Vinci system was used to perform an ultrasound-guided nerve block with a Tuohy needle and perineural catheter with an ultrasound phantom. This feasibility study demonstrated that the da Vinci system, already utilized for surgical indications and handling surgical instruments, was able to grasp and manipulate a 21-gauge 90-mm needle; additionally, the platform allowed for sufficient dexterity to attach a syringe (luer-lock) to the injection portion of the needle. Furthermore, the stimulating portion of the needle was attached to the peripheral nerve stimulator without difficulty. While the ultrasound probe required manual placement on the target, the high-frequency probe was stabilized by the robotic platform.

The Magellan system is a robotic platform uniquely devised and utilized for peripheral nerve blockade, which may be a less expensive option than other systems as this is a dedicated nerve block platform. The cost of a robotic arm is approximately $50,000.[26] This Canadian system is a multicomponent platform: a robotic arm, joystick controller, nerve block, and needle with an ultrasound device. Dedicated control software is used to guide the system that allows for remote performance of nerve blocks.

The robotic arm is the JACO (Kinova Robotics), which is an assistive robotic device that has been utilized for performing activities of daily living. The weight of the carbon fiber device is 5 kg. The arm can be configured to right or left side, which can be customized to physician comfort and preference. The arm has six degrees of motion with a reach of 35.4 inches with two fingers and an opposing "thumb." Additionally, the operator can control the speed of the arm via three settings: low (0.15 m/s), medium (0.075 m/s), and high (0.0425 m/s). Safety mechanisms are built into the system to prevent insertion of the needle beyond a preset depth.

A benefit of this platform is that the arm is mounted via a console at the bedside that allows close proximity of the interventionalist.[26] The sciatic nerve at the popliteal fossa was the target of researchers in this evaluation of patients undergoing surgery with sciatic nerve block. This study evaluated 13 patients receiving a total of 16 blocks who underwent testing with identification of the sciatic nerve by a manual approach.

From an ergonomic and logistical standpoint, the Magellan system was placed at the head. The robot was then used to place a tuohy needle and inject 35 ml of 0.25 percent bupivacaine via an out-of-plane ultrasound technique targeting the nerve sheath, but avoiding intraneural injection. The administration of medication was performed manually, with aspiration intermittently after every 5 ml of administration. In this study, all 16 blocks were found to be successful with a mean time of just over 3 min for the block; no complications were noted. Ultrasound guidance alone was used to facilitate the nerve block without nerve stimulation.

Future Directions

Surgical robotics have advanced every surgical subspecialty. Technical enhancements improve operative access, suturing, and range of motion of tissue manipulation. An improvement that has noticeably enhanced surgical approaches to robot-assisted procedures is via the addition of laparoscopic single-site surgery (LESS) to the surgical armamentarium. The development of LESS has allowed for a single port to access surgical targets, thereby decreasing surgical scar, improving tissue healing, and lesser tissue pain. This platform would also be of benefit to anesthesiologists as accessing surgical targets via a single port would have a smaller "footprint" and allow for triangulation of tissues. These benefits are coupled with improved surgical access and dexterity that the robotic platform provides.[4,5]

Another future arena for robotic surgery is in the resection of head and neck malignancies.[27] Due to the increase in cases of oropharyngeal cancers, linked to the predilection of human papillomavirus to the

Table 22.1 Surgical operating platforms

Platform	Comment
da Vinci (Intuitive Surgical)	Most commonly used platform; patent to expire in 2016
RAVEN (University of Washington/University of California)	Remote platform with Linux operating system
SPIDER (Transenterix)	Single-port laparoscopy with flexible instruments
SURGIBOT (Transenterix)	Portable robotic system; allows for surgeon to be at bedside vs remote

oropharynx, there is an incidence in the number of patients presenting for surgical resection. Robotic surgery has been advocated for resection of these tumors via a transoral approach. Innovations in urologic surgery include increased use of robotics via the LESS platform. Hepatobiliary surgery has advanced with the integration of the robotic approach.[28] This study evaluated patients who underwent robot-assisted liver surgery (ROBR) and compared surgical outcomes with laparoscopic liver resection (LAPR). The rate of major hepatectomy was higher in the LAPR approach, while a parenchyma-sparing approach was used in the ROBR. The rate of conversion to open was higher in the ROBR group versus the LAPR approach. In addition, the ROBR group had a higher mean blood loss. The authors opined, however, that despite the higher blood loss and conversion to open surgery rates, the robotic approach allows for increased dexterity and access to poorly accessible targets, particularly superiorly and posteriorly located liver tumors. More authors have corroborated this benefit.[29] A significant benefit with the introduction and refinement of the robotic approach is the ability to provide resection with parenchymal preservation.

Robotics and image-guided percutaneous endovascular repair are increasingly utilized in vascular surgery. These minimally invasive techniques increase the surgeon's precision and dexterity and consequently are replacing the traditional open techniques and greatly reducing the associated comorbidities. Endovascular repair is the first-line treatment for an abdominal aortic aneurysm.[30] The Sensei robotic system has been utilized for catheter guidance for cardiac applications. The Niobe system is a stereotactic magnetic navigation system used for catheter guidance and cardiac ablation.[31]

Numerous robotic systems are being developed, which could compete with the near-universally utilized da Vinci platform with the patent expiring in 2016 (Table 22.1). The Raven I and Raven II robots are prototype systems that incorporate the advantages of the da Vinci system – remotely controlled platform with enhanced dexterity, which can facilitate minimally invasive surgery. The Raven and evolving Raven II systems are Linux-based operating platforms and have a network-integrated researcher who can interact with the robot in real time. This is an advancement from current systems in that updates and support can occur during surgery, rather than before and after the surgical procedure.[32] TransEnterix developed the SPIDER surgical system, which uses flexible instruments to facilitate single-port laparoscopic surgery.[33] Presumably with the flexible instrument system, more inaccessible targets may be reached with more pliable instruments. The SurgiBot, also produced by TransEnxterix, is a portable robotic laparoscopic system in the evolution of the SPIDER technology and is currently being FDA-tested. The portable SurgiBot has a smaller footprint, thus allowing the surgeon to operate at the bedside within the sterile field. It requires less ancillary staff support and utilizes novel flexible instrumentation, which may reduce the number of incisions and improve structural access.[34]

Summary

Robotic surgery has advanced from being an adjunctive device to an integrated and fundamental technology for operative patient care. Costs of devices are

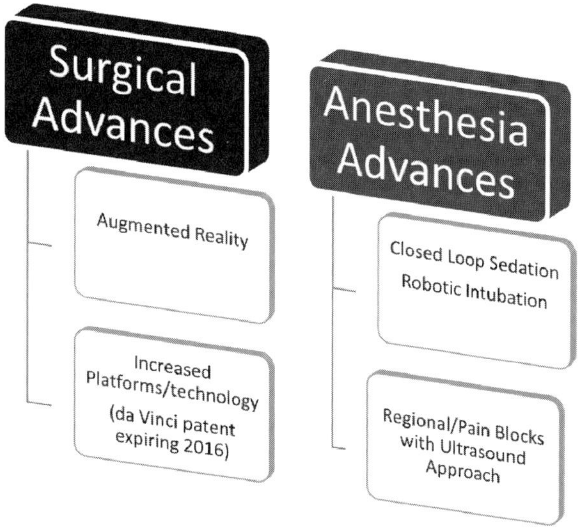

Figure 22.2 Future directions in surgery and anesthesia

decreasing along with smaller platforms for bedside procedures. Along with advancements in the surgical area came developments in the anesthesia world (see Figure 22.2). From closed-loop systems designed to allow drug delivery in a precise, algorithmic fashion to the use of robotics for interventional procedures, the robot serves to advance patient care. The October 2010 robotic surgery in Canada involving a robotic anesthesiology device may be a foreshadowing of the future of the operative environment.

References

1. Lanfranco AR, Castellanos AE, Desai JP, Meyers WC. Robotic surgery: a current perspective. *Annals of Surgery*. 2004;239(1):14–21.
2. Steinberg PL, Merguerian PA, Bihrle W III, Heaney JA, Seigne JD. A da Vinci robot system can make sense for a mature laparoscopic prostatectomy program. *Journal of the Society of Laparoendoscopic Surgeons / Society of Laparoendoscopic Surgeons*. 2008;12(1):9–12.
3. Macario A. What does one minute of operating room time cost? *Journal of Clinical Anesthesia*. 2010;22(4):233–6.
4. Autorino R, Kaouk JH, Stolzenburg JU, et al. Current status and future directions of robotic single-site surgery: a systematic review. *European Urology*. 2013;63(2):266–80.
5. Barret E, Sanchez-Salas R, Ercolani M, et al. Robotic-assisted laparoendoscopic single-site surgery (R-LESS) in urology: an evidence-based analysis. *Minerva urologica e nefrologica = The Italian Journal of Urology and Nephrology*. 2011;63(2):115–22.
6. Ahmed K, Khan R, Mottrie A, et al. Development of a standardised training curriculum for robotic surgery: a consensus statement from an international multidisciplinary group of experts. *BJU International*. 2015;116(1):93–101.
7. Romero V, Akpinar H, Smith JJ III, Assimos DG. Changing patterns in iatrogenic ureteral injuries. *Reviews in Urology*. 2011;13(4):e179–83.
8. Hsu RL, Kaye AD, Urman RD. Anesthetic challenges in robotic-assisted urologic surgery. *Reviews in Urology*. 2013;15(4):178–84.
9. Kaye AD, Vadivelu N, Ahuja N, Mitra S, Silasi D, Urman RD. Anesthetic considerations in robotic-assisted gynecologic surgery. *The Ochsner Journal*. 2013;13(4):517–24.
10. Campos J, Ueda K. Update on anesthetic complications of robotic thoracic surgery. *Minerva Anestesiologica*. 2014;80(1):83–8.
11. Wang W, Li J, Wang S, Su H, Jiang X. System design and animal experiment study of a novel minimally invasive surgical robot. *The International Journal of Medical Robotics + Computer Assisted Surgery*. 2015
12. Shuhaiber JH. Augmented reality in surgery. *Archives of Surgery (Chicago, IL: 1960)*. 2004;139(2):170–4.
13. Hughes-Hallett A, Pratt P, Mayer E, et al. Intraoperative ultrasound overlay in robot-assisted partial nephrectomy: first clinical experience. *European Urology*. 2014;65(3):671–2.
14. Nakamura K, Naya Y, Zenbutsu S, et al. Surgical navigation using three-dimensional computed tomography images fused intraoperatively with live video. *Journal of Endourology/Endourological Society*. 2010;24(4):521–4.
15. Zhu E, Hadadgar A, Masiello I, Zary N. Augmented reality in healthcare education: an integrative review. *PeerJ*. 2014;2:e469.
16. Wehbe M, Giacalone M, Hemmerling TM. Robotics and regional anesthesia. *Current Opinion in Anaesthesiology*. 2014;27(5):544–8.
17. Hemmerling TM, Taddei R, Wehbe M, Zaouter C, Cyr S, Morse J. First robotic tracheal intubations in humans using the Kepler intubation system. *British Journal of Anaesthesia*. 2012;108(6):1011–6.
18. Hemmerling TM, Wehbe M, Zaouter C, Taddei R, Morse J. The Kepler intubation system. *Anesthesia and Analgesia*. 2012;114(3):590–4.
19. Hemmerling TM, Terrasini N. Robotic anesthesia: not the realm of science fiction any more. *Current Opinion in Anaesthesiology*. 2012;25(6):736–42.
20. Shah SB. McSleepy, da Vinci, Kepler Intubation System et al. *Indian Journal of Anaesthesia*. 2013;57(1):101–2.
21. Pambianco DJ, Whitten CJ, Moerman A, Struys MM, Martin JF. An assessment of computer-assisted personalized sedation: a sedation delivery system to administer propofol for gastrointestinal endoscopy. *Gastrointestinal Endoscopy*. 2008;68(3):542–7.
22. Manberg PJ, Vozella CM, Kelley SD. Regulatory challenges facing closed-loop anesthetic drug infusion devices. *Clinical Pharmacology and Therapeutics*. 2008;84(1):166–9.
23. Cleary K, Stoianovici D, Patriciu A, Mazilu D, Lindisch D, Watson V. Robotically assisted nerve and facet blocks: a cadaveric study. *Academic Radiology*. 2002;9(7):821–5.
24. Cleary K, Watson V, Lindisch D, et al. Precision placement of instruments for minimally invasive procedures using a "needle driver" robot. *The International Journal of Medical Robotics + Computer Assisted Surgery*. 2005;1(2):40–7.

25. Tighe PJ, Badiyan SJ, Luria I, Boezaart AP, Parekattil S. Technical communication: robot-assisted regional anesthesia: a simulated demonstration. *Anesthesia and Analgesia*. 2010;111(3):813–6.

26. Hemmerling TM, Taddei R, Wehbe M, Cyr S, Zaouter C, Morse J. Technical communication: first robotic ultrasound-guided nerve blocks in humans using the Magellan system. *Anesthesia and Analgesia*. 2013;116(2):491–4.

27. de Almeida JR, Genden EM. Robotic surgery for oropharynx cancer: promise, challenges, and future directions. *Current Oncology Reports*. 2012;14(2):148–57.

28. Troisi RI, Patriti A, Montalti R, Casciola L. Robot assistance in liver surgery: a real advantage over a fully laparoscopic approach? Results of a comparative bi-institutional analysis. *The International Journal of Medical Robotics + Computer Assisted Surgery*. 2013;9(2):160–6.

29. Tranchart H, Ceribelli C, Ferretti S, Dagher I, Patriti A. Traditional versus robot-assisted full laparoscopic liver resection: a matched-pair comparative study. *World Journal of Surgery*. 2014;38(11):2904–9.

30. de Ruiter QM, Moll FL, van Herwaarden JA. Current state in tracking and robotic navigation systems for application in endovascular aortic aneurysm repair. *Journal of Vascular Surgery*. 2015;61(1):256–64.

31. Antoniou GA, Riga CV, Mayer EK, Cheshire NJ, Bicknell CD. Clinical applications of robotic technology in vascular and endovascular surgery. *Journal of Vascular Surgery*. 2011;53(2):493–9.

32. Gong Y, Hu D, Hannaford B, Seibel EJ. Accurate three-dimensional virtual reconstruction of surgical field using calibrated trajectories of an image-guided medical robot. *Journal of Medical Imaging (Bellingham, Wash.)*. 2014;1(3):035002.

33. Haber GP, Autorino R, Laydner H, et al. SPIDER surgical system for urologic procedures with laparoendoscopic single-site surgery: from initial laboratory experience to first clinical application. *European Urology*. 2012;61(2):415–22.

34. Rieder E, Martinec DV, Cassera MA, Goers TA, Dunst CM, Swanstrom LL. A triangulating operating platform enhances bimanual performance and reduces surgical workload in single-incision laparoscopy. *Journal of the American College of Surgeons*. 2011;212(3):378–84.

Index